Zebrafish Models for Development and Disease 2.0

Zebrafish Models for Development and Disease 2.0

Editors

James A. Marrs
Swapnalee Sarmah

MDPI • Basel • Beijing • Wuhan • Barcelona • Belgrade • Manchester • Tokyo • Cluj • Tianjin

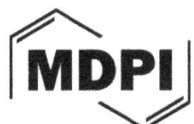

Editors
James A. Marrs
Indiana University-Purdue
University Indianapolis
USA

Swapnalee Sarmah
Indiana University-Purdue
University Indianapolis
USA

Editorial Office
MDPI
St. Alban-Anlage 66
4052 Basel, Switzerland

This is a reprint of articles from the Special Issue published online in the open access journal *Biomedicines* (ISSN 2227-9059) (available at: https://www.mdpi.com/journal/biomedicines/special_issues/Zebrafish_2).

For citation purposes, cite each article independently as indicated on the article page online and as indicated below:

LastName, A.A.; LastName, B.B.; LastName, C.C. Article Title. *Journal Name* **Year**, *Volume Number*, Page Range.

ISBN 978-3-0365-5459-4 (Hbk)
ISBN 978-3-0365-5460-0 (PDF)

© 2022 by the authors. Articles in this book are Open Access and distributed under the Creative Commons Attribution (CC BY) license, which allows users to download, copy and build upon published articles, as long as the author and publisher are properly credited, which ensures maximum dissemination and a wider impact of our publications.

The book as a whole is distributed by MDPI under the terms and conditions of the Creative Commons license CC BY-NC-ND.

Contents

About the Editors . . . . **vii**

James A. Marrs and Swapnalee Sarmah
The Genius of the Zebrafish Model: Insights on Development and Disease
Reprinted from: *Biomedicines* 2021, 9, 577, doi:10.3390/biomedicines9050577 1

Amina M. Fallata, Rachael A. Wyatt, Julie M. Levesque, Antoine Dufour, Christopher M. Overall and Bryan D. Crawford
Intracellular Localization in Zebrafish Muscle and Conserved Sequence Features Suggest Roles for Gelatinase A Moonlighting in Sarcomere Maintenance
Reprinted from: *Biomedicines* 2019, 7, 93, doi:10.3390/biomedicines7040093 5

Md Ruhul Amin, Kazi T. Ahmed and Declan W. Ali
Early Exposure to THC Alters M-Cell Development in Zebrafish Embryos
Reprinted from: *Biomedicines* 2020, 8, 5, doi:10.3390/biomedicines8010005 21

Yin-Sir Chung, Brandon Kar Meng Choo, Pervaiz Khalid Ahmed, Iekhsan Othman and Mohd. Farooq Shaikh
Orthosiphon stamineus Proteins Alleviate Pentylenetetrazol-Induced Seizures in Zebrafish
Reprinted from: *Biomedicines* 2020, 8, 191, doi:10.3390/biomedicines8070191 37

Lisa M. Barnhill, Hiromi Murata and Jeff M. Bronstein
Studying the Pathophysiology of Parkinson's Disease Using Zebrafish
Reprinted from: *Biomedicines* 2020, 8, 197, doi:10.3390/biomedicines8070197 63

Petrus Siregar, Stevhen Juniardi, Gilbert Audira, Yu-Heng Lai, Jong-Chin Huang, Kelvin H.-C. Chen, Jung-Ren Chen and Chung-Der Hsiao
Method Standardization for Conducting Innate Color Preference Studies in Different Zebrafish Strains
Reprinted from: *Biomedicines* 2020, 8, 271, doi:10.3390/biomedicines8080271 77

Swapnalee Sarmah, Marilia Ribeiro Sales Cadena, Pabyton Gonçalves Cadena and James A. Marrs
Marijuana and Opioid Use during Pregnancy: Using Zebrafish t o G ain U nderstanding of Congenital Anomalies Caused by Drug Exposure during Development
Reprinted from: *Biomedicines* 2020, 8, 279, doi:10.3390/biomedicines8080279 97

Fiorency Santoso, Ali Farhan, Agnes L. Castillo, Nemi Malhotra, Ferry Saputra, Kevin Adi Kurnia, Kelvin H.-C. Chen, Jong-Chin Huang, Jung-Ren Chen and Chung-Der Hsiao
An Overview of Methods for Cardiac Rhythm Detection in Zebrafish
Reprinted from: *Biomedicines* 2020, 8, 329, doi:10.3390/biomedicines8090329 115

Laura Massoz, Marie Alice Dupont and Isabelle Manfroid
Zebra-Fishing for Regenerative Awakening in Mammals
Reprinted from: *Biomedicines* 2021, 9, 65, doi:10.3390/biomedicines9010065 139

Lindy K. Brastrom, C. Anthony Scott, Kai Wang and Diane C. Slusarski
Functional Role of the RNA-Binding Protein Rbm24a and Its Target *sox2* in Microphthalmia
Reprinted from: *Biomedicines* 2021, 9, 100, doi:10.3390/biomedicines9020100 157

About the Editors

James A. Marrs

James A. Marrs (Professor of Biology) studies developmental and cell biology using the zebrafish to model birth defects, disease and developmental disorders.

Swapnalee Sarmah

Swapnalee Sarmah (Assistant Research Professor of Biology) has studied zebrafish developmental genetics, birth defects, disease models and developmental defects.

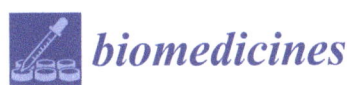

Editorial

The Genius of the Zebrafish Model: Insights on Development and Disease

James A. Marrs * and Swapnalee Sarmah

Department of Biology, Indiana University—Purdue University Indianapolis, 723 West Michigan, Indianapolis, IN 46202, USA; ssarmah@iu.edu
* Correspondence: jmarrs@iu.edu; Tel.: +1-317-278-0031

Citation: Marrs, J.A.; Sarmah, S. The Genius of the Zebrafish Model: Insights on Development and Disease. *Biomedicines* **2021**, *9*, 577. https://doi.org/10.3390/biomedicines9050577

Received: 19 April 2021
Accepted: 6 May 2021
Published: 20 May 2021

Publisher's Note: MDPI stays neutral with regard to jurisdictional claims in published maps and institutional affiliations.

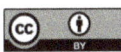

Copyright: © 2021 by the authors. Licensee MDPI, Basel, Switzerland. This article is an open access article distributed under the terms and conditions of the Creative Commons Attribution (CC BY) license (https:// creativecommons.org/licenses/by/ 4.0/).

The zebrafish is an outstanding and inexpensive vertebrate model system for biomedical research. The embryos develop externally allowing experimental access treatments; are transparent allowing for microscopy visualization; develop rapidly; and have outstanding genetic and genomic resources. The zebrafish model was first developed to study neural development, and this tradition continues. A large-scale mutagenesis screen propelled the zebrafish model rapidly forward to become the modern research platform we see today. Creative approaches using the zebrafish were developed to study toxicology, disease etiology, behavioral neuroscience and regenerative biology. Using these experimental foundations, the contributions found in this Special Issue of Biomedicines illustrate the power and potential of the zebrafish.

Due to evolutionary conservation among vertebrate organisms, animal models provide insight into disease processes that cannot be obtained by studying human patients. The genetic conservation between vertebrates allows scientists to evaluate consequences of mutations in disease etiology. There is an art to developing a useful disease model for biomedical research, and the zebrafish are being used at an increasing frequency to evaluate disease development and consequences. The genetic resources are being developed in the zebrafish, and it has been an established model system to determine the etiology of genetic disorders caused by damaging mutations in protein-coding genes. The result of the Human Genome Project led to the recognition of single-nucleotide polymorphisms (SNPs) that increase or decrease the risk for a given disease. Patients' genomic analyses have identified many clinically relevant mutations in the noncoding regions of the human genome which likely disrupt functions of cis-regulatory elements (CREs). A review by Mann and Bhatia [1] highlights the utility of the zebrafish for studying mutations in non-coding regions of the genome. The zebrafish offer low maintenance cost, short generation times, imaging approaches and transgenic technology which can be exploited to evaluate functional consequences of noncoding region mutations.

A couple of reviews discuss how the zebrafish are used to study heart disease models. Giardoglou and Beis [2] discuss the utility of the zebrafish in examining the heart and vasculature. The zebrafish heart shares features with the human heart not found in other models, and consequently, disease models share similarities in pathophysiological consequences with the human conditions. They also highlight the use of genome-wide association studies (commonly referred to as GWAS) to identify genetic variants (multiple loci and SNPs associated with coronary artery disease and cardiomyopathies) and the use of the zebrafish to dissect functional defects and validate candidate causal genes that emerge from GWAS analyses. Santoso et al. [3] review the methodology used to study cardiac rhythm in the zebrafish. There are experimental challenges associated with a small aquatic organism, but methods are continually improving to detect cardiac rhythm in both embryonic and adult zebrafish. The authors discuss current methodologies including the dynamic pixel change method, kymography, laser confocal microscopy, artificial intelligence and electrocardiography (ECG). The authors also provide perspectives on advances like imaging technology and artificial intelligence that are applied to studies of cardiac rhythm.

Parkinson's disease genes and effects of environmental toxins have been uncovered in recent years. Barnhill et al. [4] review the use of the zebrafish as a model of Parkinson's disease. Individual genes and the zebrafish models affecting the progression of a Parkinson's disease phenotype are discussed. These genes point to protein aggregation, protein degradation, mitochondrial dysfunction, synapse dysfunction, inflammation and cell death pathways. Environmental assaults are also studied in the zebrafish, which fit into similar pathophysiological pathways as the genetic defects.

Two research articles provide fundamental insight into biological processes that affect muscle and eye conditions. Fallata et al. [5] examined gelatinase A (a matrix metalloproteinase) expression and activity in muscles, which participates in myosin degradation. They showed that gelatinase A has poorly recognized signal sequences and conserved phosphorylation sites, which may regulate its enzymatic activity within the sarcomere. The gelatinase A enzyme has not been characterized in specific diseases, but the authors discussed the physiological role, and the evidence suggests potential roles in disease and injury.

An exciting study by Brastrom et al. [6] produced a model of microphthalmia (small eye phenotype) caused by mutations in the human RBM24 gene, an RNA-binding protein. This RNA-binding protein regulates the gene most commonly affected in microphthalmia patients, SOX2. The experiments showed that overexpression of the zebrafish Sox2 protein suppresses the microphthalmia phenotype, supporting the posttranscriptional role for the Rbm24 protein in binding and targeting the *sox2* mRNA.

Neuroscience of the zebrafish is at the foundation of this model organism due to the transparency of embryos allowing neural development visualization. Neuroscience functional changes can be studied using animal behavior analysis. Since fish have very different lives from humans, the analysis of fish behavior is challenging. Progress is being made with the study of zebrafish behavior and correlating fish behavior with that of humans. Zebrafish behavior is being correlated with neural development, electrophysiology and other aspects of neurobiology. A series of articles in this Special Issue of Biomedicines address neuroscience and behavior.

A review article by Basnet et al. [7] discussed the uses of the zebrafish model to evaluate and screen neuroactive drugs. They highlight the studies of the brain–behavior connection and the types of behavior assays that can be used with the zebrafish. Finally, they review studies of neuroactive drugs and toxicants that produce behavior defects in the zebrafish. The review is an excellent primer for the zebrafish behavior model, which is a growing model with outstanding potential.

Using adult zebrafish, Chung et al. [8] use a pentylenetetrazol (PTZ)-induced epileptic seizure model to evaluate anti-convulsive activities of a protein extract from a medicinal plant, *Orthosiphon stamineus*. Intraperitoneal injection of the protein extract decreased seizures and altered neurotransmitter levels in zebrafish brains. Proteomic analysis of zebrafish brains showed differential expression of proteins, particularly a regulator of the trans-SNARE complex that affects neurotransmitter exocytosis. The findings suggest potential mechanisms of antiepileptic drug action that could be further studied.

Two articles describe the development of methodology to evaluate visual responses using the zebrafish. Color preference is a useful behavioral parameter, but Siregar et al. [9] note that there are some apparent contradictions in the literature using this assay. Thus, they test several variables (light source position, light intensity, gender, age, strain, etc.) in order to standardize the method. This is a very useful study that will help the zebrafish community generate results from different laboratories that can be compared to one another. We expect that such standardization and harmonization of methodology will be completed for many assays as the zebrafish model grows.

Optomotor response is a common assay used for animal behavior, and it is an important assay used for the zebrafish. Branstrom et al. [10] produced a simple optomotor assay platform that can be performed with a tablet computer and a cell phone camera. The authors validate the assay using mutant and morpholino knockdown zebrafish larvae that disrupt the visual system. This clever and reproducible assay can be set up without expensive equipment and performed at relatively high throughput.

Regenerative medicine research grows because of the potential to treat defects and diseases that are intractable to current medical technology. The potential of these therapies is huge, but one must temper this excitement with the realization that basic research is needed to learn how the powerful potential can be controlled and applied.

Massoz et al. [11] reviewed the regenerative potential of the zebrafish and its use in the study of potential disease treatments. They focused on important targets for regenerative medicine, heart, liver, pancreas, spinal cord, brain and retina, which are the subject of numerous zebrafish studies. The authors note that it may be a long, difficult path to produce regenerative medicine therapeutics, but basic research using the zebrafish will help facilitate this journey to producing efficacious and safe treatments.

Our laboratory, in collaboration with colleagues from Lilly Research Laboratories, examined [12] the effects of a small-molecule Wnt signaling pathway activator on zebrafish caudal fin regeneration. Fin rays are bony structures, and fin regeneration is a useful model for bone growth and repair. Our studies illustrate that zebrafish fin regeneration is a potent platform to study bone healing and characterize drugs that stimulate regenerative potential.

Recreational drug use and abuse is a public health problem, and exposure to drugs during pregnancy is growing due to the ongoing opioid crisis and marijuana legalization. In a review from our laboratory and colleagues from Brazil [13], experiments using the zebrafish to model effects of marijuana and opioid exposure during development were discussed. The effects of exposure to these drugs during pregnancy are less severe than ethanol exposure and are poorly understood. However, growing evidence indicates that there are lasting defects caused by marijuana and opioid exposure. Our review discusses the zebrafish endocannabinoid and opioid signaling system in the zebrafish and the use of this model for understanding the drug exposure-associated developmental defects and identifying treatments.

Amin et al. [14] examined the effects of embryo exposure to the intoxicating ingredient in marijuana, THC, on the nervous system and muscle development. THC exposure during early development affected the Mauther cell, a large neuron that helps control the escape response in the zebrafish and related organisms. THC-exposed zebrafish also exhibited changes in muscle cells. Swimming behavior was affected by THC exposure, showing that there are significant consequences of THC exposure during development that are evident in the zebrafish model.

An impressive and diverse set of articles are found in the Special Issue of Biomedicines "Zebrafish Models for Development and Disease" that represent a significant scope of the zebrafish research arena. The common themes of the Special Issue include neuroscience, behavioral analysis, disease models and regenerative biology. These topics bridge the foundations of the zebrafish model with the areas that are growing in the field, like behavior and regeneration. The zebrafish model still has potential to spare. The model is used to test ecological toxicology, evolutionary biology, cancer biology and many other topics. There is still untapped potential of the zebrafish model that will be exploited in the future. Efforts to use the zebrafish to screen for new therapeutics are ongoing, but it seems clear that there is still room for growth. The CRISPR/Cas9 gene editing technology makes new powerful experimental models. For example, humanizing genes in the zebrafish for use in drug discovery is now a real possibility. Certainly, there are limits to the zebrafish model, but as Albert Einstein said, "Everybody is a genius. But if you judge a fish by its ability to climb a tree, it will live its whole life believing that it is stupid." We can look forward to more genius coming from the zebrafish model!

Author Contributions: Writing—original draft preparation, J.A.M. and S.S.; writing—review and editing, J.A.M. and S.S.; funding acquisition, J.A.M. and S.S. All authors have read and agreed to the published version of the manuscript.

Funding: This work was supported by NIH/NIAAA 1 R21 AA026711.

Institutional Review Board Statement: No human subjects.

Informed Consent Statement: Not applicable.

Data Availability Statement: Not applicable.

Conflicts of Interest: The authors declare no conflict of interest. The funders had no role in the writing of the manuscript, or in the decision to publish.

References

1. Mann, A.; Bhatia, S. Zebrafish: A Powerful Model for Understanding the Functional Relevance of Noncoding Region Mutations in Human Genetic Diseases. *Biomedicines* 2019, *7*, 71. [CrossRef]
2. Giardoglou, P.; Beis, D. On Zebrafish Disease Models and Matters of the Heart. *Biomedicines* 2019, *7*, 15. [CrossRef] [PubMed]
3. Santoso, F.; Farhan, A.; Castillo, A.L.; Malhotra, N.; Saputra, F.; Kurnia, K.A.; Chen, K.H.; Huang, J.C.; Chen, J.R.; Hsiao, C.D. An Overview of Methods for Cardiac Rhythm Detection in Zebrafish. *Biomedicines* 2020, *8*, 329. [CrossRef] [PubMed]
4. Barnhill, L.M.; Murata, H.; Bronstein, J.M. Studying the Pathophysiology of Parkinson's Disease Using Zebrafish. *Biomedicines* 2020, *8*, 197. [CrossRef] [PubMed]
5. Fallata, A.M.; Wyatt, R.A.; Levesque, J.M.; Dufour, A.; Overall, C.M.; Crawford, B.D. Intracellular Localization in Zebrafish Muscle and Conserved Sequence Features Suggest Roles for Gelatinase A Moonlighting in Sarcomere Maintenance. *Biomedicines* 2019, *7*, 93. [CrossRef] [PubMed]
6. Brastrom, L.K.; Scott, C.A.; Wang, K.; Slusarski, D.C. Functional Role of the RNA-Binding Protein Rbm24a and Its Target sox2 in Microphthalmia. *Biomedicines* 2021, *9*, 100. [CrossRef] [PubMed]
7. Basnet, R.M.; Zizioli, D.; Taweedet, S.; Finazzi, D.; Memo, M. Zebrafish Larvae as a Behavioral Model in Neuropharmacology. *Biomedicines* 2019, *7*, 23. [CrossRef] [PubMed]
8. Chung, Y.S.; Choo, B.K.M.; Ahmed, P.K.; Othman, I.; Shaikh, M.F. Orthosiphon stamineus Proteins Alleviate Pentylenetetrazol-Induced Seizures in Zebrafish. *Biomedicines* 2020, *8*, 191. [CrossRef] [PubMed]
9. Siregar, P.; Juniardi, S.; Audira, G.; Lai, Y.H.; Huang, J.C.; Chen, K.H.; Chen, J.R.; Hsiao, C.D. Method Standardization for Conducting Innate Color Preference Studies in Different Zebrafish Strains. *Biomedicines* 2020, *8*, 271. [CrossRef] [PubMed]
10. Brastrom, L.K.; Scott, C.A.; Dawson, D.V.; Slusarski, D.C. A High-Throughput Assay for Congenital and Age-Related Eye Diseases in Zebrafish. *Biomedicines* 2019, *7*, 28. [CrossRef] [PubMed]
11. Massoz, L.; Dupont, M.A.; Manfroid, I. Zebra-Fishing for Regenerative Awakening in Mammals. *Biomedicines* 2021, *9*, 65. [CrossRef] [PubMed]
12. Sarmah, S.; Curtis, C.; Mahin, J.; Farrell, M.; Engler, T.A.; Sanchez-Felix, M.V.; Sato, M.; Ma, Y.L.; Chu, S.; Marrs, J.A. The Glycogen Synthase Kinase-3beta Inhibitor LSN 2105786 Promotes Zebrafish Fin Regeneration. *Biomedicines* 2019, *7*, 30. [CrossRef] [PubMed]
13. Sarmah, S.; Sales Cadena, M.R.; Cadena, P.G.; Marrs, J.A. Marijuana and Opioid Use during Pregnancy: Using Zebrafish to Gain Understanding of Congenital Anomalies Caused by Drug Exposure during Development. *Biomedicines* 2020, *8*, 279. [CrossRef] [PubMed]
14. Amin, M.R.; Ahmed, K.T.; Ali, D.W. Early Exposure to THC Alters M-Cell Development in Zebrafish Embryos. *Biomedicines* 2020, *8*, 5. [CrossRef] [PubMed]

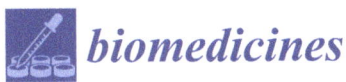

Article

Intracellular Localization in Zebrafish Muscle and Conserved Sequence Features Suggest Roles for Gelatinase A Moonlighting in Sarcomere Maintenance

Amina M. Fallata [1], Rachael A. Wyatt [1], Julie M. Levesque [1], Antoine Dufour [2,3], Christopher M. Overall [3] and Bryan D. Crawford [1,*]

1. Department of Biology, University of New Brunswick, Fredericton, NB E3B 5A3, Canada; afallata-404@hotmail.com (A.M.F.); r.a.wyatt@unb.ca (R.A.W.); jl395146@gmail.com (J.M.L.)
2. Department of Physiology & Pharmacology, University of Calgary, Calgary, AB T2N 4N1, Canada; antoine.dufour@ucalgary.ca
3. Department of Oral Biological and Medical Sciences and Centre for Blood Research, University of British Columbia, Vancouver, BC V6T 1Z4, Canada; chris.overall@ubc.ca
* Correspondence: bryanc@unb.ca

Received: 7 November 2019; Accepted: 25 November 2019; Published: 29 November 2019

Abstract: Gelatinase A (Mmp2 in zebrafish) is a well-characterized effector of extracellular matrix remodeling, extracellular signaling, and along with other matrix metalloproteinases (MMPs) and extracellular proteases, it plays important roles in the establishment and maintenance of tissue architecture. Gelatinase A is also found moonlighting inside mammalian striated muscle cells, where it has been implicated in the pathology of ischemia-reperfusion injury. Gelatinase A has no known physiological function in muscle cells, and its localization within mammalian cells appears to be due to inefficient recognition of its N-terminal secretory signal. Here we show that Mmp2 is abundant within the skeletal muscle cells of zebrafish, where it localizes to the M-line of sarcomeres and degrades muscle myosin. The N-terminal secretory signal of zebrafish Mmp2 is also challenging to identify, and this is a conserved characteristic of gelatinase A orthologues, suggesting a selective pressure acting to prevent the efficient secretion of this protease. Furthermore, there are several strongly conserved phosphorylation sites within the catalytic domain of gelatinase A orthologues, some of which are phosphorylated in vivo, and which are known to regulate the activity of this protease. We conclude that gelatinase A likely participates in uncharacterized physiological functions within the striated muscle, possibly in the maintenance of sarcomere proteostasis, that are likely regulated by kinases and phosphatases present in the sarcomere.

Keywords: Gelatinase A; Mmp2; zebrafish; sarcomere; myosin; proteostasis; phosphorylation; TAILS; secretion

1. Introduction

Matrix metalloproteinases (MMPs) are a complex family of about two dozen zinc-dependent proteases classically known for their roles in extracellular matrix (ECM) remodeling during development and disease, particularly in the contexts of inflammation and tumor biology [1–7]. They are broadly classified on the basis of their substrate specificities and structures into 'Collagenases' (MMPs 1, 8, 13, and 18), 'Gelatinases' (MMPs 2 and 9), 'Metalloelastase' (MMP12), 'Stromelysins' (MMPs 3, 10, and 11), 'Matrilysins' (MMPs 7 and 26), 'Enamelysin' (MMP20), 'Epilysin' (MMP28), 'Membrane Type MMPs' (MMPs 14, 15, 16, 17, 24, and 25), and 'Other MMPs' (MMPs 19, 21, 23, and 27) [3]. MMPs are generally localized to the extracellular space via type I secretion [8], regardless of whether they are secreted or membrane-type MMPs, with the exception of MMP23. Classical type I secretion via recognition of an N-terminal signal peptide targets other MMPs to the endoplasmic reticulum during translation, whereas MMP23 enters the ER/Golgi network post-translationally (i.e., it undergoes type II secretion), and is presented on the cell surface with its carboxyl end facing extracellularly [9]. MMPs are released into the extracellular environment or presented on the cell surface as inactive zymogens, and require the removal of an N-terminal propeptide (through the activity of pro-protein convertases or other proteases, including other MMPs) in order to become active [3,10]. Importantly, this irreversible post-translational proteolytic activation is emerging as one of, if not *the* most important level at which MMP activity is regulated, making the many reports focusing on changes in expression at the mRNA level difficult to interpret, as the biologically relevant activity is not well correlated with mRNA levels [11]. Novel approaches that focus on this post-translational activation (e.g., [12]) provide exciting opportunities to understand the regulation of MMP activity in vivo better. Once active, MMPs cleave a wide variety of extracellular matrix (ECM) and non-matrix proteins, including cell adhesion molecules, solute carriers, membrane receptors, and signaling molecules, and participate in a myriad of pathological and cell biological processes above and beyond matrix remodeling [3,6,13–15]. In addition to these well-established and undeniably important extracellular functions, many MMPs are also detected intracellularly in a variety of mammalian cell types [16–18]. They have been found in the cytosol [19–22], within the nucleus [20,23,24], and within mitochondria [19,22]. The mechanism(s) resulting in intracellular localization and the roles they play in these contexts remains poorly understood.

Gelatinase A (in humans the gelatinase A protein is called MMP-2, in mice it is referred to as MMP2, and in zebrafish as Mmp2; we have endeavored to be consistent with the naming conventions of the organisms in question, and have used 'gelatinase A' as the generic descriptor) is among the best-studied of the MMPs, and it is present nearly ubiquitously in embryonic and adult tissues of all vertebrates that have been examined. Surprisingly, mice deficient for MMP2 are viable and exhibit only subtle phenotypes (reviewed in [25]). However, anti-sense mediated knockdown of Mmp2 in zebrafish results in dramatic perturbations of embryonic development [26]. This is likely due to a combination of reduced redundancy between MMPs in zebrafish and their more rapid development providing less opportunity for compensatory mechanisms to mitigate the loss of Mmp2 activity [27]. Gelatinase A is among the MMPs found intracellularly [19,21,22,28], and it has been the focus of significant attention in the context of ischemia/reperfusion injury in cardiac muscle [29–32]. In human and murine myocytes, immunogold localization suggests it is concentrated in the sarcomeres at the Z-discs [19,22]. In human cells, MMP-2 protein accumulates intracellularly due to a poorly recognized N-terminal secretory signal; replacement of this sequence with a stronger signal sequence results in dramatically more efficient secretion, and N-terminal addition of the MMP-2 secretory signal to proteins otherwise efficiently targeted to the secretory pathway results in a dramatic reduction in the efficiency of this targeting [21].

Like research into their extracellular functions, investigations into intracellular functions of MMPs (including gelatinase A), have focused primarily on their pathological activities. In the context of mammalian cardiac muscle, ischemia/reperfusion events result in the production of reactive oxygen species (ROS), which can directly or indirectly modify the sulfhydryl group of the cysteine switch present in the autoinhibitory propeptide of gelatinase A, activating the protease [33]. Once activated, gelatinase A degrades several sarcomeric proteins, resulting in loss of contractility [31,34]. The upshot of this is that inhibition of gelatinase A activity is a promising avenue for mitigating the damage of ischemia/reperfusion injury in a clinical setting [30–32], but the question of why this potentially dangerous protease accumulates within the myocytes in the first place – i.e., what, if any, physiological functions does gelatinase A have in the sarcomere – remains unaddressed.

As well as cardiac muscle, gelatinase A has recently been detected in mammalian skeletal muscle [22,28]. Curiously, for an ostensibly extracellular enzyme, its proteolytic activity is subject to regulation by phosphorylation [35–37]. While extracellular kinases exist, and there are other examples of proteins with extracellular functions that are modulated by phosphorylation [38,39], the vast majority of kinases and phosphatases function intracellularly, and the sensitivity of mammalian gelatinase A to this type of regulation is surprising in the absence of any known intracellular function. It has been suggested that the inefficient secretion and susceptibility to regulation by phosphorylation of mammalian MMP2 may be 'evolutionary spandrels'; quirks of this particular protease that have arisen as a result of unrelated adaptive changes that lack sufficient negative consequence to drive strong selection against them. If this were the case, we would not expect to find intracellular localization and/or phosphorylation of gelatinase A orthologues conserved across distantly related species. Here we begin to address these questions by examining the localization of Mmp2 in developing zebrafish embryos, and by analyzing the conservation of sequence features relating to the targeting of the protease to the type I secretory pathway and its phosphorylation by kinases.

We find that zebrafish Mmp2 is distinctly localized within the skeletal muscle cells of both embryos and adults, but at the M-lines rather than Z-discs, and only after sarcomerogenesis is complete. The N-terminal secretory signals of gelatinase A orthologues are consistently poorly recognized as such across a broad phylogenetic array of taxa, suggesting a selective pressure to maintain an intracellular pool of the protease. Furthermore, there are several strongly conserved phosphorylation sites suggesting the existence of an undiscovered intracellular system of kinases and phosphatases that regulate the activity of gelatinase A within the sarcomere. Finally, we observe that the protein most notably protected from proteolysis by the inhibition of MMP activity in zebrafish embryos is muscle myosin heavy chain, suggesting that sarcomeric proteins are genuine MMP substrates in vivo and that the Mmp2 we detect in the M-lines of embryonic skeletal muscle is likely degrading this component of thick filaments under normal physiological conditions. Taken together, this data suggests there is an ancient and conserved role for gelatinase A in the regulated turnover of sarcomeric proteins in vertebrates.

2. Experimental Section

2.1. Zebrafish Husbandry

Embryos were collected by natural spawning from adult wildtype (Tübingen) zebrafish maintained on a 14 h light: 10 h dark schedule in a flow-through system at between 26 °C and 28.5 °C, and staged according to [40]. Embryos were raised in standard Embryo Rearing Medium (ERM: 13 mM NaCl, 0.5 mM KCl, 0.02 mM Na_2HPO_4, 0.04 mM KH_2PO_4, 1.3 mM $CaCl_2$, 1.0 mM $MgSO_4$, and 4.2 mM $NaHCO_3$, pH 7.4) at 28 °C, dechorionated manually using fine forceps, and either fixed at the desired stage in Dent's fixative (80% methanol, 20% dimethyl sulfoxide (DMSO)) overnight at 4 °C, or homogenized as described below. Adult tissues were obtained by selecting healthy individuals (both male and female), sacrificing by MS-222 overdose, and dissection on ice. Dissected tissues were fixed in Dent's fixative as above. All work with zebrafish was done with the approval and under the supervision of the University of New Brunswick's Animal Care Committee (ACC Protocols 10013 (approved May 14, 2010), 11016 (approved May 16, 2011), 12013 (approved May 10, 2012), 13001, 13013 (May 13, 2013) and 14014 (approved May 7, 2014)), in accordance with the Canadian Council on Animal Care Guidelines.

2.2. Immunofluorescence and Cryosectioning

Samples were washed with PBSTx (0.1% Triton X-100 in Phosphate-Buffered Saline (PBS: 137 mM NaCl, 2.7 mM KCl, 20 mM phosphate pH 7.3)) five times for five minutes to remove fixative, blocked in blocking buffer (5% bovine serum albumin (BSA) in PBSTx) overnight at 4 °C, and incubated with primary antibodies; rabbit anti-zebrafish-Mmp2 (Anaspec catalog #55111, Freemont, CA, USA) and mouse anti-α-actinin (Sigma, catalog #A7811, Oakville, ON Canada), diluted (1:1000) in blocking buffer overnight at 4 °C. Samples were washed another five times for five minutes with PBSTx and then incubated with fluorescent conjugated secondary antibodies (Alexa-488 conjugated goat anti-rabbit IgG, as well as Alexa-633 conjugated goat anti-mouse IgG (Invitrogen, Carlsbad CA, USA) in samples processed for double labeling) diluted (1:1000) in blocking buffer overnight at 4 °C. After the final incubation, they were again washed with PBSTx, five times for five minutes each, and imaged using a Leica SP2 laser scanning confocal microscope (Leica, Wetzlar, Germany) with 20 × 0.7 NA water immersion and 63 × 1.4 NA oil immersion lenses.

For cryosectioning, 72 hours post-fertilization (hpf) zebrafish embryos were processed for double-labeling immunofluorescence as described above, washed in PBSTx, and embedded in 2.3 M sucrose dissolved in PBS overnight at 4 °C. The following day, the embedded embryos were frozen with liquid nitrogen and cut into 500 nm ultrathin sections using a Leica Ultracut T ultramicrotome. Sections were mounted on poly-L-Lysine coated glass slides and imaged as described above.

Images were assembled, and scale bars added using FIJI [41], and overlapping confocal stacks were projected stitched for the composite image shown in Figure 1A using the pairwise stitching plugin [42].

2.3. Immunoblotting

Embryos were collected at specified stages, dechorionated, and anesthetized in 0.4 mg/mL buffered tricaine before being homogenized in TRIzol (Thermo Fisher Scientific, Waltham, MA, USA) and stored at −20 °C. Homogenates were thawed on ice, centrifuged to remove insoluble debris, and protein separated from nucleic-acid containing fractions, according to the manufacturers directions. Protein pellets were solubilized in SDS-PAGE sample buffer (45 mM Tris pH 6.8, 10% glycerol, 1% SDS, 0.01% bromophenol blue, 50 mM DTT) and concentration was determined by BCA assays (Pierce, Rockford IL, USA). Three-hundred and fifty µg of protein from each stage was resolved on a 12% acrylamide gel, transferred to PVDF membrane, and the membrane incubated in blocking buffer (PBS with 0.1% Tween-20 (PBSTw) and 5% w/v skim milk powder) for 2 h at RT with gentle agitation. Membranes were probed with anti-zebrafish-Mmp2 (Anaspec, Freemont, CA, USA) diluted at 1:5000 in blocking buffer overnight at 4 °C. Unbound antibody was removed with three ten minute washes in PBSTw with gentle agitation at room temperature, and bands were visualized by incubating for 2 h at RT with HRP-conjugated goat anti-rabbit IgG (Invitrogen, Carlsbad, CA, USA) diluted 1:10000 in blocking buffer, followed by three ten minute washes in PBSTw and detection using Pierce™ ECL Plus Western Blotting Substrate (ThermoFisher Scientific).

2.4. Analysis of Signal Peptides

Gene records for MMPs were retrieved from the NCBI Genbank database via keyword searches. The set of the longest protein sequences from each gene record were curated manually to include only sequences for which the gene symbol indicates an MMP. The sequence sets for each MMP, and the vitronectin control, were then aligned using MUltiple Sequence Comparison by Log-Expectation (MUSCLE 3.8.31 [43]), and the alignment was trimmed in AliView [44] to include only entries with highly conserved sequences in the first two dozen amino acids to avoid annotation errors in starting position or isoforms with divergent start positions. Sequences were removed from the analysis if they had gaps in the first fifteen amino acids, or if their start position was divergent from the consensus. The resulting set of sequences were processed using SignalP 4.1 [45] and mean S scores for each protein were graphed using R [46–48].

2.5. Phosphorylation Score Analysis

Phosphorylation scores for all orthologues of gelatinase A were predicted using NetPhos [49,50]. A multiple sequence alignment calculated using MUSCLE [43] was used to create a gap-map to translate the locations of possible phosphorylation sites (exported with the position in the amino acid sequence) from sequence coordinates into alignment coordinates and then back into the coordinates of a reference sequence (in this case the *Danio rerio* sequence). Sites were then restricted to those with scores higher than 0.65 and conservation in at least 97% of sequences (202 sequences out of 208).

2.6. Terminal Amine Isotopic Labeling of Substrates (TAILS)

TAILS identification of MMP substrates was performed as previously described [51]. Briefly, 2000 embryos were reared at 28 °C in ERM until 24 hpf, manually dechorionated with fine forceps, and then split into groups of 1000 and incubated at 28 °C with 3 µM phenanthroline (Sigma) or DMSO (vehicle) controls until 48 hpf and flash-frozen in liquid nitrogen. Proteomes were prepared as previously described, and their quality verified by SDS-PAGE. Proteomes were reduced and alkylated, and primary amines were labeled using 40 mM formaldehyde and 20 mM cyanoborohydride, using heavy ($^{13}CD_2O$ and $NaBD_3CN$) isotopically labeled reagents in the control reactions, and light ($^{12}CH_2O$ and $NaBH_3CN$) in the MMP-inhibited proteome, at 37 °C overnight. Labeled proteomes were precipitated with ice cold methanol, resolubilized in 50 mM HEPES pH 7.5, and digested with 5 µg of Trypsin Gold (Promega) overnight at 37 °C. Completion of trypsin digestion was verified by SDS-PAGE, and the peptides with newly generated amino-termini were removed by coupling to amine-reactive polymer, leaving only labeled N-terminal peptides from the original proteomes free in solution. Peptides were collected by filtration using 10 kD cut-off ultrafiltration (Amicon), pooled and acidified to pH 3 using formic acid, and bound to C_{18} stage tips before analysis by mass spectrometry using an LTQvelos Orbitrap as previously described [52]. Peptides were identified using MaxQuant (1.4.1.2) and the zebrafish UniProt (FASTA, 2014, *Danio rerio*) database. Peptides with a heavy:light ratio >3 were identified as amino termini significantly enriched in the control proteome, and therefore being representative of substrates protected by inhibition of MMPs.

3. Results

3.1. Mmp2 is Expressed after Gastrulation and Accumulates Intracellularly at the M-Lines of Skeletal Muscle Sarcomeres

Previous studies of *mmp2* expression in zebrafish embryos using in situ hybridization and RT-PCR suggested ubiquitous expression from early cleavage (1.5 h post-fertilization (hpf)) onwards [26], but no data on the distribution of the protein in zebrafish embryos has been published. Immunoblots of whole embryo homogenates probed with an antibody against zebrafish Mmp2 reveal little expression prior to the completion of gastrulation and the onset somitogenesis (~12 hpf), consistent with publicly available RNAseq data (http://www.ebi.ac.uk/gxa/experiments/E-ERAD-475). Both transcript and protein increase in abundance until about 72 hpf (Figure 1). Indirect immunofluorescence reveals broad, indistinct immunoreactivity starting during segmentation (data not shown). As the embryo develops, Mmp2 becomes increasingly abundant in the skeletal musculature, exhibiting apparently sarcomeric staining at high magnifications (Figure 1A and B). Strong immunoreactivity is also apparent associated with the posterior tip of the notochord, actinotrichia of the fins, neuromasts, mesenchymal cells in the head and eyes, and some axonal projections in the eyes and musculature. These axonal projections are not immunoreactive with the sensory neuron-specific antibody Zn-12 [53], suggesting they are likely a subset of motor-afferents (Figure S1).

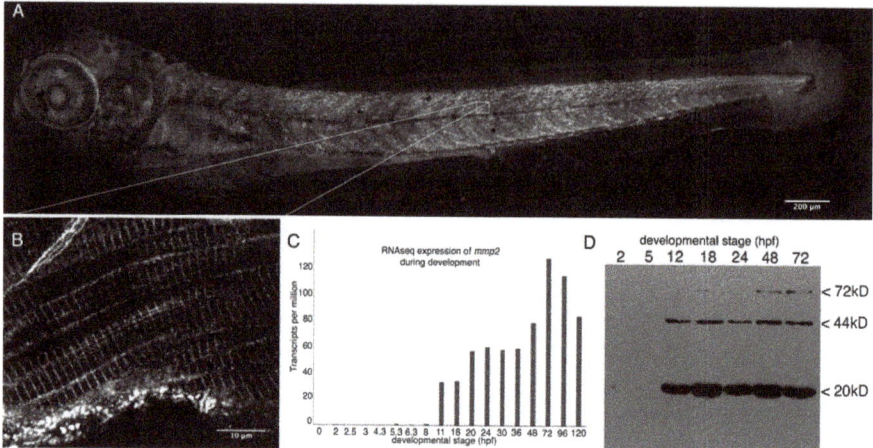

Figure 1. Mmp2 is expressed ubiquitously from early development and accumulates in a striated pattern within the skeletal muscle. (**A**) Composite confocal projections of a 72 hpf embryo stained with anti-Mmp2 exhibiting labeling throughout the embryo with notable accumulation in the skeletal muscle (scale bar = 200 µm). (**B**) High magnification view of a single confocal section through the trunk musculature (indicated by the inset) showing strong labeling of the myotome boundary (upper left corner), and striated staining in myofibrils (scale bar = 10 µm). (**C**) RNASeq data showing absolute abundance of *mmp2* transcripts in embryos from fertilization to five days post-fertilization (dpf). (**D**) Immunoblot of whole embryo homogenates (350 µg per lane) made from 2 hpf (cleavage), 5 hpf (50% epiboly), 12 hpf (early somitogenesis), 18 hpf (late somitogenesis), 24 hpf (prim-5), 48 hpf (long pec), and 72 hpf (protruding mouth) embryos probed with anti-Mmp2. Immunoreactivity is detected in embryos after 12 h of development, with bands at the expected mobility for full-length Mmp2 (72 kD) and stronger bands at 44 and 20 kD, which combine to give the expected size for activated Mmp2 (64 kD).

Double immunofluorescence using an antibody against the Z-disc component α-actinin reveals Mmp2 immunoreactivity in distinct bands localized precisely between the α-actinin-positive Z-discs, corresponding with the M-line of the sarcomeres, in both embryonic and adult skeletal muscle (Figure 2). Consistent with M-line localization, Mmp2 immunoreactivity co-localizes with myosin heavy chain labeled with mAb F59 [54] (Figure S2). The dimensions of the confocal voxels in these micrographs have an axial resolution of 0.617 µm (calculated using https://svi.nl/NyquistCalculator), which is substantially less than the diameter of an adult myofibril (>10 µm), but uncomfortably close to the diameter of an embryonic myofibril (~1 µm). It is therefore theoretically possible that the Mmp2 immunoreactivity in the embryonic musculature could be superficial, rather than genuinely intracellular. To eliminate this possibility, we repeated the α-actinin/Mmp2 double immunofluorescence on ultrathin (500 nm) cryosections of skeletal muscle from 72 hpf embryos, thereby physically eliminating the possibility of superficial staining artifactually appearing between α-actinin immunoreactive Z-discs. Again, we observe robust Mmp2 immunoreactivity precisely between α-actinin positive Z-discs (Figure 2C). In all three preparations, the intensity of Mmp2 immunoreactivity correlates negatively with the intensity of α-actinin staining (correlation coefficients of −0.537, −0.496, and −0.649 in the confocal images of embryonic, adult, and cryosectioned embryonic muscle, respectively). This demonstrates unequivocally that Mmp2 protein accumulates at the M-lines of zebrafish skeletal muscle.

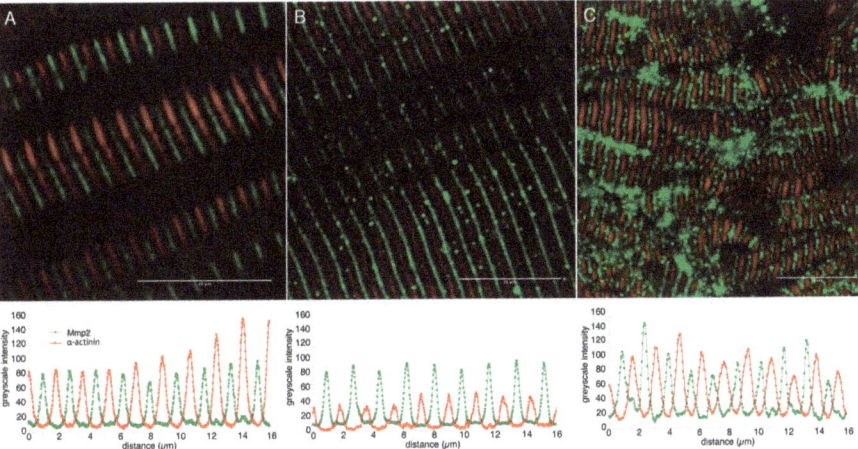

Figure 2. Mmp2 is localized between Z-discs in sarcomeres of embryonic and adult muscle. Confocal micrographs of skeletal muscle from 72 hpf embryos (**A**) or adults (**B**), and 500 nm thick cryosection of 72 hpf skeletal muscle (**C**) stained with anti-α-actinin (**red**) and anti-Mmp2 (**green**). Greyscale intensity profiles of both channels along a line drawn perpendicular to the sarcomeres are shown below each micrograph. Mmp2 immunoreactivity occurs at regularly spaced intervals precisely between the α-actinin-labeled Z-discs. Scale bars = 10 µm.

3.2. Mmp2 Accumulates at M-Lines Subsequent to Sarcomere Assembly

The skeletal musculature of vertebrates is derived from mesodermal somites, which form in zebrafish embryos starting around 11 hpf, with functionally contractile musculature arising around 18 hpf [40,55]. Since Mmp2 protein begins to accumulate prior to muscle cell differentiation and sarcomere formation, we wondered if the concentration of this protease in the sarcomeres begins before or after the assembly of the Z-discs from Z-bodies, during early sarcomereogenesis [56]. α-actinin/Mmp2 double immunofluorescence of the differentiating myofibrils in the trunk of 24 hpf embryos reveals the formation of nascent Z-discs in the periphery of early multi-nucleate myofibrils, but Mmp2 immunoreactivity remains roughly homogeneous within these cells at this stage, showing no strong correlation or anticorrelation with α-actinin immunoreactivity (correlation coefficient of 0.334) (Figure 3), suggesting that whatever role Mmp2 plays, its accumulation does not precede sarcomere formation.

3.3. Gelatinase A Orthologues have poorly Recognized Signal Sequences

The apparent abundance of Mmp2 within the skeletal muscle cells of the zebrafish embryos and adults led us to wonder if the zebrafish Mmp2 protein has an inefficiently recognized secretory signal peptide, as is the case in the human MMP-2 [21]. SignalP 4.1 is a software neural network trained to recognize class I secretory signals in eukaryotic proteins using known secreted proteins [45]. It is used routinely to identify secreted proteins in zebrafish and other vertebrates [57]. SignalP outputs C, S, Y, and D scores, representing predicted signal peptide cleavage sites, overall 'signal peptideness', a combined cleavage site prediction, and a final type I secretory protein 'discrimination score', respectively [45]. The zebrafish Mmp2 protein has an N-terminal secretory signal, but like the human MMP-2 protein, this sequence is barely recognizable by SignalP (zebrafish Mmp2 S_{mean} = 0.795; human MMP-2 S_{mean} = 0.845; typical secreted proteins have S_{mean} scores > 0.9), suggesting that, as is the case in mammals, a significant proportion of the Mmp2 protein produced in zebrafish cells escapes recognition by the signal recognition particle and is retained in the cytosol after translation. Given that the secretory signal is removed from the N-terminus of the protein as it is translocated through the Sec61 complex [58], the sequence of this part of the protein cannot affect the folding or activity of the rest of the molecule once it enters the secretory pathway. So it is difficult to imagine any selective pressures that would prevent this sequence converging on an efficiently recognized secretory signal unless there are advantageous physiological processes that require gelatinase A within the cell (where this N-terminal sequence would be retained). We tested this hypothesis by comparing the S scores of 208 gelatinase A orthologues to those of orthologues of an extracellular matrix protein that is efficiently secreted (vitronectin) and those of all other secreted MMPs, including orthologues of MMP23, which undergoes type II secretion and therefore lacks a conserved N-terminal secretory signal (Figure 4). As expected, orthologues of vitronectin have consistently well-recognized signal sequences, and orthologues of MMP23 have N-termini without recognizable signal sequences. Interestingly, while almost all other secreted MMPs have easily recognizable signal sequences, orthologues of gelatinase A (and MMP21) have consistently less recognizable N-terminal secretory signals. This suggests that there are selective pressures acting against efficient secretion of gelatinase A and MMP21.

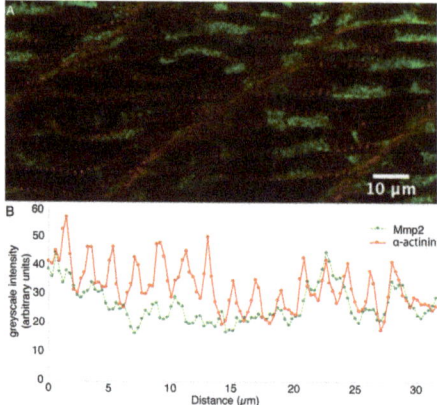

Figure 3. Sarcomeric Mmp2 begins to accumulate subsequent to the assembly of Z-disks. (**A**) Confocal section through the trunk musculature of a 24 hpf embryo posterior to the yolk extension, at the position at which myofibrils are differentiating. (**B**) Sarcomeric α-actinin (**red**) is beginning to become apparent as Z-bodies in the periphery of differentiating myocytes, but Mmp2 immunoreactivity (**green**) remains roughly homogeneously distributed. Greyscale intensity profiles of both channels along a line drawn through the periphery of a differentiating myocyte are shown below the micrograph. Scale bar = 10 μm.

3.4. Gelatinase A has Conserved Phosphorylation Sites that Regulate its Enzymatic Activity

Consistent with it having unrecognized intracellular functions, the proteolytic activity of gelatinase A is regulated by phosphorylation [35]. NetPhos 4.1 predicts both generic and kinase-specific phosphorylation sites in eukaryotic proteins [49,50], and several of the sites it identifies in human MMP-2 have been empirically verified [37]. Of the gelatinase A sequences currently known, there are five predicted phosphorylation sites that are conserved in all 208 orthologues (Figure 5). Two of these are sites that have been empirically verified as being phosphorylated in vivo, and all of them occur within the catalytic domain of the protein. There are five more sites that are conserved in 99% of sequences, and another three that are conserved in 97% of gelatinase A sequences. The extremely strong conservation of these known and predicted phosphorylation sites suggests they are under functional constraint, implying the existence of regulatory kinases and phosphatases that modulate the activity of this protease in an intracellular context.

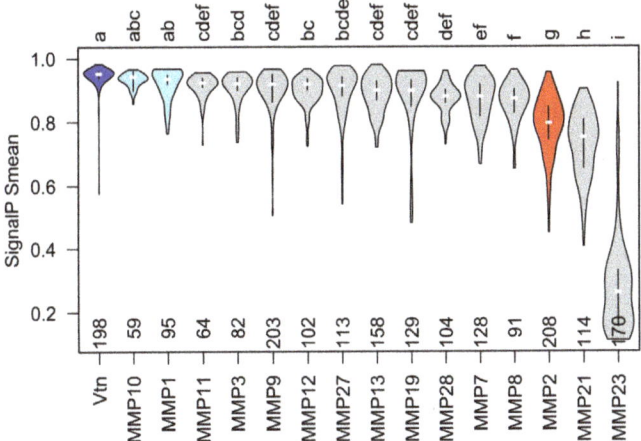

Figure 4. The secretory signal peptide of gelatinase A orthologues is consistently and significantly less likely to be recognized than that of most other type-I secreted proteins. Violin plots of mean 'S' scores of the N-terminal secretory signals from orthologues of vitronectin (Vtn) and all secreted MMPs. MMPs with mean S score statistically indistinguishable from vitronectin are shown in blue. Mean S scores for orthologues of gelatinase A (red) are significantly lower than those of vitronectin and other secreted MMPs apart from MMP21 and MMP23, which undergoes type II secretion and therefore, does not have an N-terminal secretory signal. Statistically, indistinguishable groups are indicated with letters at the top of the plot, and the number of orthologues of each protein analyzed is indicated along the x-axis.

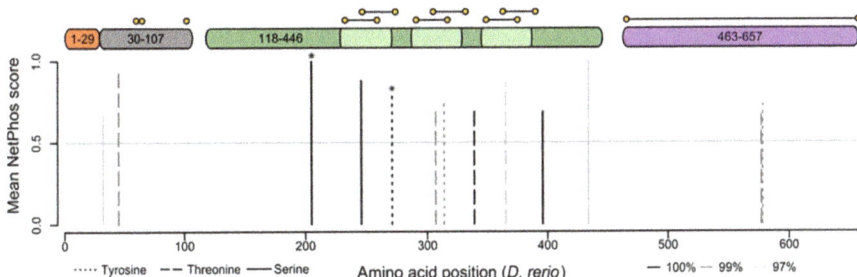

Figure 5. Gelatinase A orthologues have highly conserved phosphorylation sites. Putative serine (solid lines), threonine (dashed lines), and tyrosine (dotted lines) phosphorylation sites conserved in 100% (**black**), 99% (**dark grey**), or 97% (**light grey**) of gelatinase A orthologues are shown with respect to a structural schematic of the gelatinase A protein, illustrating the signal sequence (1–29 (**orange**)), propeptide (30–107 (**grey**)), catalytic domain (118–446 (**green**)) with fibronectin-like repeats (light green), and hemopexin-like domain (463–657 (**purple**)). Cysteines are indicated with yellow spots, connected by horizontal lines if they are predicted to participate in intramolecular disulfide bonds. Conserved residues that have been empirically demonstrated to be phosphorylated in vivo in the human protein are indicated with asterisks.

3.5. Myosin is a Target of Metalloproteinases in Zebrafish Embryos in vivo

A longstanding problem in MMP biology has been the identification of genuine substrates in vivo [59–62]. Recently, terminal amino isotopic labeling of substrates (TAILS) has been used to quantitatively compare the abundance of novel N-termini between proteomes of samples collected under conditions with and without the activity of (a) specific protease(s), in order to generate 'degradomes' that allow the identification of proteins that are genuine targets of the protease(s) in question [51]. We used TAILS to compare the degradomes of 48 hpf zebrafish embryos in the presence or absence of the broad-spectrum MMP inhibitor phenanthroline [63]. We were able to identify 321 peptides using the zebrafish UniProt database, 49 of which exhibited heavy/light ratios greater than 3, indicating they are likely targets of proteases inhibited by phenanthroline (Data S1). A disproportionately high 24% (12/49) of these are fragments of myosin, four of which have isoleucine, leucine, or valine in the P1' position characteristic of gelatinase A cleavage sites [64] (Table 1). Thus, it appears that myosin is a genuine physiological target of MMPs in vivo, and it is likely that Mmp2 contributes at least some if not all, of the relevant proteolytic activity targeting this primary component of the thick sarcomeric filaments.

Table 1. Myosin peptides represent 24% of significant hits in TAILS after inhibition of metalloproteinases in 48 hpf zebrafish embryos. (Bold indicates P1' residues typical of Gelatinase A substrates).

Myosin Peptide	P1' Residue	Normalized H/L Ratio
DLEESTLQHEATAAALR	Asp	8.3856
IEELEEELEAER	**Ile**	7.6228
ELETEIEAEQR	Glu	6.6756
ADLSRELEEISER	Ala	4.6963
VRELESEVEAEQR	**Val**	4.4234
TLEDQLSEIKSKNDENLR	Thr	3.4527
VQLELNQVKSEIDR	**Val**	3.4453
LEDEEEINAELTAKKR	**Leu**	3.3276
ELESEVEAEQR	Glu	3.1041
ADIAESQVNKLR	Ala	3.0920
EQFEEEQEAKAELQR	Glu	3.0497
QLEEKEALVSQLTR	Gln	3.0294

4. Discussion

Gelatinase A is well known for its roles in ECM remodeling during development and wound healing, and as a central player in a wide variety of pathologies such as tumor metastasis and fibrosis of various tissues [65]. It also has key roles in complement activation [66] and in the regulation of chemokine and cytokine signaling in vivo [6,7]. In addition to these extracellular roles, Gelatinase A functions as an intracellular enzyme [16], but the mechanism(s) by which it becomes resident intracellularly and its function(s) in this context remain poorly understood. Why this potentially dangerous protease is not secreted more efficiently, thereby protecting cells from its inappropriate intracellular activation, is a mystery. Mutations in the sequence encoding the N-terminal secretory signal cannot affect the function of the protein once it enters the secretory pathway as the signal sequence is removed during translation [8,57], so one would expect the signal sequence of any protein that functions exclusively extracellularly to converge on one that is easily recognized by the signal recognition particle. This appears to be true for most secreted proteins, including most MMPs, but not for orthologues of gelatinase A.

The N-terminal secretory signal of human MMP-2 is inefficiently recognized, and secretion of MMP-2 can be dramatically improved by mutating this sequence such that it is better recognized by the signal recognition particle [21]. This is not an idiosyncrasy of the human protein; we observe that orthologues of gelatinase A across a broad phylogenetic array of taxa have N-terminal secretory signals that are consistently difficult to recognize, suggesting that there is a selective pressure that maintains this curious inefficiency, effectively splitting the production of gelatinase A protein between the outside and the inside of cells expressing this gene. Consistent with this, in the zebrafish Mmp2 protein is present within the myocytes of embryonic and adult skeletal muscle, demonstrating that this is a general feature of striated muscle cells and not a peculiarity of mammalian cardiac myocytes or mammalian cells in general. It is difficult to envision a scenario in which it would be advantageous to maintain a portion of any protein, let alone a potentially dangerous protease, within the cell if there were no adaptive functions for that molecule to fulfill within the cell, especially when mutations that increase the efficiency of secretion do not require changes to the sequence of the mature protein.

We detect Mmp2 at the M-lines of sarcomeres in skeletal muscle, and our TAILS data demonstrates that the myosin of thick filaments found in the M-band is degraded by MMPs—likely including Mmp2—under normal physiological conditions. This inconsistency with previous reports localizing mammalian MMP2 to Z-discs [19,22], may represent a genuine difference between cardiac and skeletal myocytes, or between mammalian and teleost myocytes, or both. Alternatively, this may represent an aspect of the functional regulation of gelatinase A activity; it may shuttle between these locations, similarly to the shuttling between the Z-disc and A-band exhibited by the myosin chaperones Unc45b and Hsp90 [67]. It is tempting to speculate that such changes in the localization of gelatinase A might be regulated by changes in its phosphorylation status.

Gelatinase A purified from mammalian cells is definitely phosphorylated, and while we may speculate on how its phosphorylation status may alter its localization, there is no doubt that phosphorylation profoundly alters its enzymatic activity [35–37]. This is likely true of zebrafish Mmp2, and the conservation of verified and putative phosphorylation sites suggests it is likely true of all gelatinase A orthologues. While ATP is generally not abundant extracellularly, extracellular kinases do exist and tissue inhibitor of matrix metalloproteinases 2 (TIMP-2) is phosphorylated in vivo [38,68,69]. So we cannot rule out the possibility that the phosphorylation of gelatinase A functions to regulate its extracellular activity. However, the most abundant extracellular kinases phosphorylate serine within SxE motifs [69], and none of the putative or known phosphorylation sites in gelatinase A match this pattern, nor are there known examples of other extracellular proteases that are regulated by phosphorylation.

The M-band of the sarcomere is rich in kinases and phosphatases that are known to function in regulating the turnover of sarcomeric proteins [70], although the specific mechanisms they regulate remain somewhat obscure. This suggests to us that gelatinase A may play a role in maintaining the proteostasis of the sarcomere, possibly contributing to the complex system mediating recycling of surplus and damaged components of the thick filament during muscle cell development and in response to exhaustive exercise [71–73]. The phosphorylation status of gelatinase A may therefore indicate the physiological status of the myocyte, and the zebrafish is emerging as an excellent model system for investigating these sorts of questions regarding muscle cell development and physiology [74,75].

The extracellular functions of gelatinase A and other MMPs remain important research questions, but we must not neglect the intracellular functions of these proteins or consider them only in pathological contexts [18]. Understanding the normal physiological mechanisms in which these molecules participate, their molecular regulation, their development, and their evolutionary origins will undoubtedly provide insights that are valuable in treating the pathologies that arise as a result of their misregulation. There is clearly selective pressure on orthologues of gelatinase A and MMP21 to maintain an intracellular pool of these proteases; Mmp2 is consistently present in the sarcomeres of striated muscle from fish to mammals, and sarcomeric proteins are predominant in the zebrafish MMP degradome in vivo. Taken together with the conservation of putative and empirically verified phosphorylation sites that regulate this proteolytic activity (and possibly localization) of this protease, we conclude that gelatinase A likely plays an important unrecognized role in the physiology of striated muscle that deserves more thorough investigation.

Supplementary Materials: Supplementary materials can be found at http://www.mdpi.com/2227-9059/7/4/93/s1.

Author Contributions: B.D.C. conceived and designed the experiments, performed TAILS experiments, prepared figures, and wrote the manuscript. A.M.F. helped design experiments, performed experiments illustrated in Figures 2–4, and helped with manuscript preparation. J.M.L. performed experiments illustrated in Figure 1. R.A.W. helped design and performed the bioinformatic analyses, prepared Figures 4 and 5, and edited the manuscript. A.D. helped with the design and execution of the TAILS experiment, analysis of TAILS data, and edited the manuscript. C.M.O. graciously hosted B.D.C., contributed reagents, helped with the design and analysis of the TAILS experiment.

41. Schindelin, J.; Arganda-Carreras, I.; Frise, E.; Kaynig, V. Fiji: An open-source platform for biological-image analysis. *Nature* **2012**, *9*, 676–682. [CrossRef]
42. Preibisch, S.; Saalfeld, S.; Tomancak, P. Globally Optimal Stitching of Tiled 3D Microscopic Image Acquisitions. *Bioinformatics* **2009**, *25*, 1463–1465. [CrossRef]
43. Edgar, R.C. MUSCLE: A multiple sequence alignment method with reduced time and space complexity. *BMC Bioinform.* **2004**, *5*, 113. [CrossRef] [PubMed]
44. Larsson, A. AliView: A fast and lightweight alignment viewer and editor for large data sets. *Bioinformatics* **2014**, *30*, 3276–3278. [CrossRef] [PubMed]
45. Petersen, T.N.; Brunak, S.; Von Heijne, G.; Nielsen, H. SignalP 4.0: Discriminating signal peptides from transmembrane regions. *Nat. Methods* **2011**, *8*, 785–786. [CrossRef] [PubMed]
46. R Core Team. *R: A Language and Environment for Statistical Computing*; R Foundation for Statistical Computing: Vienna, Austria, 2017; Available online: https://www.R-project.org/ (accessed on 10 February 2019).
47. Adler, D.; Kelly, S.T. Vioplot: Violin Plot. R Package Version 0.3.2. 2018. Available online: https://github.com/TomKellyGenetics/vioplot (accessed on 10 February 2019).
48. De Mendiburu, F. agricolae: Statistical Procedures for Agricultural Research. R package version 1.3-0. 2019. Available online: https://CRAN.R-project.org/package=agricolae (accessed on 10 February 2019).
49. Blom, N.; Gammeltoft, S.; Brunak, S. Sequence- and structure-based prediction of eukaryotic protein phosphorylation sites. *J. Mol. Biol.* **1999**, *294*, 1351–1362. [CrossRef] [PubMed]
50. Blom, N.; Sicheritz-Ponten, T.; Gupta, R.; Gammeltoft, S.; Brunak, S. Prediction of post-translational glycosylation and phosphorylation of proteins from the amino acid sequence. *Proteomics* **2004**, 1633–1649. [CrossRef]
51. Kleifeld, O.; Doucet, A.; Keller, U.A.D.; Prudova, A.; Schilling, O.; Kainthan, R.K.; E Starr, A.; Foster, L.J.; Kizhakkedathu, J.N.; Overall, C.M. Isotopic labeling of terminal amines in complex samples identifies protein N-termini and protease cleavage products. *Nat. Biotechnol.* **2010**, *28*, 281–288. [CrossRef]
52. Huesgen, P.F.; Lange, P.F.; Rogers, L.D.; Solis, N.; Eckhard, U.; Kleifeld, O.; Goulas, T.; Gomis-Rüth, F.X.; Overall, C.M. LysargiNase mirrors trypsin for protein C-terminal and methylation-site identification. *Nat. Methods* **2015**, *12*, 55–58. [CrossRef]
53. Metcalfe, W.K.; Myers, P.Z.; Trevarrow, B.; Bass, M.B.; Kimmel, C.B. Primary neurons that express the L2/HNK-1 carbohydrate during early development in the zebrafish. *Development* **1990**, *110*, 491–504.
54. Miller, J.B. Slow and fast myosin heavy chain content defines three types of myotubes in early muscle cell cultures. *J. Cell Biol.* **1985**, *101*, 1643–1650. [CrossRef]
55. Goody, M.F.; Carter, E.V.; Kilroy, E.A.; Maves, L.; Henry, C.A. "Muscling" Throughout Life: Integrating Studies of Muscle Development, Homeostasis, and Disease in Zebrafish. *Curr. Top. Dev. Biol.* **2017**, *124*, 197–234. [CrossRef]
56. Kontrogianni-Konstantopoulos, A.; Ackermann, M.A.; Bowman, A.L.; Yap, S.V.; Bloch, R.J. Muscle giants: Molecular scaffolds in sarcomerogenesis. *Physiol. Rev.* **2009**, *89*, 1217–1267. [CrossRef] [PubMed]
57. Klee, E.W. The zebrafish secretome. *Zebrafish* **2008**, *5*, 131–138. [CrossRef] [PubMed]
58. Nyathi, Y.; Wilkinson, B.M.; Pool, M.R. Co-translational targeting and translocation of proteins to the endoplasmic reticulum. *BBA—Mol. Cell Res.* **2013**, *1833*, 2392–2402. [CrossRef] [PubMed]
59. Overall, C.M.; Kleifeld, O. Tumour microenvironment—Opinion: Validating matrix metalloproteinases as drug targets and anti-targets for cancer therapy. *Nat. Rev. Cancer* **2006**, *6*, 227–239. [CrossRef] [PubMed]
60. Butler, G.S.; Overall, C.M. Updated biological roles for matrix metalloproteinases and new "intracellular" substrates revealed by de-gradomics. *Biochemistry* **2009**, *48*, 10830–10845. [CrossRef]
61. Auf dem Keller, U.; Schilling, O. Proteomic techniques and activity-based probes for the system-wide study of proteolysis. *Biochimie* **2010**, *92*, 1705–1714. [CrossRef]
62. Prudova, A.; auf dem Keller, U.; Butler, G.S.; Overall, C.M. Multiplex N-terminome analysis of MMP-2 and MMP-9 substrate degradomes by iTRAQ-TAILS quantitative proteomics. *Mol. Cell. Proteom.* **2010**, *9*, 894–911. [CrossRef]
63. Ellis, T.R.; Crawford, B.D. Experimental Dissection of Metalloproteinase Inhibition-Mediated and Toxic Effects of Phenanthroline on Zebrafish Development. *Int. J. Mol. Sci.* **2016**, *17*, 1503. [CrossRef]

64. Eckhard, U.; Huesgen, P.F.; Schilling, O.; Bellac, C.L.; Butler, G.S.; Cox, J.H.; Dufour, A.; Goebeler, V.; Kappelhoff, R.; Keller, U.A.D.; et al. Active site specificity profiling of the matrix metalloproteinase family: Proteomic identification of 4300 cleavage sites by nine MMPs explored with structural and synthetic peptide cleavage analyses. *Matrix Biol.* **2016**, *49*, 37–60. [CrossRef]
65. Henriet, P.; Emonard, H. Matrix metalloproteinase-2: Not (just) a "hero" of the past. *Biochimie* **2019**, *166*, 223–232. [CrossRef]
66. Auf dem Keller, U.; Prudova, A.; Eckhard, U.; Fingleton, B.; Overall, C.M. Systems-Level Analysis of Proteolytic Events in Increased Vascular Permeability and Complement Activation in Skin Inflammation. *Sci. Signal.* **2013**, *6*. [CrossRef] [PubMed]
67. Etard, C.; Roostalu, U.; Strähle, U. Shuttling of the chaperones Unc45b and Hsp90a between the A band and the Z line of the myofibril. *J. Cell Biol.* **2008**, *180*, 1163–1175. [CrossRef] [PubMed]
68. Cui, J.; Xiao, J.; Tagliabracci, V.S.; Wen, J.; Rahdar, M.; Dixon, J.E. A secretory kinase complex regulates extracellular protein phosphorylation. *elife* **2015**, *4*, e06120. [CrossRef] [PubMed]
69. Yalak, G.; Ehrlich, Y.H.; Olsen, B.R. Ectoprotein kinases and phosphatases: An emerging field for translational medicine. *J. Transl. Med.* **2014**, *12*, 165. [CrossRef] [PubMed]
70. Hu, L.Y.; Ackermann, M.A.; Kontrogianni-Konstantopoulos, A. The sarcomeric M- region: A molecular command center for diverse cellular processes. *BioMed Res. Int.* **2015**, *2015*, 714197. [CrossRef] [PubMed]
71. Carlisle, C.; Prill, K.; Pilgrim, D. Chaperones and the Proteasome System: Regulating the Construction and Demolition of Striated Muscle. *Int. J. Mol. Sci.* **2018**, *19*, 32. [CrossRef]
72. Carmeli, E.; Moas, M.; Lennon, S.; Powers, S.K. High intensity exercise increases expression of matrix metalloproteinases in fast skeletal muscle fibres. *Exp. Physiol.* **2008**, *90*, 613–619. [CrossRef]
73. Rullman, E.; Norrbom, J.; Stromberg, A.; Wagsater, D.; Rundqvist, H.; Haas, T.; Gustafsson, T. Endurance exercise activates matrix metalloproteinases in human skeletal muscle. *J. Appl. Physiol.* **2009**, *106*, 804–812. [CrossRef]
74. Maves, L. Recent advances using zebrafish animal models for muscle disease drug discovery. *Expert Opin. Drug Discov.* **2014**, *9*, 1033–1045. [CrossRef]
75. Talbot, J.; Maves, L. Skeletal muscle fiber type: Using insights from muscle developmental biology to dissect targets for susceptibility and resistance to muscle disease. *Wiley Interdiscip. Rev. Dev. Biol.* **2016**, *5*, 518–534. [CrossRef]

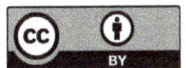

© 2019 by the authors. Licensee MDPI, Basel, Switzerland. This article is an open access article distributed under the terms and conditions of the Creative Commons Attribution (CC BY) license (http://creativecommons.org/licenses/by/4.0/).

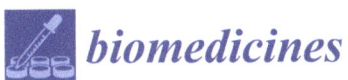

Article

Early Exposure to THC Alters M-Cell Development in Zebrafish Embryos

Md Ruhul Amin [1], Kazi T. Ahmed [1] and Declan W. Ali [1,2,*]

1. Department of Biological Sciences, CW-405 Biological Sciences Bldg., University of Alberta, Edmonton, AB T6G 2E9, Canada; mdruhul@ualberta.ca (M.R.A.); ktahmed@ualberta.ca (K.T.A.)
2. Neuroscience and Mental Health Institute, University of Alberta, Edmonton, AB T6G 2E1, Canada
* Correspondence: declan.ali@ualberta.ca; Tel.: +1-780-492-6094

Received: 16 October 2019; Accepted: 31 December 2019; Published: 4 January 2020

Abstract: Cannabis is one of the most commonly used illicit recreational drugs that is often taken for medicinal purposes. The psychoactive ingredient in cannabis is Δ^9-Tetrahydrocannabinol (Δ^9-THC, hereafter referred to as THC), which is an agonist at the endocannabinoid receptors CB_1R and CB_2R. Here, we exposed zebrafish embryos to THC during the gastrulation phase to determine the long-term effects during development. We specifically focused on reticulospinal neurons known as the Mauthner cells (M-cell) that are involved in escape response movements. The M-cells are born during gastrulation, thus allowing us to examine neuronal morphology of neurons born during the time of exposure. After the exposure, embryos were allowed to develop normally and were examined at two days post-fertilization for M-cell morphology and escape responses. THC treated embryos exhibited subtle alterations in M-cell axon diameter and small changes in escape response dynamics to touch. Because escape responses were altered, we also examined muscle fiber development. The fluorescent labelling of red and white muscle fibers showed that while muscles were largely intact, the fibers were slightly disorganized with subtle but significant changes in the pattern of expression of nicotinic acetylcholine receptors. However, there were no overt changes in the expression of nicotinic receptor subunit mRNA ascertained by qPCR. Embryos were allowed to further develop until 5 dpf, when they were examined for overall levels of movement. Animals exposed to THC during gastrulation exhibited reduced activity compared with vehicle controls. Together, these findings indicate that zebrafish exposed to THC during the gastrula phase exhibit small changes in neuronal and muscle morphology that may impact behavior and locomotion.

Keywords: cannabinoids; Mauthner; motor neurons; muscle; NMJ; CNS

1. Introduction

THC (Δ^9-Tetrahydrocannabinol) is the main psychotropic ingredient in the plant *Cannabis sativa*. THC binds to and activates two distinct classes of G-protein coupled receptors: cannabinoid receptors 1 (CB_1R) and cannabinoid receptors 2 (CB_2R) [1]. CB_1Rs are localized to the central nervous system (CNS) [2–4], whereas CB_2Rs are mainly associated with the peripheral nervous system, the immune system [5,6], the digestive and reproductive systems, and to a small extent the CNS [7–9]. In chicks and mice, CB_1R protein expression occurs even before the onset of neuronal development [10] and increases in a location-specific manner [11]. In rats, the offspring of mothers that were exposed to THC during gestation show different locomotor and exploratory behavior compared with controls [12], and in humans, prenatal exposure to THC leads to increased incidences of tremors and startle behaviors [13]. Significant evidence has been accumulated to show that prenatal or embryonic exposure to cannabinoids alters a range of behaviors, physiological processes, and gene expression, in large part because it appears to affect the normal functioning of the endocannabinoid (eCB) system. With regard to CNS development, the eCB system has been shown to regulate neural progenitor proliferation, specification, and migration (Reviewed in [14]), axonal growth, pathfinding and fasciculation [3,15], and the development of appropriate synaptic activity [16].

In zebrafish, CB_1Rs are highly expressed in the hindbrain where they are associated with reticulospinal neurons [3]. In fact, zebrafish express both CB_1Rs and CB_2Rs in the embryonic stages of development [17]. CB_1R expression appears low in early development prior to 24 hpf but increases as development proceeds, whereas CB_2R expression follows the reverse pattern, with high levels prior to 24 hpf and lower relative levels thereafter [17]. The knockdown of CB_1R expression with morpholino antisense oligonucleotides, or block of CB_1Rs with the receptor blocker AM251 alters patterns of axonal growth [3]. These findings prompted us to ask whether early exposure to THC alters the development of the primary reticulospinal neurons in the zebrafish hindbrain, the Mauthner cell (M-cell). We specifically focused on M-cell morphology and aspects of locomotion associated with M-cell function, such as the escape response to touch. M-cell neurons first appear around 8–9 h post fertilization (hpf) in the middle of the developmental period known as gastrulation. In zebrafish, gastrulation occurs from 5.25 hpf to 10.75 hpf [18]. At this stage, three germ layers are formed (ectoderm, mesoderm, and endoderm) and primary neurons, including M-cells appear. Shortly after their birth, the M-cells project an axon contralaterally and caudally down the spinal cord to the tail region [19]. As each M-cell projects down the cord, it forms synapses with primary motor neurons which innervate the white muscle fibers of the trunk [19].

We had previously found that zebrafish embryos exposed to THC during gastrulation exhibited altered fast escapes in response to acoustic but not mechanosensitive stimuli [20], indicating a possible deficit with M-cell form or function. Our results from the present study indicate that M-cells are largely intact following exposure to THC during gastrulation and that there appears to be minor but significant changes to neuronal morphology. Moreover, muscle morphology and locomotor responses are also impacted by exposure to THC.

2. Experimental Section

2.1. Animal Care and Exposure to THC

The fish used in this study were wild type zebrafish (*Danio rerio*) embryos of the Tubingen Longfin (TL) strain that were maintained at the University of Alberta Aquatic Facility. All animal housing and experimental procedures in this study were approved by the Animal Care and Use Committee at the University of Alberta (AUP #00000816) and adhered to the Canadian Council on Animal Care guidelines for humane animal use. For breeding, 3–5 adults, usually consisting of 3 females and 2 males, were placed in breeding tanks the evening before eggs were required. The following morning, fertilized eggs were collected from the breeding tanks, usually within 30 min of fertilization. Embryos and larvae were housed in incubators on a 12 h light/dark cycle, and set at 28.5 °C. Embryos were exposed to egg water (EW; 60 mg/mL Instant Ocean) containing either 6 mg/L THC (diluted from a stock solution obtained from Sigma; Δ^9-Tetrahydrocannabinol solution 1.0 mg/mL in methanol) or equivalent amounts of methanol during the period of gastrulation, which occurs between 5.25 hpf and 10.75 hpf. The exposure medium was then replaced at 10.75 hpf with 25 mL of fresh EW. Embryos were washed several times in EW and then incubated in fresh EW until further experiments at 48 hpf. For immunohistochemical studies, pigment formation was blocked by adding 0.003% phenylthiourea (PTU) dissolved in egg water at 24 hpf. The dose of THC (6 mg/L) was selected based on our previous work identifying critical concentration that affects survival and embryonic development [20].

2.2. Immunohistochemistry

Embryos (2 dpf) were fixed in 2% paraformaldehyde for 1–2 h and washed with 0.1 M phosphate buffered saline (PBS) every 15 min for 2 h. The preparations were then permeabilized for 30 min in 4% Triton-X 100 containing 2% BSA and 10% goat serum. Tissues were incubated for 48 h at 4 °C in either mouse monoclonal anti-3A10 (Developmental Studies Hybridoma Bank, Iowa City, IA, USA) (1:250) which targets neurofilaments associated with M-cell [21] or anti-RMO44 (Thermo Fisher Scientific, Waltham, MA, USA) (1:250) which labels several types of reticulospinal neurons. Tissues were also incubated in anti-F59 which targets myosin heavy chain (Developmental Studies Hybridoma Bank, 1:50) isoform of red muscle fibers [22] or anti-F310 (Developmental Studies Hybridoma Bank, 1:100) that targets myosin light chain 1 and 3f of white muscle fibers [23]. Tissues were washed in PBS twice every 15 min for 2–3 h and then incubated for 4 h at room temperature in the secondary antibody, Alexa Fluor®488 goat anti-mouse IgG or Alexa Fluor®555 goat anti-mouse IgG, (Molecular Probes, Thermo Fisher Scientific), at a dilution of 1:1000. The embryos were then washed for 7 h with PBS and mounted in MOWIOL mounting media. For the labelling of nicotinic acetylcholine receptors (nAChRs), embryos at 2 dpf were permeabilized as previously stated and incubated with 100 nM Alexa-488 conjugated α-bungarotoxin (Molecular Probes, Thermo Fisher Scientific) for 4 h at room temperature. Embryos were then washed for 7 h with PBS and mounted in MOWIOL mounting media. All embryos were imaged on a Zeiss LSM 710 confocal microscope (CA, USA) and photographed under a 40x objective. Images were compiled using Zeiss LSM Image Browser software and are shown as maximum intensity z-stack compilations. Measurements of the images were done using Image J (ImageJ 1.51r, National Institutes of Health, Bethesda, MD, USA).

2.3. Escape Response in 2 dpf Embryos

Escape responses of 2 dpf embryos were tested and recorded as previously described [24]. Briefly, 2 dpf embryos were immobilized in 2% low-melting point agarose (LMPA; Sigma-Aldrich; St. Louis, MO, USA) dissolved in embryo medium. LMPA was cut away from the embryo's trunk and tails allowing them to move, while the heads remained embedded in the gel. Embryo media was added to the petri dish to ensure that the embryos remained immersed in solution. Borosilicate glass micropipettes were pulled, filled with solution and then positioned close to embryo's otolith without touching the embryo. Embryos were stimulated using a 15 ms pulse of phenol red (Sigma-Aldrich) dissolved in embryo media ejected from a Picospritzer II (General Valve Corporation, Cambridge, MA, USA). Embryonic responses were recorded for about 900 ms following the stimulus using an AOS video camera (AOS S-PRI 1995; 1250 FPS; shutter speed: 800 µs) mounted on a dissecting microscope. The video-recordings were analyzed using a Motion Analysis Software, ProAnalyst®(Xcitex Inc., Cambridge, MA, USA).

2.4. qPCR of nAChR Subunits

To analyze the expression of different nAChR subunits, mRNA was extracted from whole embryos (n = 30–50 embryos, N = 5 batches) using a Trizol reagent according to manufacturer protocol. The concentration and purity of the RNA was determined by NanoDrop spectrophotometry (Thermo Fisher Scientific). A Maxima First Strand cDNA Synthesis kit (Thermo Fisher Scientific) was used to synthesize cDNA from 1 µg of the mRNA stocks according to the manufacturer's protocol. cDNA was diluted to 1:40 in 1 × TE buffer for real-time PCR reaction. TaqMan gene expression assays (Thermo Fisher Scientific) for zebrafish *chrna*1, *chrng* and *chrne* that were previously validated [25] were reused for qPCR reaction.

Quantitative real-time PCR was carried out with the 7500 Fast system (Applied Biosystems). For each reaction (10 µL), 5 µL of 2 × TaqMan Gene Expression Mastermix, 0.5 µL of 20 × TaqMan Gene Expression Assay, and 2.5 µL of Nuclease-free water was added to 2 µL of cDNA diluted to 1:40. The thermal profile included a holding step of 50 °C for 2 min followed by another holding step of 95 °C for 10 min, and 40 cycles including denature at 95 °C for 5 s and anneal/extend at 60 °C for 1 min. All samples were run in triplicate and the threshold cycle (Ct) was determined automatically by SDS software (Applied Biosystems). Outliers possibly originating from inaccurate pipetting were omitted and Ct values were averaged. Housekeeping gene Beta -actin (*actb*1) was used as internal control for our calculation. Comparative Ct Method (DDCt) was used for data representation using vehicle control as calibrator. No template controls (NTC) were included for each assay in every plate as negative control.

2.5. Locomotor Activity in 5 dpf Larva

To track locomotor activities, individual 5 dpf larvae were placed in a single well of a 96-well plate, then video-taped, and the data analysed according to previously published procedures [26,27]. Larvae were gently positioned in the centre of wells containing 150 μL egg water, pH 7.0 and 48 wells were used each time from a 96 well plate in our study (Costar #3599). Prior to video recording, larvae were acclimated in the well plate for 60 min. Plates were placed on top of an infrared backlight source and a Basler GenlCaM (Basler acA 1300-60) scanning camera with a 75 mm f2.8 C-mount lens, provided by Noldus (Wageningen, Netherlands) was used for individual larval movement tracking.

EthoVision ®XT-11.5 software (Noldus) was used to quantify activity (%), velocity (mm/s), swim bouts frequency and cumulative duration of swim bouts for one hour. To exclude background noise, ≥0.2 mm was defined as active movement. Activity was defined as % pixel change within a corresponding well between samples (motion was captured by taking 25 samples/frames per second) as reported previously [27].

2.6. Statistics

All values are reported as means ± SEM (standard error of the mean). Significance was determined using a non-parametric *t*-test between vehicle and treated group followed by Mann-Whitney analysis where appropriate ($p < 0.05$). Comparisons between multiple groups were done by one-way ANOVA followed by a Tukey post-hoc multiple comparisons test. Statistical analysis was done using the statistical software built in to GraphPad prism.

3. Results

3.1. THC Exposure Reduces Axonal Diameter of M-Cell

In a previous study, we found that zebrafish embryos exposed to THC from 1–10 mg/L exhibited morphological and neuronal changes that ranged from no effect at the lower concentrations, to disorganized neuronal morphology and alterations in responses to sound at the higher concentrations [20]. In the present study we continue our work by examining the morphology of M-cells following exposure to the primary psychoactive ingredient in cannabis, THC. We exposed zebrafish embryos to 6 mg/L THC as we had done previously and compared these embryos with vehicle controls (0.6% methanol). An immunohistochemical analysis of M-cell morphology was performed at 2 dpf with anti-3A10. Embryos exposed to THC exhibited M-cells that were largely similar to controls but appeared disheveled and possessed slightly thinner and wispier looking axons (Figure 1A–E). The diameter of the M-cell body was unchanged ($p > 0.05$; $n = 8$–10) (Figure 1C), whereas the M-cell axon diameter was significantly smaller in the treated group compared with controls ($p < 0.05$). Specifically, the M-cell diameter in the control group was 2.0 ± 0.1 μm ($n = 8$) while it was 1.5 ± 0.1 μm ($n = 11$) in the THC treated group (Figure 1F). To confirm these findings, we performed an additional immunohistochemical analysis of the M-cells by labelling reticulospinal neurons using the anti-RMO44 antibody. We found that there was an overall reduction in the intensity of the fluorescent labelling of many neurons in the THC-treated animals compared with controls (Figure 1G,J). The diameter of the M-cell body remained unchanged (Figure 1I); however, the diameter of the M-cell axon was significantly smaller (1.2 ± 0.06 μm, $n = 9$) in the treated group compared with vehicle controls (1.8 ± 0.1 μm, $n = 7$) ($p < 0.05$) (Figure 1L). These results, obtained using two distinct and independent antibodies, strongly suggest that the M-cells exhibit small but significant changes following exposure to 6 mg/L THC in the gastrulation stage.

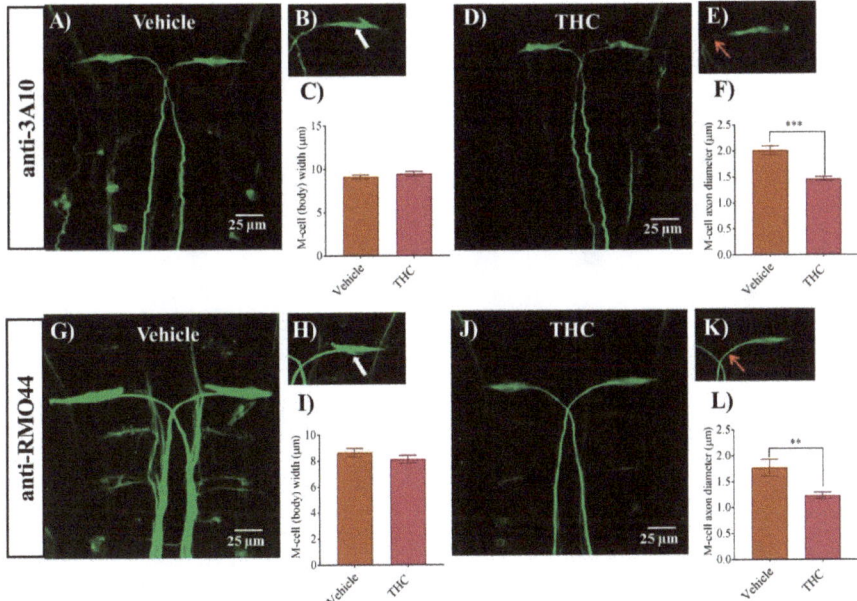

Figure 1. Δ^9-Tetrahydrocannabinol (THC) exposure reduces M-cell axonal diameter. (**A,G**) Immunolabeling of M-cells with anti-3A10 and anti-RMO44 in a vehicle-treated embryo; (**B,H**) Higher magnification of M-cell body and axon of vehicle-treated embryos. White arrow shows the cell body of the M-cell. (**C,I**) Bar graph of the width of an M-cell body in vehicle and THC treated embryos. (**D,J**) Immunolabeling of M-cells with anti-3A10 and anti-RMO44 in a THC-treated (6 mg/L) embryo; (**E,K**) Higher magnification of M-cell body and axon of a THC-treated embryo. Red arrow points to the proximal axon immediately anterior to the decussation point. (**F,L**) Bar graph of the diameter of M-cell axons slightly anterior to the decussation point in vehicle and THC-treated embryos. ** Significantly different from vehicle control, $p < 0.005$. *** significantly different from vehicle control, $p < 0.001$.

3.2. Escape Response Properties Were Altered Due to THC Exposure

To determine if the properties of the escape response had been altered by exposure to THC, we recorded the C-bend following a mechanosensitive stimulus to the head of 2 dpf embryos. The C-bend response rate between the two groups was similar and there were no overt differences between the treatments. However, the angle of the C-bend was significantly greater in the THC treated animals compared with vehicle controls (Figure 2A; $p < 0.05$; $n = 7$–13). Analysis of the maximum speed and acceleration showed no significant differences in these parameters (Figure 2B,C; $p > 0.05$; $n = 7$–13). Further, the time to maximum bend of the trunk was greater in the THC treated animals (Figure 2D, $p < 0.05$; $n = 7$–13), likely because the bend angle was greater.

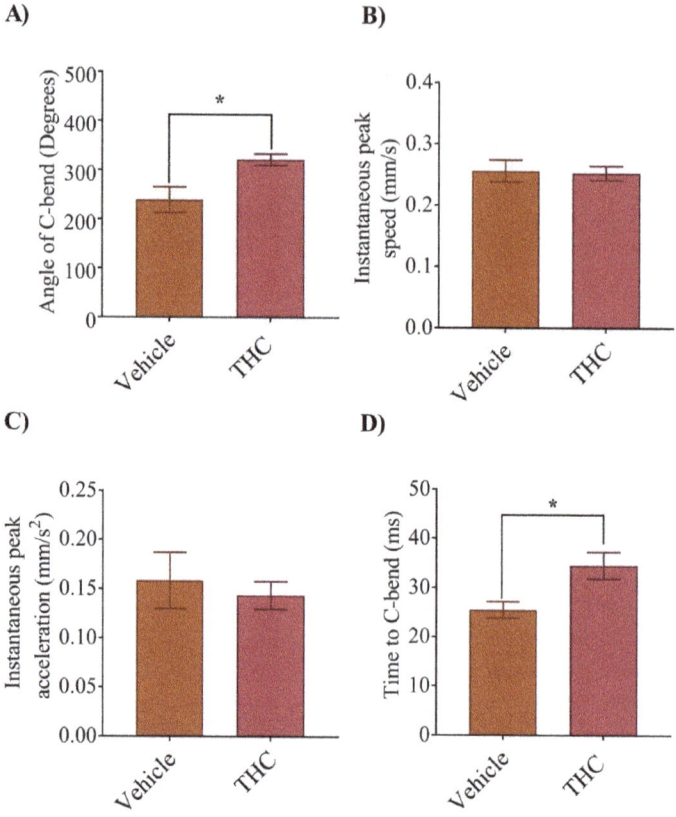

Figure 2. Exposure to THC during gastrulation alters escape response parameters. Analysis and quantification of C-bend parameters was carried out at 2 dpf. Zebrafish embryos exhibit a C-bend in response to a jet of water directed at the head just behind the eyes. (**A**) Bar graph shows the maximum angle of bend for vehicle and THC-treated (6 mg/L) embryos. (**B**) Shows the instantaneous peak speed (mm/s) during c-bend. (**C**) Shows the instantaneous peak acceleration during C-bend. (**D**) Bar graph showing the time for the tail to bend to the maximum angle. * Significantly different from vehicle control, $p < 0.05$.

3.3. White and Red Muscle Fibers Appear Thinner and Slightly Disorganized in THC Treated Embryos

To determine if the small changes in the C-bend escape response could be accounted for by properties of the muscle fibers, we performed an immunohistochemical analysis of the trunk muscles in conjunction with labelling of the nicotinic receptors using fluorescently tagged α- bungarotoxin. The trunk muscles of embryonic and larval zebrafish embryos are composed of a single layer of outer red muscles and several layers of inner white muscles [28]. The outer red muscle of vehicle control animals developed in an orderly fashion with clear and precise boundaries between the trunk segments (Figure 3). The α-bungarotoxin labelling of nAChRs in untreated animals was neatly aligned at the segmental boundaries (Figure 3A–C) as described in previous studies [29,30]. However, embryos treated with THC exhibited thinner individual muscle fibers (Figure 3E) that appeared less tightly packed, with larger spaces in between the fibers and unclear segmental boundaries. The diameter of THC treated red muscle fiber was reduced to 5.1 ± 0.2 μm from control values of 6.3 ± 0.3 μm in vehicle exposed fibers (Figure 3G, $p < 0.05$; $n = 24$–34). However, the lengths of the fibers remained unchanged (Figure 3H). Moreover, the nAChR expression, that was largely confined to the segmental boundaries, was somewhat disorganized (Figure 3D–F).

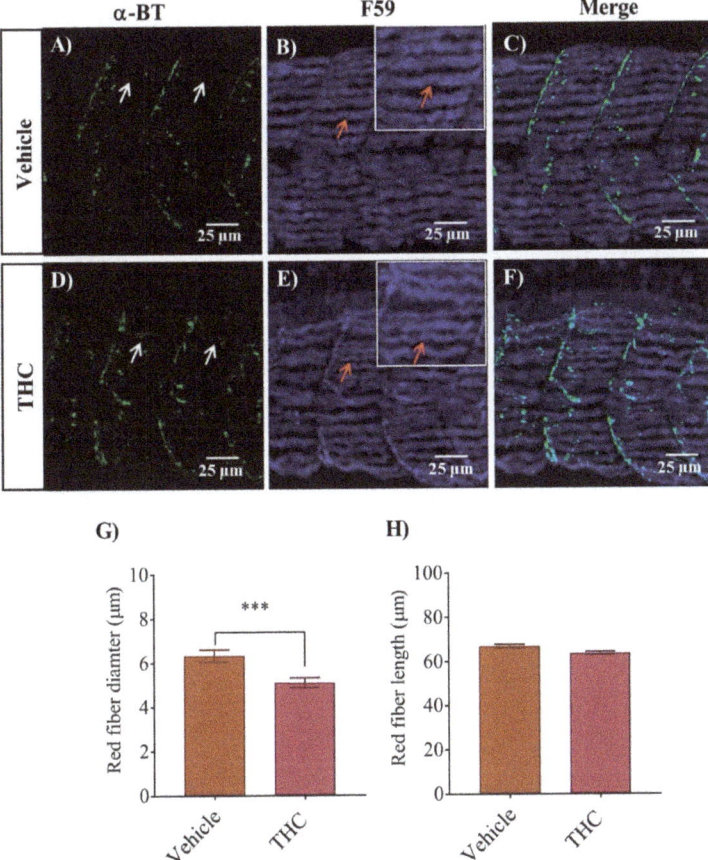

Figure 3. Co-labeling of red muscle fibers and nAChRs using anti-F59 and Alexa 488 conjugated α-bungarotoxin respectively. (**A**) α-Bungarotoxin labelled nAChRs associated with red muscle fibers in vehicle-treated embryos. (**B**) Anti-F-59 labelled muscle fibers. Red arrows point to the edge of a muscle fiber. Inset shows muscle fibers at higher magnification to better determine the size of the fiber. (**C**) Merged image showing the co-labeled red muscle fiber and nAChR in vehicle-treated animals. (**D**) α-bungarotoxin labelled nAChRs associated with red muscle fibers in THC-treated (6 mg/L) embryos. White arrow shows the cluster of nAChRs. (**E**) Anti-F59 labelled muscle fibers. Red arrows point to the edge of a muscle fiber. Inset shows muscle fibers at higher magnification to better determine the size of the fiber. (**F**) Merged image showing the co-labeled red muscle fiber and nAChR in THC-treated animals. (**G**) Bar graph showing the diameter of red fibers for vehicle and THC treated embryos and (**H**) Measurement of red fiber length. *** significantly different from vehicle control, $p < 0.001$.

A similar analysis of the white fibers using the F310 antibody combined with α-bungarotoxin labelling of nAChRs provided a similar result (Figure 4). The white fiber diameter for control embryos was 7.8 ± 0.3 μm (Figure 4G), whereas it decreased to 4.6 ± 0.3 μm for THC treated embryo muscle fibers (Figure 4G, $p < 0.05$; $n = 18$–22). We did not observe any significant changes in the length of individual fibers (Figure 4H). The white fibers exhibited periodic regions of disorganization with intermittent nAChR expression (Figure 4D–F). Further, the labelling of α-bungarotoxin showed more condensed nAChR that was also disorganized (Figure 4D).

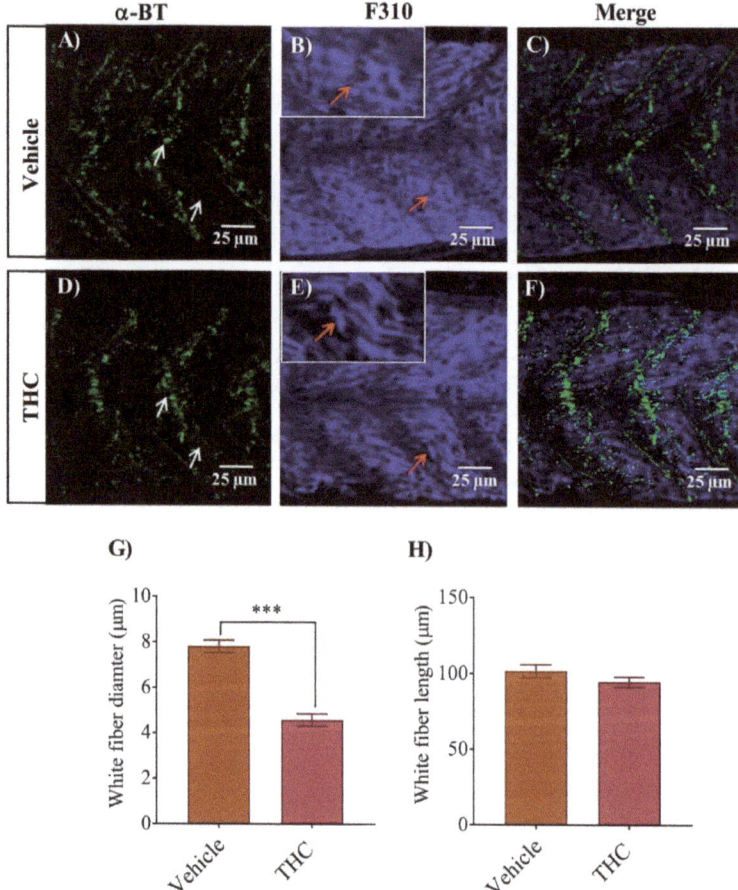

Figure 4. Co-labeling of white muscle fibers and nAChRs using anti-F310 and Alexa 488 conjugated α-bungarotoxin respectively. (**A**) α-Bungarotoxin labelled nAChRs associated with white muscle fibers in vehicle-treated embryos. White arrow shows clusters of nAChRs. (**B**) Anti-F-59 labelled muscle fibers. Red arrows point to the edge of a muscle fiber. Inset shows muscle fibers at higher magnification to better determine the size of the fiber. (**C**) Merged image showing the co-labeled white muscle fiber and nAChR in vehicle-treated animals. (**D**) α-bungarotoxin labelled nAChRs associated with white muscle fibers in THC-treated (6 mg/L) embryos. White arrow shows clusters of nAChRs. (**E**) Anti-F310 labelled muscle fibers. Red arrows point to the edge of a muscle fiber. Inset shows muscle fibers at higher magnification to better determine the size of the fiber. (**F**) Merged image showing the co-labeled white muscle fiber and nAChR in THC-treated animals. (**G**) Bar graph showing the diameter of white fibers for vehicle and THC treated embryos and (**H**) Measurement of white fiber length. *** significantly different from vehicle control, $p < 0.001$.

3.4. THC Does Not Alter nAChR Subunit Expression

To determine if the expression of the nAChR subunits was altered following THC exposure, we performed a semi quantitative analysis of the mRNA for the $α1$, $γ$ and $ε$ subunits in relation to the β subunit. However, we found no significant differences in the relative expression of the nAChR subunits (Figure 5A–C) suggesting that differences in nAChR subunits expression do not occur as a result of early THC exposure in our experimental paradigm.

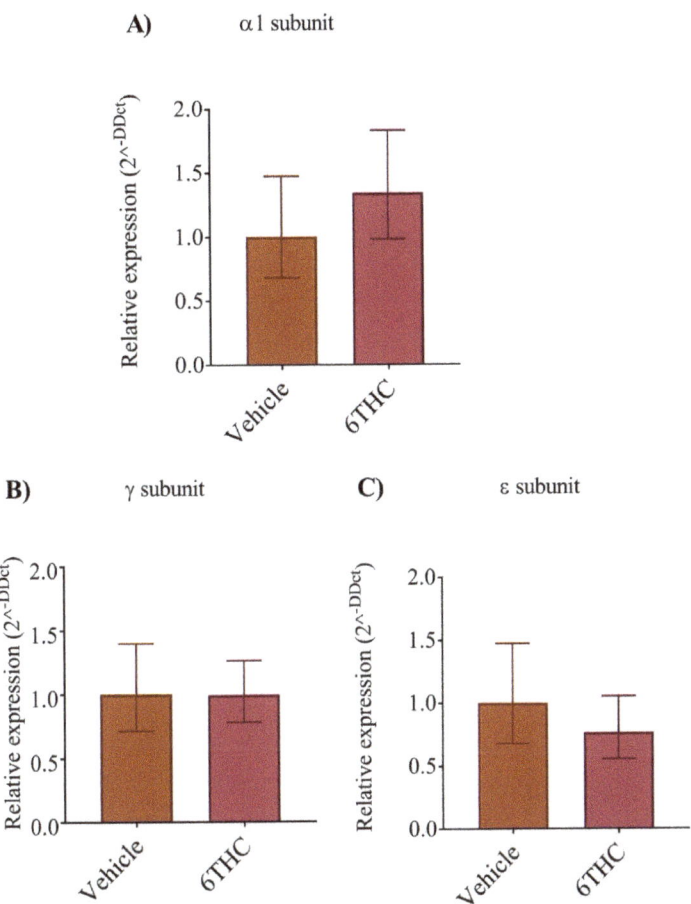

Figure 5. The relative levels of nAChR subunits (α1, γ and ε) mRNAs were analyzed by real-time qPCR. The relative expression was measured from vehicle control and THC treated embryos using expression in vehicle control as calibrator. (**A**) The relative level of α1 nAChR expression from vehicle and THC treated embryos. (**B**,**C**) The relative expression of γ and ε, respectively. Data are expressed as the mean ± SE for individual groups ($n = 5$).

3.5. THC Exposure Alters the Locomotion at 5dpf

Lastly, we allowed the animals to develop until they were 5 dpf, at which age they actively swim to feed. This allowed us to determine if exposure to THC affected their basal level of activity. We found that all aspects of their movement were altered by THC treatment during gastrulation (Figure 6A–D). For instance, the mean distance swam changed from 3200 ± 620 mm/hr in the controls ($n = 77$) to 960 ± 170 mm/h in the THC treated animals (Figure 6A, $n = 77$; $p < 0.001$). The mean velocity fell from 0.70 ± 0.08 mm/s ($n = 77$) to 0.22 ± 0.03 mm/s ($n = 79$) (Figure 6B, $p < 0.001$), the mean activity fell from 0.073% ($n = 84$) to 0.015% ($n = 84$) (Figure 6C, $p < 0.001$) and the movement frequency fell from 635 ± 72 ($n = 74$) to 247 ± 44 ($n = 74$) (Figure 6D, $p < 0.001$). Taken together, these findings suggest that cannabinoid treatment during gastrulation affected neuronal morphology to a small degree, as well as the development of muscle fibers and various aspects of locomotion. These results are consistent with our previous study and suggest that developing organisms exposed to THC may experience subtle alterations in development.

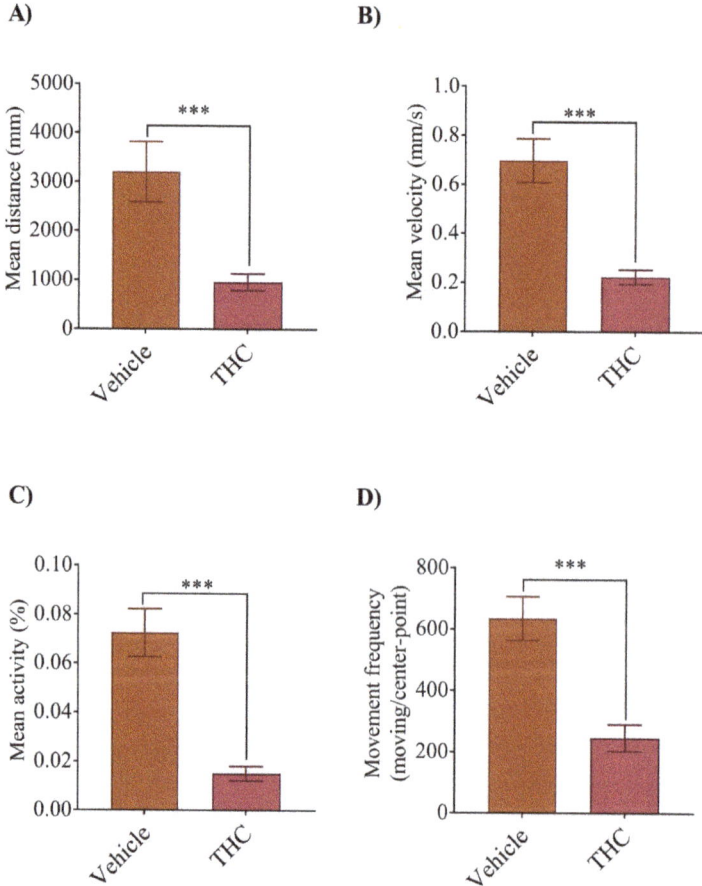

Figure 6. THC exposure affects free swimming activity (locomotion) of zebrafish embryos at 5 dpf. Bar graphs display changes in larval mean distance moved (**A**), mean velocity (in mm/s for one hour) (**B**), mean activity (% rate for one hour) (**C**), and frequency of swim bouts within one hour (**D**). *** significantly different from vehicle control, $p < 0.001$.

4. Discussion

In the present study we asked whether M-cells exposed to THC at the time of their (cellular) birth (during gastrulation) experience deficits in axonal projections, or if zebrafish embryos exhibit changes in escape response properties. Multiple reports provide convincing data to show that the eCB system, particularly the CB_1Rs, play a role in the differentiation of neural progenitor cells [31,32], the proper development of axonal projections and in neurite outgrowth [3,14–16,33,34]. Our findings suggest that brief exposure to THC subtly alters some aspects of M-cell morphology such as size and shape, although their axonal projections appear to be largely intact and project normally. There were minor changes in the C-start response to touch such as the angle of the C-bend. Finally, muscle fiber development was impacted to a small degree and overall activity levels were reduced.

Cannabis has been characterized as the most commonly used illicit drug in pregnant women [35] to reduce morning sickness. Moreover, in North America, there has been an increase in the cannabis use among women of reproductive age [36]. THC is the main psychoactive ingredient in cannabis and an increase in the potency and content of THC has been reported over the last 25 years [37]. Even though cannabis is used by pregnant women to reduce morning sickness there is relatively little information on the effects of cannabinoids on embryonic organisms during early development. In our research we focus on exposure to cannabinoids at some of the earliest developmental time points when the nervous system starts to form from the ectodermal tissue of the gastrula. In zebrafish, this is also the time when the M-cells first appear, around 8–9 hpf [19]. At this developmental time point, cannabinoid receptor expression is low, but mRNA coding for both CB_1Rs and CB_2Rs can be detected as early as the start of gastrulation [17]. In fact, in chick embryos CB_1Rs are present from the earliest stages of neuronal life and in the developing chick they first appear in the CNS as early as the birth of the first neurons [38]. In embryonic organisms CB_1R agonists and antagonists are capable of altering axonal growth [15], and signaling through the endocannabinoid system has been shown to play chemo-attractive and chemo-repulsive roles in developing cortex [39,40]. Several reports show an interaction between the endocannabinoid system and growth factors during early development. For instance, in cerebellar neurons CB_1R activation linked to FGF receptor activity influences neurite outgrowth, while CB_1R interaction with TrKB receptors in cortical interneurons is required for interneuron migration and specification [39]. Thus, the endocannabinoid system has the ability to control neuronal migration and differentiation by regulating growth factor activity. The endocannabinoid system has also been shown to modulate the expression of neurotransmitters in the basal ganglia that are involved in movement such as GABA and glutamate [7]. Others have shown that morpholino knockdown of CB_1R in zebrafish leads to aberrant axonal growth and fasciculation of reticulospinal neurons in the hindbrain [3]. Our perturbation of the eCB system via exposure to THC did not yield similar results to these earlier studies, but we exposed animals to significantly high levels of THC so that the eCB system could be overstimulated, and we did so for only 5 h around the time of neuronal birth, whereas morpholino oligonucleotides are often functional for up to 4-5 days.

Blood plasma concentrations of THC can peak as high as 0.25 mg/L during the smoking of a single cannabis cigarette [41]. In our study, we exposed the embryos to 6 mg/L of THC while they were still in the egg casing, and it is difficult to ascertain exactly what concentration of THC equilibrates in the neuronal tissue of the gastrula. Moreover, recent analysis shows that the THC content of cannabis has increased up to 20-fold over the last 15–20 years [37,42,43]. It has been estimated that approximately 0.1%–10% of toxicants typically cross the chorion [44,45], suggesting that concentrations as low as 0.006–0.6 mg/L may be directly exposed to the embryonic neuronal tissue. Hence, we believe that the concentrations of THC (6 mg/L) used in this study may be within the physiological range experienced during cannabis use.

Cannabinoid receptors are largely localized to the plasma membrane, but they have also been shown to be associated with the endoplasmic reticulum (ER), endosomes, lysosomes, mitochochondria (mt) [17]. As a general rule CB_1Rs are highly localized to the CNS while CB_2Rs are mainly found outside of the CNS in systems such as the immune and digestive systems. At the subcellular level, mitochondrially expressed CB_1Rs are found in axon terminals and dendrites of neurons. CB_2Rs have been reported in neuronal and glial cells in the cortex, hippocampus and substantia nigra of rat brain [46,47]. In neurons, CB_2Rs are present in the cell body and dendrites, and are therefore typically localized to presynaptic regions [46,47]. CB_2Rs are also associated with the rough ER, Golgi apparatus and dendrites. In zebrafish, CB_1R expression, determined by in situ hybridization, is localized to the pre-optic areas at 24 hpf and the telencephalon, tegmentum, hypothalamus and anterior hindbrain by 48 hpf [17,48]. In contrast, CB_2R mRNA expression in zebrafish brain was relatively weak and appeared to be limited primarily to the rostral portion of the pituitary [49,50].

In this study, we investigated whether exposure to THC alters locomotion in zebrafish embryos and larvae. In particular, we set out to examine touch evoked-escape response in 2 dpf animals but also investigated locomotion in older 5 dpf larvae. While the escape response is driven by reticulospinal neuronal activity (M-cell, Mid2cm, Mid3cm neurons), swimming is generated by networks of neurons in spinal cord including excitatory & inhibitory interneurons (Ins), primary and secondary motor neurons and muscle fibers. Escape response and free swimming can be categorized as fast (>30 Hz) and slow frequency (<30 Hz) swimming respectively. Fast frequency escape responses involve the relay of sensory information to M-cells, which in turn excites a CPG network of neurons in the spinal cord that activates muscle fibers. During fast swimming, more dorsal MNs (both primary and secondary) become recruited and activated than ventral MNs. White fibers are active during fast swimming frequency but not in slow swimming. In contrast, only the most ventral MNs are active during slow swimming. The red fibers are active during slow swimming and become deactivated during faster swimming frequency. Slow frequency free swimming begins to appear at 3 dpf which last only few seconds as it consists of occasional swimming episodes. By 4 dpf, embryos exhibit beat and glide locomotion and by 5 dpf they swim more frequently. Beat-and-glide fashion consists of swim bouts, periods of rhythmic tail movement, and alternate period of rest.

The immunolabelling of muscle showed that exposure to THC resulted in smaller red and white fibers that appeared disorganized compared with vehicle controls. Zebrafish red and white trunk muscles arise from two completely separate precursor cell populations [51,52]. The red fibers are pioneer cells that migrate to the surface of the trunk where they form a single layer of muscle that becomes innervated by secondary motor neurons [52]. The white fibers develop from lateral pre-somitic cells and constitute a separate population of cells that can be identified via distinct morphological and genetic features [51]. CB_2Rs are known to be associated with embryonic stem cells but it is unclear if cannabinoid receptors are found on muscle precursors. Cannabinoids are highly lipophilic substances and may actually remain associated with cell membranes long after the exposure time frame has elapsed. If so, then this might suggest that the effects of cannabinoids may continue long after direct exposure has ended.

In our previous study [20], we investigated the branching pattern of primary and secondary MNs involved in the CPG network. In the current study, we wanted to examine whether exposure to THC altered additional components of the network including M-cells, and then secondarily, if white and red fiber morphology was altered. Our findings show that THC exposure reduced the diameter of M-cell axons and resulted in smaller, more loosely packed, and slightly disorganized architecture of red fiber and white fiber. These findings are consistent with other studies that show that exposure to neurotoxic substances induces changes in skeletal muscle organization and composition, and disrupts the normal sarcomeric pattern, alters glycoprotein composition, and damages mitochondria [49]. While some of our findings appear to be minor, such as the small reduction in M-cell axon diameter, we believe that the key element to take note of is that a brief exposure to THC during embryological development may impact organismal growth, form, and function, and therefore, even only minor changes may have significant physiological consequences.

Author Contributions: M.R.A., K.T.A. and D.W.A. conceived and designed the experiments; M.R.A. and K.T.A. performed the experiments and analyzed the data; M.R.A. and D.W.A. wrote the paper. All authors have read and agreed to the published version of the manuscript.

Funding: This research was funded by the Natural Sciences and Engineering Research Council of Canada (NSERC) grant number 2016-04695 to Declan W. Ali.

Acknowledgments: This research was supported by the Natural Sciences and Engineering Research Council of Canada Discovery Grant to Declan W. Ali. Funds were not received to cover the costs of open access publishing.

Conflicts of Interest: The authors declare no conflict of interest. The founding sponsors had no role in the design of the study; in the collection, analyses, or interpretation of data; in the writing of the manuscript, and in the decision to publish the results.

References

1. Pertwee, R.G. Ligands that target cannabinoid receptors in the brain: From THC to anandamide and beyond. *Addict. Biol.* **2008**, *13*, 147–159. [CrossRef] [PubMed]
2. Herkenham, M.; Lynn, A.B.; Little, M.D.; Johnson, M.R.; Melvin, L.S.; de Costa, B.R.; Rice, K.C. Cannabinoid receptor localization in brain. *Proc. Natl. Acad. Sci. USA* **1990**, *87*, 1932–1936. [CrossRef] [PubMed]
3. Watson, S.; Chambers, D.; Hobbs, C.; Doherty, P.; Graham, A. The endocannabinoid receptor, CB1, is required for normal axonal growth and fasciculation. *Mol. Cell. Neurosci.* **2008**, *38*, 89–97. [CrossRef] [PubMed]
4. Kano, M.; Ohno-Shosaku, T.; Hashimotodani, Y.; Uchigashima, M.; Watanabe, M. Endocannabinoid-mediated control of synaptic transmission. *Physiol. Rev.* **2009**, *89*, 309–380. [CrossRef] [PubMed]
5. Smita, K.; Sushil Kumar, V.; Premendran, J.S. Anandamide: An update. *Fundam. Clin. Pharmacol.* **2007**, *21*, 1–8. [CrossRef]
6. Pandey, R.; Mousawy, K.; Nagarkatti, M.; Nagarkatti, P. Endocannabinoids and immune regulation. *Pharmacol. Res.* **2009**, *60*, 85–92. [CrossRef]
7. Benarroch, E. Endocannabinoids in basal ganglia circuits: Implications for Parkinson disease. *Neurology* **2007**, *69*, 306–309. [CrossRef]
8. Stempel, A.V.; Stumpf, A.; Zhang, H.Y.; Ozdogan, T.; Pannasch, U.; Theis, A.K.; Otte, D.M.; Wojtalla, A.; Racz, I.; Ponomarenko, A.; et al. Cannabinoid Type 2 Receptors Mediate a Cell Type-Specific Plasticity in the Hippocampus. *Neuron* **2016**, *90*, 795–809. [CrossRef]
9. Liu, Q.R.; Canseco-Alba, A.; Zhang, H.Y.; Tagliaferro, P.; Chung, M.; Dennis, E.; Sanabria, B.; Schanz, N.; Escosteguy-Neto, J.C.; Ishiguro, H.; et al. Cannabinoid type 2 receptors in dopamine neurons inhibits psychomotor behaviors, alters anxiety, depression and alcohol preference. *Sci. Rep.* **2017**, *7*, 17410. [CrossRef]
10. Psychoyos, D.; Vinod, K.Y.; Cao, J.; Xie, S.; Hyson, R.L.; Wlodarczyk, B.; He, W.; Cooper, T.B.; Hungund, B.L.; Finnell, R.H. Cannabinoid receptor 1 signaling in embryo neurodevelopment. *Birth Defects Res. B Dev. Reprod. Toxicol.* **2012**, *95*, 137–150. [CrossRef]
11. Buckley, N.E.; Hansson, S.; Harta, G.; Mezey, E. Expression of the CB1 and CB2 receptor messenger RNAs during embryonic development in the rat. *Neuroscience* **1998**, *82*, 1131–1149. [CrossRef]
12. Navarro, M.; Rubio, P.; de Fonseca, F.R. Behavioural consequences of maternal exposure to natural cannabinoids in rats. *Psychopharmacology* **1995**, *122*, 1–14. [CrossRef] [PubMed]
13. Morris, C.V.; DiNieri, J.A.; Szutorisz, H.; Hurd, Y.L. Molecular mechanisms of maternal cannabis and cigarette use on human neurodevelopment. *Eur. J. Neurosci.* **2011**, *34*, 1574–1583. [CrossRef] [PubMed]
14. Harkany, T.; Guzman, M.; Galve-Roperh, I.; Berghuis, P.; Devi, L.A.; Mackie, K. The emerging functions of endocannabinoid signaling during CNS development. *Trends Pharmacol. Sci.* **2007**, *28*, 83–92. [CrossRef]
15. Williams, E.J.; Walsh, F.S.; Doherty, P. The FGF receptor uses the endocannabinoid signaling system to couple to an axonal growth response. *J. Cell Biol.* **2003**, *160*, 481–486. [CrossRef]
16. Bernard, C.; Milh, M.; Morozov, Y.M.; Ben-Ari, Y.; Freund, T.F.; Gozlan, H. Altering cannabinoid signaling during development disrupts neuronal activity. *Proc. Natl. Acad. Sci. USA* **2005**, *102*, 9388–9393. [CrossRef]
17. Oltrabella, F.; Melgoza, A.; Nguyen, B.; Guo, S. Role of the endocannabinoid system in vertebrates: Emphasis on the zebrafish model. *Dev. Growth Differ.* **2017**, *59*, 194–210. [CrossRef]
18. Kimmel, C.B.; Ballard, W.W.; Kimmel, S.R.; Ullmann, B.; Schilling, T.F. Stages of embryonic development of the zebrafish. *Dev. Dyn.* **1995**, *203*, 253–310. [CrossRef]
19. Kimmel, C.B.; Sessions, S.K.; Kimmel, R.J. Morphogenesis and synaptogenesis of the zebrafish Mauthner neuron. *J. Comp. Neurol.* **1981**, *198*, 101–120. [CrossRef]
20. Ahmed, K.T.; Amin, M.R.; Shah, P.; Ali, D.W. Motor neuron development in zebrafish is altered by brief (5-hr) exposures to THC ((9)-tetrahydrocannabinol) or CBD (cannabidiol) during gastrulation. *Sci. Rep.* **2018**, *8*, 10518. [CrossRef]
21. Hatta, K. Role of the floor plate in axonal patterning in the zebrafish CNS. *Neuron* **1992**, *9*, 629–642. [CrossRef]
22. Miller, J.B.; Crow, M.T.; Stockdale, F.E. Slow and fast myosin heavy chain content defines three types of myotubes in early muscle cell cultures. *J. Cell Biol.* **1985**, *101*, 1643–1650. [CrossRef] [PubMed]
23. Kok, F.O.; Oster, E.; Mentzer, L.; Hsieh, J.C.; Henry, C.A.; Sirotkin, H.I. The role of the SPT6 chromatin remodeling factor in zebrafish embryogenesis. *Dev. Biol.* **2007**, *307*, 214–226. [CrossRef] [PubMed]
24. Shan, S.D.; Boutin, S.; Ferdous, J.; Ali, D.W. Ethanol exposure during gastrulation alters neuronal morphology and behavior in zebrafish. *Neurotoxicol. Teratol.* **2015**, *48C*, 18–27. [CrossRef] [PubMed]

25. Ahmed, K.T.; Ali, D.W. Nicotinic acetylcholine receptors (nAChRs) at zebrafish red and white muscle show different properties during development. *Dev. Neurobiol.* **2016**, *76*, 916–936. [CrossRef] [PubMed]
26. Baraban, S.C.; Taylor, M.R.; Castro, P.A.; Baier, H. Pentylenetetrazole induced changes in zebrafish behavior, neural activity and c-fos expression. *Neuroscience* **2005**, *131*, 759–768. [CrossRef] [PubMed]
27. Leighton, P.L.A.; Kanyo, R.; Neil, G.J.; Pollock, N.M.; Allison, W.T. Prion gene paralogs are dispensable for early zebrafish development and have nonadditive roles in seizure susceptibility. *J. Biol. Chem.* **2018**, *293*, 12576–12592. [CrossRef]
28. Waterman, R.E. Development of the lateral musculature in the teleost, Brachydanio rerio: A fine structural study. *Am. J. Anat.* **1969**, *125*, 457–493. [CrossRef]
29. Lefebvre, J.L.; Jing, L.; Becaficco, S.; Franzini-Armstrong, C.; Granato, M. Differential requirement for MuSK and dystroglycan in generating patterns of neuromuscular innervation. *Proc. Natl. Acad. Sci. USA* **2007**, *104*, 2483–2488. [CrossRef]
30. Park, J.Y.; Mott, M.; Williams, T.; Ikeda, H.; Wen, H.; Linhoff, M.; Ono, F. A single mutation in the acetylcholine receptor delta-subunit causes distinct effects in two types of neuromuscular synapses. *J. Neurosci. Off. J. Soc. Neurosci.* **2014**, *34*, 10211–10218. [CrossRef]
31. Palazuelos, J.; Ortega, Z.; Diaz-Alonso, J.; Guzman, M.; Galve-Roperh, I. CB2 cannabinoid receptors promote neural progenitor cell proliferation via mTORC1 signaling. *J. Biol. Chem.* **2012**, *287*, 1198–1209. [CrossRef] [PubMed]
32. Xapelli, S.; Agasse, F.; Sarda-Arroyo, L.; Bernardino, L.; Santos, T.; Ribeiro, F.F.; Valero, J.; Braganca, J.; Schitine, C.; de Melo Reis, R.A.; et al. Activation of type 1 cannabinoid receptor (CB1R) promotes neurogenesis in murine subventricular zone cell cultures. *PLoS ONE* **2013**, *8*, e63529. [CrossRef] [PubMed]
33. Diaz-Alonso, J.; Aguado, T.; Wu, C.S.; Palazuelos, J.; Hofmann, C.; Garcez, P.; Guillemot, F.; Lu, H.C.; Lutz, B.; Guzman, M.; et al. The CB(1) cannabinoid receptor drives corticospinal motor neuron differentiation through the Ctip2/Satb2 transcriptional regulation axis. *J. Neurosci. Off. J. Soc. Neurosci.* **2012**, *32*, 16651–16665. [CrossRef] [PubMed]
34. Galve-Roperh, I.; Chiurchiu, V.; Diaz-Alonso, J.; Bari, M.; Guzman, M.; Maccarrone, M. Cannabinoid receptor signaling in progenitor/stem cell proliferation and differentiation. *Prog. Lipid Res.* **2013**, *52*, 633–650. [CrossRef]
35. McCabe, J.E.; Arndt, S. Demographic and substance abuse trends among pregnant and non-pregnant women: Eleven years of treatment admission data. *Matern. Child Health J.* **2012**, *16*, 1696–1702. [CrossRef]
36. Brown, Q.L.; Sarvet, A.L.; Shmulewitz, D.; Martins, S.S.; Wall, M.M.; Hasin, D.S. Trends in Marijuana Use Among Pregnant and Nonpregnant Reproductive-Aged Women, 2002–2014. *JAMA* **2017**, *317*, 207–209. [CrossRef]
37. Mehmedic, Z.; Chandra, S.; Slade, D.; Denham, H.; Foster, S.; Patel, A.S.; Ross, S.A.; Khan, I.A.; ElSohly, M.A. Potency trends of Delta9-THC and other cannabinoids in confiscated cannabis preparations from 1993 to 2008. *J. Forensic Sci.* **2010**, *55*, 1209–1217. [CrossRef]
38. Begbie, J.; Doherty, P.; Graham, A. Cannabinoid receptor, CB1, expression follows neuronal differentiation in the early chick embryo. *J. Anat.* **2004**, *205*, 213–218. [CrossRef]
39. Berghuis, P.; Dobszay, M.B.; Wang, X.; Spano, S.; Ledda, F.; Sousa, K.M.; Schulte, G.; Ernfors, P.; Mackie, K.; Paratcha, G.; et al. Endocannabinoids regulate interneuron migration and morphogenesis by transactivating the TrkB receptor. *Proc. Natl. Acad. Sci. USA* **2005**, *102*, 19115–19120. [CrossRef]
40. Berghuis, P.; Rajnicek, A.M.; Morozov, Y.M.; Ross, R.A.; Mulder, J.; Urban, G.M.; Monory, K.; Marsicano, G.; Matteoli, M.; Canty, A.; et al. Hardwiring the brain: Endocannabinoids shape neuronal connectivity. *Science* **2007**, *316*, 1212–1216. [CrossRef]
41. Huestis, M.A. Human cannabinoid pharmacokinetics. *Chem. Biodivers.* **2007**, *4*, 1770–1804. [CrossRef] [PubMed]
42. Zhang, F.; Qin, W.; Zhang, J.P.; Hu, C.Q. Antibiotic toxicity and absorption in zebrafish using liquid chromatography-tandem mass spectrometry. *PLoS ONE* **2015**, *10*, e0124805. [CrossRef] [PubMed]
43. Brox, S.; Ritter, A.P.; Kuster, E.; Reemtsma, T. A quantitative HPLC-MS/MS method for studying internal concentrations and toxicokinetics of 34 polar analytes in zebrafish (Danio rerio) embryos. *Anal. Bioanal. Chem.* **2014**, *406*, 4831–4840. [CrossRef] [PubMed]
44. Brusco, A.; Tagliaferro, P.A.; Saez, T.; Onaivi, E.S. Ultrastructural localization of neuronal brain CB2 cannabinoid receptors. *Ann. N. Y. Acad. Sci.* **2008**, *1139*, 450–457. [CrossRef]

45. Onaivi, E.S.; Ishiguro, H.; Gu, S.; Liu, Q.R. CNS effects of CB2 cannabinoid receptors: Beyond neuro-immuno-cannabinoid activity. *J. Psychopharmacol.* **2012**, *26*, 92–103. [CrossRef]
46. Lam, C.S.; Rastegar, S.; Strahle, U. Distribution of cannabinoid receptor 1 in the CNS of zebrafish. *Neuroscience* **2006**, *138*, 83–95. [CrossRef]
47. Rodriguez-Martin, I.; de Velasco, E.M.F.; Rodriguez, R.E. Characterization of cannabinoid-binding sites in zebrafish brain. *Neurosci. Lett.* **2007**, *413*, 249–254. [CrossRef]
48. Rodriguez-Martin, I.; Herrero-Turrion, M.J.; de Velasco, E.M.F.; Gonzalez-Sarmiento, R.; Rodriguez, R.E. Characterization of two duplicate zebrafish Cb2-like cannabinoid receptors. *Gene* **2007**, *389*, 36–44. [CrossRef]
49. Avallone, B.; Agnisola, C.; Cerciello, R.; Panzuto, R.; Simoniello, P.; Creti, P.; Motta, C.M. Structural and functional changes in the zebrafish (Danio rerio) skeletal muscle after cadmium exposure. *Cell Biol. Toxicol.* **2015**, *31*, 273–283. [CrossRef]
50. Devoto, S.H.; Melancon, E.; Eisen, J.S.; Westerfield, M. Identification of separate slow and fast muscle precursor cells in vivo, prior to somite formation. *Development* **1996**, *122*, 3371–3380.
51. Stickney, H.L.; Barresi, M.J.; Devoto, S.H. Somite development in zebrafish. *Dev. Dyn.* **2000**, *219*, 287–303. [CrossRef]
52. Westerfield, M.; McMurray, J.V.; Eisen, J.S. Identified motoneurons and their innervation of axial muscles in the zebrafish. *J. Neurosci. Off. J. Soc. Neurosci.* **1986**, *6*, 2267–2277. [CrossRef]

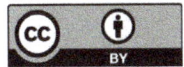

© 2020 by the authors. Licensee MDPI, Basel, Switzerland. This article is an open access article distributed under the terms and conditions of the Creative Commons Attribution (CC BY) license (http://creativecommons.org/licenses/by/4.0/).

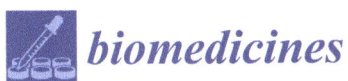

Article

Orthosiphon stamineus Proteins Alleviate Pentylenetetrazol-Induced Seizures in Zebrafish

Yin-Sir Chung [1,2], Brandon Kar Meng Choo [1], Pervaiz Khalid Ahmed [3,4], Iekhsan Othman [1,2] and Mohd. Farooq Shaikh [1,*]

1. Neuropharmacology Research Laboratory, Jeffrey Cheah School of Medicine and Health Sciences, Monash University Malaysia, Bandar Sunway 47500, Malaysia; chung.yinsir@monash.edu (Y.-S.C.); Brandon.Choo@monash.edu (B.K.M.C.); Iekhsan.Othman@monash.edu (I.O.)
2. Liquid Chromatography-Mass Spectrometry (LCMS) Platform, Jeffrey Cheah School of Medicine and Health Sciences, Monash University Malaysia, Bandar Sunway 47500, Malaysia
3. School of Business, Monash University Malaysia, Bandar Sunway 47500, Malaysia; pervaiz.ahmed@monash.edu
4. Global Asia in the 21st Century (GA21), Monash University Malaysia, Bandar Sunway 47500, Malaysia
* Correspondence: farooq.shaikh@monash.edu

Received: 4 June 2020; Accepted: 30 June 2020; Published: 2 July 2020

Abstract: The anticonvulsive potential of proteins extracted from *Orthosiphon stamineus* leaves (OSLP) has never been elucidated in zebrafish (*Danio rerio*). This study thus aims to elucidate the anticonvulsive potential of OSLP in pentylenetetrazol (PTZ)-induced seizure model. Physical changes (seizure score and seizure onset time, behavior, locomotor) and neurotransmitter analysis were elucidated to assess the pharmacological activity. The protective mechanism of OSLP on brain was also studied using mass spectrometry-based label-free proteomic quantification (LFQ) and bioinformatics. OSLP was found to be safe up to 800 µg/kg and pre-treatment with OSLP (800 µg/kg, i.p., 30 min) decreased the frequency of convulsive activities (lower seizure score and prolonged seizure onset time), improved locomotor behaviors (reduced erratic swimming movements and bottom-dwelling habit), and lowered the excitatory neurotransmitter (glutamate). Pre-treatment with OSLP increased protein Complexin 2 (Cplx 2) expression in the zebrafish brain. Cplx2 is an important regulator in the trans-SNARE complex which is required during the vesicle priming phase in the calcium-dependent synaptic vesicle exocytosis. Findings in this study collectively suggests that OSLP could be regulating the release of neurotransmitters via calcium-dependent synaptic vesicle exocytosis mediated by the "Synaptic Vesicle Cycle" pathway. OSLP's anticonvulsive actions could be acting differently from diazepam (DZP) and with that, it might not produce the similar cognitive insults such as DZP.

Keywords: *Orthosiphon stamineus*; plant-derived proteins; epilepsy; seizures; zebrafish

1. Introduction

Epilepsy is a chronic non-communicable disease of the brain that affects around 70 million people of all ages worldwide and accounts for about 1% of the global burden of disease. Epilepsy has a high prevalence and an estimated five million people are diagnosed with epilepsy each year. Epilepsy is characterized by recurrent seizures due to brief disturbances in the electrical functions of the brain. It involves brief episodes of involuntary movement that lead to changes in sensory perception, motor control, behavior, autonomic function, or sometimes loss of consciousness [1]. To date, despite having more than 30 antiepileptic drugs (AEDs) on the market [2,3], there are still difficulties in reaching the goal of treating epilepsy and its associated complications without adverse effects. Globally, epilepsy remains a public health imperative.

People with epilepsy often require lifelong treatment. AEDs are the mainstay of treatment. These conventional drugs bring about clinically worthwhile improvements but have tolerability issues due to their side effects. Many AEDs used in current mainstream clinical practice have been reported to elicit undesired neuropsychological consequences such as depression (24% lifetime prevalence), anxiety (22%), and intellectual disability, particularly in children with epilepsy (30%–40%) [1]. More than one-third of epileptic seizures are not well controlled by a single AED and often require treatment with two or more AEDs (add-on therapy) [1,2]. Furthermore, about 40%–60% of epileptic patients, accounting for both children and adults, develop neuropsychological impairments [3]. This drives a significant portion of epileptic patients to seek alternative interventions, particularly in herbal medicine [4]. Current systematic studies are reporting promising anticonvulsive activities in a constellation of medicinal plants [5,6].

Orthosiphon stamineus (OS) or *Orthosiphon aristatus var. aristatus* (OAA), also commonly known as cat's whiskers or "misai kucing," is an important medicinal plant. Choo et al. (2018) has shown that the ethanolic extract of OS, exhibited anticonvulsive activity in zebrafish Choo, Kundap [7] and Coelho et al. (2015) has demonstrated the anticonvulsant potential of rosmarinic acid in mice, which is an active chemical constituent in OS extract Coelho, Vieira [8]. Nonetheless, until now the protective potential of OS primary metabolites has not been studied, let alone its proteins. The proteins extracted from OS leaves (OSLP) may also hold valuable protective potential for central nervous system (CNS) disorders such as epilepsy. In the research of epilepsy and drug discovery, zebrafish (*Danio rerio*) has been widely recognised as an important and promising vertebrate model. Genetic profile of zebrafish shares approximately 70% similarity with human and about 84% of genes known to human diseases are also expressed in zebrafish [9,10]. This makes the zebrafish model particularly useful as a high-throughput screening system in studying mechanisms of brain functions and dysfunctions [11]. To the best of our knowledge, this is the first study on elucidating the anticonvulsive potential of proteins extracted from OSLP.

2. Experimental Section

2.1. Materials Chemicals and Apparatuses

L-Glutamic acid (Glu), Gamma-Aminobutyric acid (γ-aminobutyric acid), Pentylenetetrazol (PTZ), Diazepam (DZP), Benzocaine, complete EDTA-free protease inhibitors, phosphatase inhibitors cocktail 2, dithiothreitol (DTT), trifluoroethanol (TFE), ammonium bicarbonate (ABC), 2,3,5-triphenyltetrazolium chloride (TTC), formic acid (FA), and methanol (MeOH) of HPLC-grade were purchased from Sigma-Aldrich (St. Louis, MO, USA). Pierce®trypsin protease, Pierce® Radioimmunoprecipitation assay (RIPA) buffer of mass spec grade and Pierce®C18 mini spin columns were purchased from Thermo Scientific Pierce (Rockford, IL, USA). Protein LoBind microcentrifuge tube (Eppendorf, Enfield, CT, USA), acetonitrile (ACN), trifluoroacetic acid (TFA), indoleacetic acid (IAA) and CHAPS (Nacailai Tesque, Kyoto, Japan) of mass spec grade were from Sigma-Aldrich (St. Louis, MO, USA), Quick Start™ Bradford Protein Assay Kit from Bio-Rad (Hercules, CA, USA), Dimethylsulfoxide (DMSO) and 37% formaldehyde solution were from Friendemann Schmidt Chemical (Parkwood, Western Australia), Milli-Q ultrapure (MQUP) water from Millipore GmbH (Darmstad, Germany), acetic acid (glacial, 100%) from Merck (Darmstadt, Germany) and Phosphate buffered saline (PBS) tablets from VWR Life Science AMRESCO® (Radnor, PA, USA). Liquid nitrogen was purchased from Linde Malaysia, Hamilton syringes 25 µL (MICROLITER™ #702) from Hamilton Co. (Reno, NV, USA), 35 gauge needles (PrecisionGlide™) were from Becton, Dickinson and Company (Franklin Lakes, NJ, USA), ultrasonic cell crusher (JY88-II N, Shanghai Xiwen Biotech. Co., Ltd., Shanghai, China), Eyela SpeedVac Vacuum Concentrator (Thermo Scientific Pierce, Rockford, IL, USA), Camry High-Precision Electronic Pocket Scale (Model EHA901, Zhaoqing, China) and Classic pH Pen Tester from Yi Hu Fish Farm Trading Pte. Ltd. (Singapore). The other chemicals of analytical grade were from established suppliers worldwide.

2.2. Software and Equipment

For the behavioral study, SMART V3.0.05 tracking software (Panlab Harvard Apparatus, Barcelona, Spain) was used for the automated tracking of zebrafish swimming patterns. The video recorded using the camcorder was analyzed using the software. The water-filled tank was divided into two halves of the same size; the upper-half was marked as the top zone and the lower-half as the bottom zone as described by Kundap et al. 2017 [12].

For the neurotransmitter analysis, the solvent delivery was performed using Agilent Ultra High-Performance Liquid Chromatography (UHPLC) 1290 Series (Agilent Technologies, Santa Clara, CA, USA) consisting of Agilent 1290 Series High-Performance Autosampler, Agilent 1290 Series Binary Pump and Agilent 1290 Series Thermostatted Column Compartment; the separations were performed using Zorbax Eclipse Plus C18 (Rapid Resolution HD, 2.1 × 150.0 mm with 1.8 µM pore size reverse-phase column) (Agilent Technologies, Santa Clara, CA, USA), and coupled with Agilent 6410B Triple Quadrupole (QQQ) mass spectrometer equipped with an electrospray ionization (ESI) (Agilent Technologies, Santa Clara, CA, USA) to detect the targeted neurotransmitters.

In the protein expression study, Agilent 1200 series HPLC coupled with Agilent 6550 iFunnel Quadrupole Time of Flight (Q-TOF) LC/MS, C-18 300Å Large Capacity Chip (Agilent Technologies, Santa Clara, CA, USA) and Agilent MassHunter data acquisition software were used to identify the differentially expressed proteins (Agilent Technologies, Santa Clara, CA, USA). In addition, PEAKS®Studio software (Version 8.0, Bioinformatics Solution, Waterloo, ON, Canada) and UniProtKB (Organism: *Danio rerio*) database were used for the analysis of mass spectrometry-based label-free proteomic quantification (LFQ). Cytoscape software (Version 3.7.2 plugin BiNGO for Gene Ontology (GO) annotated information, Cytoscape Consortium, San Diego, CA, USA), Zebrafish Information Network (ZFIN) Database Information, KAAS (KEGG Automatic Annotation Server Version 2.1, Kanehisa Lab., Kyoto, Japan) and KEGG PATHWAY Database (Organism: *Danio rerio*) were used to study the functional annotations, protein-protein interactions, and systemic pathway enrichment analysis.

2.3. Zebrafish Maintenance and Housing Conditions

Adult zebrafish (*Danio rerio*; 3–4 months old) of heterogeneous strain wild-type stock (standard short-fin phenotype) were housed in the Animal Facility of Monash University Malaysia and maintained under standard husbandry conditions as follows: standard zebrafish tanks (length of 36 cm × width of 22 cm × height of 26 cm) equipped with circulating water systems to provide constant aeration, controlled water temperature between 26–28 °C and controlled water pH between 6.8–7.1. They were kept in stress-free and hygienic conditions. The zebrafish aquarium was maintained under a 250-lux light intensity with a cycle of 14-h of light to 10-h of darkness controlled by autotimer (light on at 0800 and light off at 2200). Group housing was practiced (10–12 fish per tank) with the females and males separated. The adult zebrafish were fed ad libitum three times a day (TetraMin® Tropical Flakes) and were supplemented with live brine shrimps (Artemia) purchased from Bio-Marine (Aquafauna Inc., Hawthorne, CA, USA). The adult zebrafish were allowed to acclimatize for a period of seven days to reduce stress before commencing the experiments. The Monash University Malaysia Animal Ethics Committee approved all the animal experimental procedures on 17 January 2019.

2.4. Experimental Design

2.4.1. OSLP Safety Study in Adult Zebrafish

A limit test was first performed based on a modified version of the OECD Guidelines for the Testing of Chemicals No. 203 [11,12] and the protocols of Choo et al. [10,13]. Prior to the experimental procedures, all the adult zebrafish were fasted for 24 h. Meanwhile, OSLP powder was completely dissolved in tank water (26–28 °C) and concentrations ranging from 50–1600 µg/kg of zebrafish body weight were freshly prepared. Three-month-old adult zebrafish with an average weight of 0.45–0.50 g were selected. The zebrafish were then divided into 7 groups (Table 1), with 8 fish per group ($n = 8$) as follows:

Table 1. Experimental groups in OSLP safety study.

Group	Treatment
VC	Vehicle control (tank water, i.p.)
Treatment Group a	OSLP (50 µg/kg, i.p.)
Treatment Group b	OSLP (100 µg/kg, i.p.)
Treatment Group c	OSLP (200 µg/kg, i.p.)
Treatment Group d	OSLP (400 µg/kg, i.p.)
Treatment Group e	OSLP (800 µg/kg, i.p.)
Treatment Group f	OSLP (1600 µg/kg, i.p.)

A clean observation tank was first set up and filled with 13 L of tank water (Milli-Q filtered water used for keeping the zebrafish; 26–28 °C). One zebrafish from the vehicle control (VC) group was then placed in the observation tank and its behavior was recorded for 10 min using a digital camera (Sony, Japan). After finishing recording, the zebrafish was transferred into a clean individual 1 L tank filled with the same water. This procedure was then repeated for all the other zebrafish in the VC group. For the OSLP-treated groups (II–VII), different concentrations of OSLP were injected intraperitoneally (i.p.) into the zebrafish. Before each IP injection, a zebrafish was individually immersed in anesthesia solution (30 mg/L of Benzocaine) until the cessation of movement [10,13,14]. Immediately, the zebrafish was extracted out to determine the body weight and to calculate the injection volume. The injection volume was calculated at a volume corresponding to 10 microliters per gram of body weight (modified from 15). After injection, the zebrafish was immediately transferred back to the 13 L observation tank. Then, the same recording and tank transfer procedure was repeated, as performed in the VC group. All 56 zebrafish were then kept for 96 h in their respective 1 L tanks. They were checked on every 15 min for the first two hours of exposure and every half an hour thereafter for the first day. On subsequent days, the zebrafish were checked on the morning, afternoon, and evening (3 times per day). Any zebrafish found to exhibit signs of pain, suffering, or anomaly according to our predefined monitoring sheet at any checkpoint were humanely euthanized via an overdose of benzocaine. This protocol deviates from the OECD guidelines in that it does not use mortality as the criterion to determine toxic effects due to the concerns of the MARP-Australia in using death as an endpoint.

2.4.2. Anticonvulsive Potential of OSLP in Adult Zebrafish

The anticonvulsive potential of OSLP was investigated in the pentylenetetrazol (PTZ)-induced seizure model. Seizure score and seizure onset time, were one of the primary evaluation parameters used to examine the anticonvulsive activity. Behavioral changes in the zebrafish were determined by evaluating their swimming patterns, total distance travelled (cm) and time spent in the tank (upper-half versus lower-half, s). Three-month-old adult zebrafish with an average weight of 0.45–0.50 g were selected. Prior to beginning the experiments, the zebrafish were kept in 1 L treatment tanks filled with 1 L of tank water (26–28 °C) normally used to fill the zebrafish tanks. In this study, the zebrafish were divided into 5 groups ($n = 10$) (Table 2) and procedures of experiment (Figure 1) were as follows:

Table 2. Experimental groups in the evaluation of OSLP anti-convulsive potential.

Group	Treatment
VC	Vehicle control (tank water, i.p. + tank water)
NC	Negative control (tank water + PTZ 170 mg/kg, i.p.)
PC	Positive control (DZP 1.25 mg/kg + PTZ 170 mg/kg, i.p.)
TC	Treatment control (800 µg/kg + tank water, i.p.)
O+P	OSLP-treated PTZ (800 µg/kg + PTZ 170 mg/kg, i.p.)

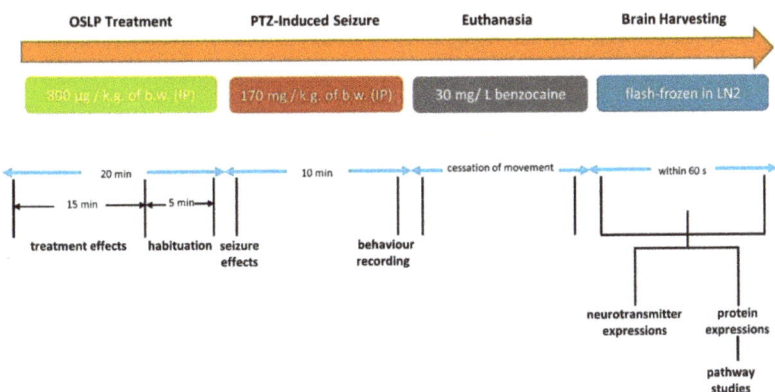

Figure 1. Shows the procedures of experiment.

All the groups were habituated in their treatment tanks for a half hour before the administration of PTZ. Before each i.p. injection, a zebrafish was individually immersed in anesthesia solution (30 mg/L of Benzocaine) until the cessation of movement. When multiple IP injections were required in tandem on the same zebrafish, the injections were given at alternating lateral ends, rather than the midline between the pelvic fins 10, 13, 14. The VC group was injected with tank water twice. The NC group was first pre-treated with tank water and then PTZ (170 mg/kg) whereas the PC group was pre-treated with diazepam (1.25 mg/kg) followed by PTZ (170 mg/kg). The TC group was injected with 800 µg/kg of OSLP and tank water. The O+P group was pre-treated with OSLP (800 µg/kg) followed by PTZ (170 mg/kg). PTZ-induced seizures lasted for approximately 10 min after the PTZ injection [10,13,14]. All the groups were then transferred to a 13 L observation tank filled three quarters of the way with water. Behavioral changes of the zebrafish were then recorded individually (10 min) with a digital camera (Sony, Japan). The PTZ injected zebrafish presented diverse seizure profiles, intensities and latency in reaching the different seizure scores and seizure onset times. In order to determine the seizure score and seizure onset time, the individual video was analyzed using a computer as per the scoring system below (Table 3) [10,13–16]:

Table 3. Seizure scoring system.

Score	Criteria
1	short swim mainly at the bottom of tank
2	increased swimming activity and high frequency of opercular movements
3	burst swimming, left and right movements as well as the erratic movements
4	circular movements

At the end of the experiment, all the groups were sacrificed. The zebrafish were euthanized with 30 mg/L of Benzocaine until the cessation of movement. The brains were then carefully harvested for neurotransmitter analysis, protein expression study and systemic pathway enrichment analysis.

2.5. Extraction of Brains from Zebrafish

At the end of the behavioral studies, the zebrafish brains were carefully harvested from the zebrafish skulls and kept in a sterile Petri dish. Each brain was then immediately transferred into a sterile, pre-chilled 2.0 mL microtube and was flash-frozen in liquid nitrogen (LN_2) before storing them at −152 °C until further analysis.

2.6. Brain Neurotransmitter Analysis Using Nanoflow Liquid Chromatography Coupled with Tandem Mass Spectrometry (Nanoflow-ESI-LC-MS/MS)

The levels of neurotransmitters in the brains, namely gamma-aminobutyric acid (GABA) and glutamate (Glu) were estimated using LC-MS/MS with modifications [13,14,17]. All experiments were performed in 3 independent biological replicates.

A mother stock of neurotransmitter standards was prepared by mixing GABA and Glu in methanol, MQUP water and 0.1% formic acid, to make up a final concentration of 1 mg/mL. Next, serial dilution was performed to prepare 8 points of standard calibrations ranging from 6.25–1000 ng/mL. A blank (methanol, MQUP water in 0.1% formic acid) with a final concentration of 1 mg/mL was also prepared. Together with the 8 points of standard calibrations, they were used for quantifying the levels of GABA and Glu in LC-MS/MS study.

Firstly, each LN_2 flash-frozen zebrafish brain was homogenized in 1 mL ice-cold methanol/MQUP water (3:1, *vol/vol*) using an ultrasonic cell crusher (JY88-II N, Shanghai Xiwen Biotech. Co., Ltd., Shanghai, China). The homogenate was then vortex-mixed (2500 rpm, 3 m) and later incubated on an agitating shaker (4 °C, 1 h). The homogenate was then centrifuged (4 °C, 10,000× *g*, 10 min) and the supernatant was carefully transferred into a sterile 2.0 mL microtube. 100 µL of 0.1% formic acid was slowly added, vortex-mixed (2500 rpm, 3 m) and then centrifuged (4 °C, 10,000× *g*, 10 min). The supernatant was carefully transferred into a sterile insert and vial. Finally, all the brain samples were subjected to LC-MS/MS analysis.

LC-MS/MS was run on an Agilent 1290 Infinity UHPLC coupled with an Agilent 6410B Triple Quad MS/MS equipped with an electrospray ionization (ESI). The separations were performed using Zorbax Eclipse Plus C18 (Rapid Resolution HD, 2.1 × 150.0 mm with 1.8 uM pore size reverse-phase column). The flow rate was 0.3 mL/min with the mobile phase consisting of 0.1% formic acid in water (Solvent A) and acetonitrile (Solvent B). The gradient elution used was: (i) 0 min, 5% Solvent B; (ii) 0–3 min, 50% Solvent B and (iii) 3–5 min, 100% Solvent B, with one-minute post time. The injection volume was 1.0 µL per sample with the column compartment temperature and the autosampler temperature set at 25 °C and 4 °C respectively. The total run time for each injection was 5 min. ESI-MS/MS was used in positive ionization mode with a nitrogen gas temperature of 325 °C, gas flow 9 L/min, nebulizer pressure of 45 psi and the capillary voltage of 4000 V. The MS acquisition was scanned in multiple reaction monitoring (MRM) mode. A calibration range of 1.56–200 ng/mL was used for quantifying the targeted neurotransmitters, with a linear plot where $r^2 > 0.99$.

2.7. Protein Expression Profiling Using Mass Spectrometry-Based Label-Free Proteomic Quantification (LFQ)

Brains of these two groups, namely NC (injected with PTZ 170 mg/kg) and O+P (pre-treated with OSLP 800 µg/kg followed by PTZ 170 mg/kg) were subjected to tissue lysis to extract the proteins for mass spectrometry-based label-free proteomic quantification (LFQ). All experiments were performed in 4 independent biological replicates.

2.7.1. Protein Extraction from Zebrafish Brain

The zebrafish brain was lysed with 1 mL of ice-cold lysis buffer (RIPA, protease inhibitor 20% *v/v*, phosphatase inhibitor 1% *v/v*) in a sterile ProtLoBind microtube and then incubated on an orbital shaker (4 °C; 90 min). Next, the content was homogenized using an ultrasonic cell crusher, briefly centrifuged (18,000 × *g*, 4 °C; 10 min) and the supernatant produced was harvested. The supernatant extracted was collected into a new sterile ProtLoBind microtube. Protein concentration was estimated using the Quick Start™ Bradford Protein Assay as instructed by the manufacturer (Bio-Rad, Hercules, CA, USA). After that, the brain lysates were concentrated in a speed-vacuum concentrator (300 rpm; 24 h; 60 °C).

2.7.2. In-Solution Digestion of Proteins

In-solution protein digestion was carried out according to the instructions (Agilent Technologies, Santa Clara, CA, USA). Briefly, protein samples were re-suspended, denatured and reduced in 25 µL of ABC, 25 µL of TFE and 1 µL of DTT, followed by being vortex-mixed (2500 rpm, 3 m) and then heated in an oven (60 °C, 60 min). Next, the samples were alkylated in 4 µL of IAA and were incubated in the dark (60 min, r.t.). After that, 1 µL of DTT was again added to quench excessive IAA (60 min, r.t., in the dark). 300 µL of MQUP water and 100 µL of ABC were added to dilute and adjust the pH of the protein solutions (pH 7–9). Following that, 1 µL of trypsin was added and was then incubated in an oven (37 °C, 18 h, in the dark). Upon completion of incubation, 1 µL of formic acid was added to terminate the tryptic digestion. Finally, all the samples were concentrated in a speed-vacuum concentrator (300 rpm; 24 h; 60 °C, Eyela SpeedVac Vacuum Concentrator). The dry pellets were kept at −20 °C.

2.7.3. De-Salting of Proteins

De-salting of the protein sample was carried out. Each biological replicate was de-salted independently using a Pierce®C18 mini spin column as instructed (Thermo Scientific Pierce, Rockford, IL, USA), with modifications. Firstly, each mini spin column was activated in 50% ACN (repeated 3 times, r.t.) and equilibrated in 0.5% of TFA in 5% ACN (repeated 3 times, r.t.). Separately, 90 µL of crude protein was added into 30 µL of sample buffer (2% of TFA in 20%) and briefly vortexed at 2200 rpm to mix well. This step was repeated for all the protein samples. Following that, each of the protein samples was loaded onto a mini spin column and was de-salted (repeated 3 times, r.t.). Subsequently, all the protein samples were washed in 0.5% of TFA in 5% ACN (repeated 3 times, r.t.). Lastly, all the protein samples were eluted in 70% ACN (repeated 3 times, r.t.) and all the flow-through produced was collected, vacuum-concentrated (300 rpm; 24 h; 60 °C) and stored at −20 °C prior to mass spectrometry-based LFQ.

2.7.4. Mass Spectrometry-Based Label-Free Proteomic Quantification (LFQ) Using Nanoflow-ESI-LCMS/MS

De-salted peptides were loaded onto an Agilent C-18 300Å Large Capacity Chip. The column was equilibrated by 0.1% formic acid in water (Solution A) and peptides were eluted with an increasing gradient of 90% acetonitrile in 0.1% formic acid (Solution B) by the following gradient, 3%–50% Solution B from 0–30 min, 50%–95% Solution B from 30–32 min, 95% Solution B from 32–39 min and 95%–3% Solution B from 39–47 min. The polarity of Q-TOF was set at positive, capillary voltage at 2050 V, fragmentor voltage at 300 V, drying gas flow 5 L/min and gas temperature of 300 °C. The intact protein was analyzed in auto MS/MS mode from range 110–3000 m/z for MS scan and 50–3000 m/z range for MS/MS scan. The spectrum was analyzed using Agilent MassHunter data acquisition software.

2.7.5. Brain Protein and Peptide Identification by Automated de Novo Sequencing and LFQ Analysis

Protein identification by automated de novo sequencing was performed with PEAKS®Studio Version 8.0. UniProtKB (Organism: *Danio rerio*) database (http://www.uniprot.org/proteomes/UP000000437, 46,847 proteins, accessed on 14 February 2020) was used for protein identification and homology search by comparing the de novo sequence tag, with the following settings: both parent mass and precursor mass tolerance was set at 0.1 Da, carbamidomethylation was set as fixed modification with maximum missed cleavage was set at 3, maximum variable post-translational modification was set at 3, trypsin cleavage, the minimum ratio count set to 2, mass error tolerance set as 20.0 ppm and other parameters were set as default by Agilent. False discovery rate (FDR) threshold of 1% and protein score of −10lgP > 20 were applied to filter out inaccurate proteins. PEAKS® indicated that a −10lgP score of greater than 20 is of relatively high in confidence as it targets very few decoy matches above the threshold.

For LFQ analysis, the differentially expressed proteins between the NC (injected with PTZ 170 mg/kg) and O+P (pre-treated with OSLP 800 µg/kg followed by PTZ 170 mg/kg) groups were identified with the following settings: FDR threshold ≤ 1%, fold change ≥ 1, unique peptide ≥ 1, and significance score ≥ 20. PEAKSQ indicated that a significance score of greater than 20 is equivalent to significance p value < 0.01. Other parameters were set as default by Agilent.

2.8. Bioinformatics Analysis

Bioinformatics analysis (functional annotations, protein-protein interactions and systemic pathway enrichment analysis) of the differentially expressed proteins were analyzed and matched with the databases obtained from GO Consortium, ZFIN (www.zfin.org) and the KEGG PATHWAY Database (*Danio rerio*) [13]. KAAS provides functional annotation of genes by BLAST or GHOST comparisons against the manually curated KEGG GENES database. The result contains KO (KEGG Orthology) assignments (bi-directional best hit) and automatically generated KEGG pathways. The KEGG pathway maps organism-specific pathways: green boxes are hyperlinked to GENES entries by converting K numbers (KO identifiers) to gene identifiers in the reference pathway, indicating the presence of genes in the genome and also the completeness of the pathway.

2.9. Statistical Analysis

For behavioral study and neurotransmitter estimation, statistical analysis was performed using GraphPad Prism version 8.0. All data were expressed as mean ± standard error of the mean (SEM). One-way analysis of variance (ANOVA) followed with Dunnett's post-hoc test at significance levels of * $p < 0.05$, ** $p < 0.01$ and *** $p < 0.001$ against the negative control group (NC, 170 mg/kg PTZ). PEAKSQ statistical analysis (built-in statistical tool of PEAKS® software) was used in the analysis of differentially expressed proteins identified by LFQ. A significance score of 20% (equivalent to significance level of 0.01) and FDR ≤ 1% was considered statistically significant. In bioinformatics analysis, hypergeometric test followed with Benjamini and Hochberg FDR correction at p value < 0.05 (BiNGO built-in statistical tool) was used to correlate the association between functional annotation of genes and interacting proteins; the built-in statistical tool of KAAS was used to assess the possible association of interacting proteins and systemic pathways in the KEGG PATHWAY Database.

3. Results

3.1. OSLP Safety Study in Adult Zebrafish

3.1.1. Behavioral Study

Swim Path Analysis

As seen in the swim paths generated by PANLAB SMART v3.0 software, the VC group (Figure 2a) swam throughout the whole tank without showing apparent preference for any part of the tank. The OSLP-treated groups, 50, 100, 200, and 400 µg respectively, showed slight preferences for the bottom half of tank when compared to the VC group (Figure 2b–e). In comparison, the OSLP 800 µg group (Figure 2f) showed a similar swimming pattern to the VC group as they swam throughout the whole tank with no apparent preference for any part of the tank. The 1600 µg/kg dose was excluded for causing mortality after an extended duration.

3.1.2. Locomotion Parameters

For the mean total distance travelled, no significant differences (F = 1.798, $p > 0.05$) were found between the untreated VC group and all the OSLP-treated groups (50–800 µg/kg) (Figure 3a).

For another locomotion parameter, time spent in upper half of tank (s), no significant differences (F = 1.408, $p > 0.05$) were found between the untreated VC group and all the OSLP-treated groups Figure 3b, c). In a similar trend, no significant differences were also found in the mean time spent in lower half of tank, except in the OSLP 800 µg group. The zebrafish treated with OSLP 800 µg/kg spent a shorter time in the lower half of tank, 328 ± 54 s (F = 6.596, ** $p < 0.01$) than the VC group.

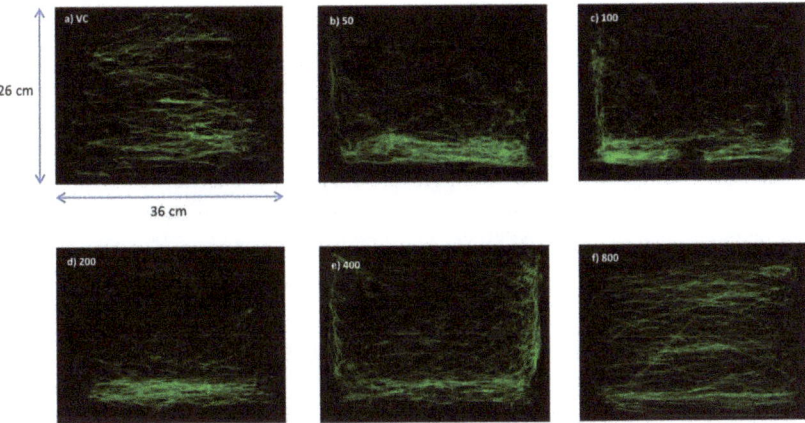

Figure 2. Representative swim paths for the corresponding 6 experimental groups ($n = 8$). (**a**) VC (tank water only, i.p.), (**b**) OSLP (50 µg/kg, i.p.), (**c**) OSLP (100 µg/kg, i.p.), (**d**) OSLP (200 µg/kg, i.p.), (**e**) OSLP (400 µg/kg, i.p.) and (**f**) OSLP (800 µg/kg, i.p.).

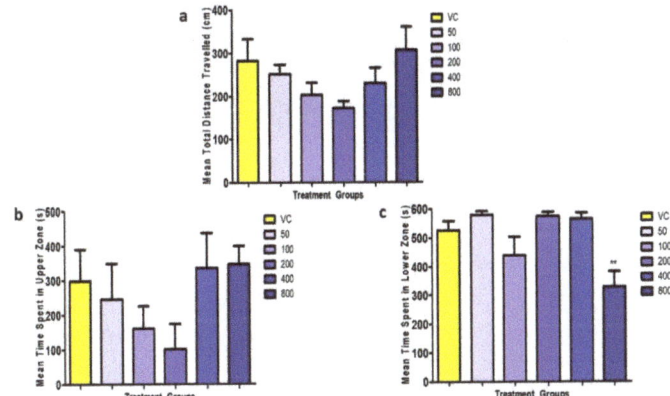

Figure 3. Mean locomotion parameters over 600 s for all the experimental groups. Figure (**a**) represents the mean total distance travelled (cm), Figure (**b**) shows the mean time spent in upper zone (s) and Figure (**c**) displays the mean time spent in lower zone (s). The data are expressed as Mean ± SEM, $n = 8$ and was analyzed using One-way ANOVA followed with Dunnett's post-hoc test at significance level of ** $p < 0.01$ against the VC group (tank water only, i.p.).

Based on the swim path analysis (Figure 2) and locomotion parameters (Figure 3), OSLP ranging from 50 to 800 µg did not result in any abnormal behavioral changes in the adult zebrafish. These doses were found to be safe for the use in adult zebrafish and did not result in any mortality or morbidity. Considering the maximum protective effects OSLP could possibly exhibit in brain at a safe concentration, 800 µg was fixed as the maximum safe starting dose. Subsequently, OSLP at 800 µg was used as the treatment dose across all further studies in this work. On the other hand, mortality in the adult zebrafish was recorded when treated with 1600 µg of OSLP. Therefore, this dose was considered as unsafe and the findings were not included in this work.

3.2. Evaluation of Anticonvulsive Potential of OSLP

3.2.1. Behavioral Study

Swim Path Analysis

The VC group (Figure 4a) managed to swim throughout the entire tank without showing apparent preference for any part of the tank. In contrast, the NC group showed a more erratic swimming pattern after the PTZ challenge, with the zebrafish dwelling at the bottom half of tank more frequently (Figure 4b). Pre-treatment with DZP (PC group) modified the post PTZ challenge swimming behavior into a swimming pattern comparable to the VC group, with roughly equal amount of time being spent at the top and bottom of the tank (Figure 4c). Pre-treatment with OSLP 800 µg (O+P) also produced a swimming pattern similar to that of the VC group, without showing apparent preference for any part of the tank (Figure 4d). The treatment control group (TC) managed to swim throughout the whole tank without showing erratic swimming pattern (Figure 4e).

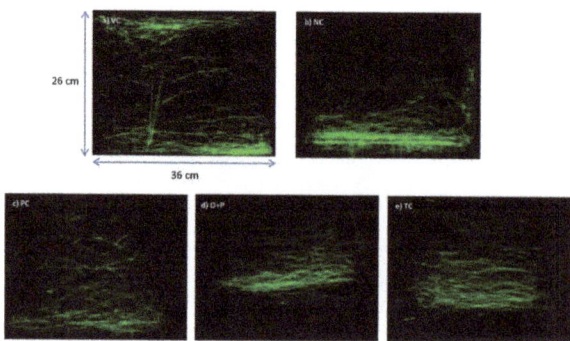

Figure 4. Representative swimming patterns for the corresponding 5 experimental groups ($n = 10$). VC ((**a**) tank water, i.p.), NC ((**b**) PTZ 170 mg/kg, i.p.), PC ((**c**) DZP 1.25 mg/kg + PTZ 170 mg/kg, i.p.), O+P ((**d**) OSLP 800 µg/kg + PTZ 170 mg/kg, i.p.) and TC ((**e**) OSLP 800 µg/kg + tank water, i.p.).

3.2.2. Seizure Score and Seizure Onset Time

The cutoff time for seizure scoring was 600 s as fish fully recovered from seizures by 600 s. Mean seizure onset time for both the VC group and TC group were set as 600 s and a maximum seizure score of zero was assigned to these groups. They did not receive any PTZ challenges and thus did not show seizures. They served only as the study controls. PTZ injection into the zebrafish resulted in diverse seizure profiles, intensities, and latency in reaching the different seizure scores and onset time.

The NC group injected with PTZ had a significant increase in seizure score to 2.8 ($F = 34.35$ *** $p < 0.001$) and had significantly prompted the seizure onset time to the lowest, 76 s ($F = 49.50$, *** $p < 0.001$), when compared to the VC group. Higher seizure score with a concurrent lower seizure onset time indicated more severe seizures in the PTZ-injected zebrafish. Treatment with 800 µg/kg of OSLP showed a significant decrease in seizure score, to 1.5 ($F = 34.35$, *** $p < 0.001$) and significantly delayed the seizure onset time to 349 s ($F = 49.50$, *** $p < 0.001$) compared to the NC group. As expected, the PC group treated with DZP also showed a significant decrease in seizure score, to < 1 ($F = 34.35$, *** $p < 0.001$) and had significantly delayed the seizure onset time to 564 s ($F = 49.50$, *** $p < 0.001$) compared to the NC group.

In this study, PTZ (170 mg/kg of b.w.) was shown to sufficiently induce seizures in the adult zebrafish, with a high seizure score and a fast seizure onset time. OSLP treatment (800 µg/kg of b.w.) was shown to reduce seizure severity, with a lower seizure score and delayed the onset time to the most serious seizure score 4 (Figure 5).

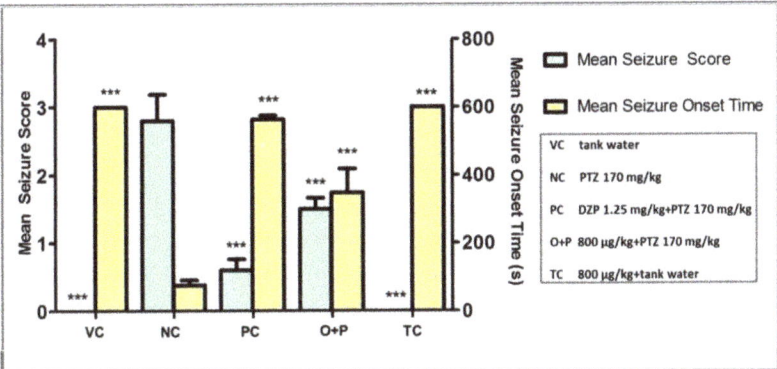

Figure 5. Mean seizure scores and mean seizure onset time (s) for the corresponding 5 experimental groups. Data are mean ± SEM. Experiments were repeated in $n = 10$, *** showed $p < 0.001$ against negative control. One-way ANOVA with Dunnett's post-hoc test. VC (tank water, i.p.), NC (PTZ 170 mg/kg, i.p.), PC (DZP 1.25 mg/kg + PTZ 170 mg/kg, i.p.), O+P (OSLP 800 µg/kg + PTZ 170 mg/kg, i.p.) and TC (OSLP 800 µg/kg + tank water, i.p.).

3.2.3. Locomotion Parameters

Mean total distance travelled of the VC group was 68±16 cm (F = 4.527, ** $p < 0.01$) and was significantly shorter than the NC group injected with PTZ (172 ± 34 cm, F = 4.527, **$p < 0.01$). The NC group travelled about a 60% longer distance than the VC group (Figure 6a). The PC group treated with DZP had mean total distance travelled of 74 ± 16 cm which was 57% shorter than the PTZ-injected group (F = 4.527, ** $p < 0.01$) (Figure 6a). This significant improvement was also comparable to the VC group (68 ± 16 cm). A reduction was also seen in the O+P group, with mean total distance travelled of 137 ± 22 cm, which was about 20% shorter than the PTZ-induced alone group (Figure 6A).

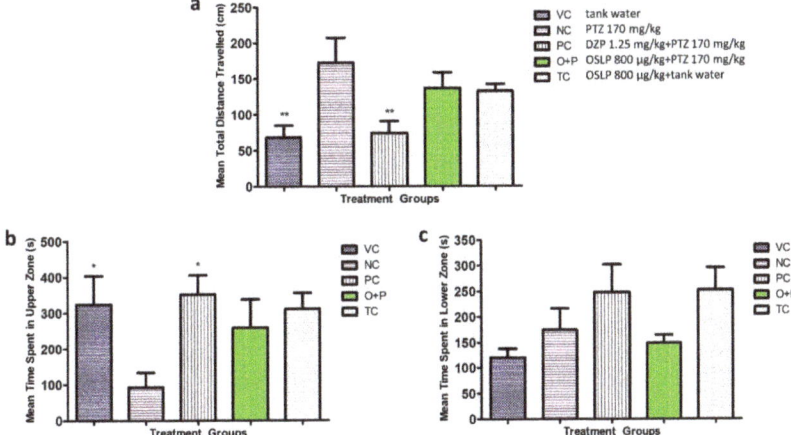

Figure 6. Mean locomotion parameters over 600 s for all the experimental groups. Figure (**a**) represents the mean total distance travelled (cm), Figure (**b**) shows the mean time spent in upper zone (s) and Figure (**c**) displays the mean time spent in lower zone (s). The data are expressed as Mean ± SEM, $n = 10$ and was analyzed using One-way ANOVA followed with Dunnett's post-hoc test at significance level of * $p < 0.05$ and ** $p < 0.01$ against the negative control group (NC, PTZ 170 mg/kg). VC (tank water, i.p.), PC (DZP 1.25 mg/kg + PTZ 170 mg/kg, i.p.), O+P (OSLP 800 µg/kg + PTZ 170 mg/kg, i.p.) and TC (OSLP 800 µg/kg + tank water, i.p.).

For the parameter of time spent in each half of the tank, only groups VC and PC showed a significant longer time spent in the upper half of tank (324 ± 80 s and 352 ± 54 s respectively, F = 2.716, * $p < 0.05$) and a visibly shorter time spent in the bottom of tank than the NC group (Figure 6b,c). The O+P group (Figure 6b) had a trend of spending a slightly longer time in the upper half of tank (259 ± 78 s) but a slightly shorter time in the bottom half (149 ± 15 s) compared to the NC group (Figure 6c).

It is also worthy to mention that the TC group had displayed a similar trend to the VC group in all three locomotion parameters (Figure 6a–c). OSLP at a dose of 800 µg/kg did not trigger any locomotor manipulations and hence, was considerably safe in the adult zebrafish (Figure 6a–c).

3.2.4. Neurotransmitter Study

Neurotransmitters in the zebrafish brains, namely GABA and glutamate (Glu) and their ratio (GABA/Glu) were evaluated (Figure 7a–c).

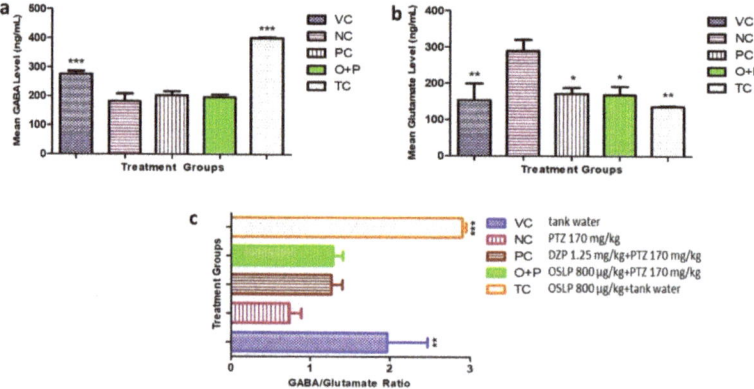

Figure 7. Mean neurotransmitter levels (ng/mL), namely GABA (**a**), glutamate (**b**) and GABA/Glu ratio (**c**) over 600 s for all the experimental groups. The data are expressed as Mean ± SEM, $n = 10$ and was analyzed using One-way ANOVA followed with Dunnett's post-hoc test at significance level of * $p < 0.05$, ** $p < 0.01$ and *** $p < 0.001$ against the negative control group (NC, PTZ 170 mg/kg). VC (tank water, i.p.), PC (DZP 1.25 mg/kg + PTZ 170 mg/kg, i.p.), O+P (OSLP 800 µg/kg + PTZ 170 mg/kg, i.p.) and TC (OSLP 800 µg/kg + tank water, i.p.).

The NC group showed a significant decrease in mean GABA levels (182 ± 26 ng/mL, *** $p < 0.001$) when compared to the VC group (276 ± 10 ng/mL, F = 37.74, *** $p < 0.001$) (Figure 7a). Mean GABA levels of the O+P group was 196 ± 9 ng/mL. Despite attaining about 7% higher GABA levels than the NC group, this treatment however did not attain statistical significance (Figure 7a). DZP treatment also brought about a slight increase in the GABA levels, to 202 ± 14 ng/mL as compared to 182 ± 26 ng/mL in the NC group ($p > 0.05$) (Figure 7a). Similarly, both PC (202 ± 14 ng/mL) and O+P (196 ± 9 ng/mL) had showed just slightly higher GABA levels than the NC group (Figure 7a).

In contrast, NC group showed a significant increase in Glu level (290 ± 30 ng/mL, F = 4.779, ** $p < 0.01$) when compared to the VC and TC groups (153 ± 46 ng/mL and 136 ± 2 ng/mL respectively, F = 4.779, ** $p < 0.01$) (Figure 7b). Meanwhile, DZP treatment brought about a significant decrease to 172 ± 16 ng/mL in the Glu levels, or about 41% lower than the NC group (F = 4.779, * $p < 0.05$) (Figure 7b). Mean Glu levels of the O+P group was 169 ± 22 ng/mL, which was 42% significantly lower than the NC group (F = 4.779, * $p < 0.05$) (Figure 7b). This outcome thus suggests that OSLP treatment could be effectively lower the Glu concentrations, normalizing it to the level comparable to those treated with DZP.

In addition, PTZ injection caused a significant decrease in the GABA/Glu ratio to <1, whereas, both VC and TC groups had a higher GABA/Glu ratio (R > 2, F = 13.81, ** $p < 0.01$ and *** $p < 0.001$, respectively) (Figure 7c). Very noteworthy is that the OSLP-treated and DZP-treated groups had a similar GABA/Glu ratio, though they did not attain statistical significance when compared to the NC (Figure 7c). It is worth mentioning that the TC group (treatment dose control) had higher GABA levels (401 ± 3 ng/mL, F = 37.74, *** $p < 0.001$) (Figure 7a) and lower Glu levels (136 ± 2 ng/mL, F = 4.779, *** $p < 0.001$) (Figure 7b) than the VC group. Also, the GABA/Glu ratio was comparable to the VC group.

3.2.5. Proteins Expression Profiling Using Mass Spectrometry-Based Label-Free Proteomic Quantification (LFQ)

LFQ profiled 29 differentially expressed proteins from the brain samples of PTZ injected zebrafish (NC group) and the OSLP-treated PTZ group (O+P). These proteins were found to be expressed at lower levels in the NC group than in the O+P group (Figure 8 and Table 4). Among them, five proteins, namely hemoglobin subunit alpha (Hbaa1, isoforms Q803Z5 and Q90487), hemoglobin subunit beta-1 (Hbba1, Q90486), fructose-bisphosphate aldolase C-B (Aldocb, Q8JH70), actin beta 2 (Actb2, A8WG05), and complexin 2 (Cplx2, E7FBR8) were found expressed at higher levels.

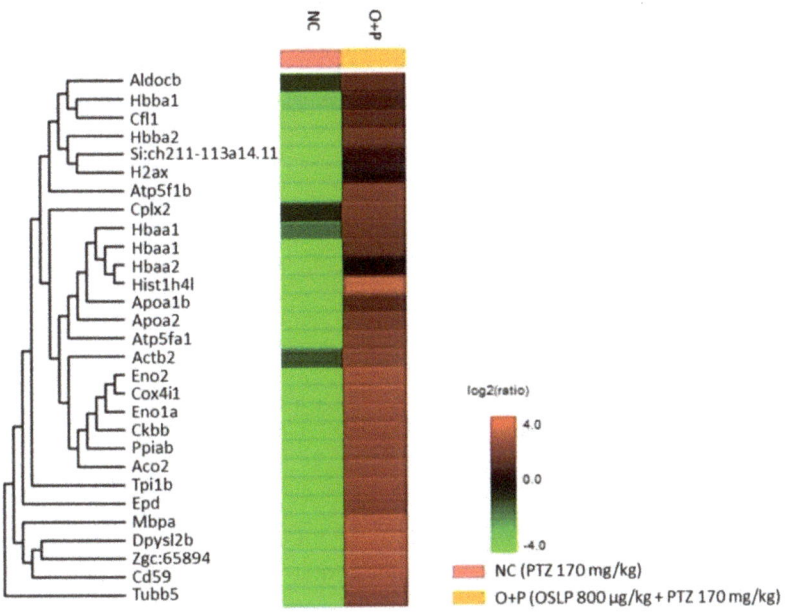

Figure 8. Heat map shows the differentially expressed proteins identified from negative control (NC, PTZ 170 mg/kg only) and O+P (OSLP 800 µg/kg + PTZ 170 mg/kg) zebrafish brains, $n = 4$, significance ≥ 20, FDR ≤ 1%, fold change ≥ 1, unique peptide ≥ 1. Protein names are listed on the left while experimental groups are indicated on top. The color key on the bottom right indicates the log2 (ratio) expression levels (green = low and red = high).

3.2.6. Bioinformatics Analysis

The differentially expressed proteins (Table 4) were searched in the ZFIN Database Information to match the gene ID. The database of InterPro Classification of Protein Families was searched for the respective protein class. The results were presented in Table 5.

Table 4. Differentially expressed proteins identified from negative control (NC, PTZ 170 mg/kg only) and O+P (OSLP 800 µg/kg + PTZ 170 mg/kg) zebrafish brains.

Uniprot Accession ID	Uniprot Protein Name	Significance (≥13)	Coverage (%)	#Peptides	#Unique	Avg. Mass	Group Profile (Ratio of NC/O+P)	ZFIN Protein
Q90487	Hemoglobin subunit alpha	200	49	12	4	15,524	0.00:1.00	Hbaa1
Q803Z5	Hemoglobin subunit alpha	200	49	12	4	15,508	1.00:255.14	Hbaa1
Q90486	Hemoglobin subunit beta-1	200	43	8	8	16,389	1.00:49.49	Hbba1
Q08BA1	ATP synthase subunit alpha	200	15	6	3	59,744	0.00:1.00	Atp5fa1
Q6PC12	Enolase 1	200	12	4	3	47,074	0.00:1.00	Eno1a
Q4VBK0	ATP synthase subunit beta	200	9	3	3	55,000	0.00:1.00	Atp5f1b
Q6ZM12	Hemoglobin beta adult 2	200	13	3	3	16,295	0.00:1.00	Hbba2
E7F2M5	CD59 molecule (CD59 blood group)	200	26	2	2	12,914	0.00:1.00	Cd59
E9QBF0	Triosephosphate isomerase	200	20	4	4	21,811	0.00:1.00	Tpi1b
Q6PC53	Peptidyl-prolyl cis-trans isomerase	200	18	3	3	17,489	0.00:1.00	Ppiab
F8W4M7	Aconitate hydratase mitochondrial	200	4	2	2	85,590	0.00:1.00	Aco2
Q8AY63	Brain-subtype creatine kinase	153.53	7	3	3	42,884	0.00:1.00	Ckbb
Q4VBT9	Cox4i1 protein	126.93	18	2	2	19,443	0.00:1.00	Cox4i1
Q8IH70	Fructose-bisphosphate aldolase C-B	126.51	12	4	4	39,259	1.00:8.14	Aldocb
Q6PE34	Tubulin beta chain	125.32	31	12	3	49,635	0.00:1.00	Zgc:65894
A0A0R4IKF0	Apolipoprotein A-Ib	112	9	2	2	30,140	0.00:1.00	Apoa1b
F8W3W8	Myelin basic protein a	110.44	63	10	2	10,776	0.00:1.00	Mbpa
A3KPR4	Histone H4	104.16	24	2	2	11,367	0.00:1.00	Hist1h4l
B3DFP9	Apolipoprotein A-II	103.56	21	2	2	15,537	0.00:1.00	Apoa2
Q5BJC7	Haemoglobin alpha adult 2	79.54	17	3	2	15,403	0.00:1.00	Hbaa2
Q8AYC4	Tubulin beta chain	76.34	39	13	2	49,826	0.00:1.00	Tubb5
R4GE02	Sich211–113a14.11	56.58	21	4	2	27,149	0.00:1.00	Sich211–113a14.11
Q7ZUY3	Histone H2AX	56.36	34	4	2	15,001	0.00:1.00	H2ax
Q6TH32	Cofilin 1	44.76	13	2	2	18,771	0.00:1.00	Cfl1
A0A2R8QZZ0	Ependymin	44.72	12	2	2	23,370	0.00:1.00	Epd
A8WG05	Actin beta 2	43.68	15	6	6	41,753	1.00:9.75	Actb2
E7FBR8	Complexin 2	43.27	24	2	2	15,094	1.00:5.64	Cplx2
A8DZ95	Dihydropyrimidinase-like 2b	43.27	6	2	2	58,285	0.00:1.00	Dpysl2b
Q6GQM9	Eno2 protein	36.01	7	2	1	46,841	0.00:1.00	Eno2

Remark: ZFIN protein nomenclatures were searched in the ZFIN Database Information (www.zfin.org) as accessed on 17/02/2020.

Table 5. Protein family of the differentially expressed proteins identified from negative control (NC, PTZ 170 mg/kg only) and O+P (OSLP 800 µg/kg + PTZ 170 mg/kg) zebrafish brains.

Protein Family	ZFIN Protein	ZFIN Gene ID
Globin domain-containing protein		
Belongs to the family of hemoglobin, alpha-type and to the subfamily of hemoglobin, pi	Hbaa1	ZDB-GENE-980526-79
	Hbaa2	ZDB-GENE-081104-38
Member of the hemoglobin, beta-type	Hbba1	ZDB-GENE-990415-18
	Hbba2	ZDB-GENE-040801-164
Plasma protein		
Member of the CD marker	Cd59	ZDB-GENE-030131-7871
Member of the apolipoprotein A/E	Apoa2	ZDB-GENE-030131-1046
Belong to the myelin basic protein	Mbpa	ZDB-GENE-030128-2
Member of the apolipoprotein A/E	Apoa1b	ZDB-GENE-050302-172
Cytoskeletal protein		
Member of the actin family	Actb2	ZDB-GENE-000329-3
Member of the beta tubulin	Tubb5	ZDB-GENE-031110-4
	Zgc:65894	ZDB-GENE-030131-7741
Enzyme protein		
Transferase		
Member of the ATP:guanido phosphotransferase protein	Ckbb	ZDB-GENE-020103-2
Member of the ATP synthase, F1 complex, beta subunit	Atp5f1b	ZDB-GENE-030131-124
Member of the mitochondrial F1-F0 ATP synthase subunit F	Atp5mf	ZDB-GENE-050309-87
Member of the ATP synthase, F1 complex, alpha subunit	Atp5fa1	ZDB-GENE-060201-1
Isomerase		
Member of the cyclophilin-type peptidyl-prolyl cis-trans isomerase	Ppiab	ZDB-GENE-030131-7459
Member of the triosephosphate isomerase	Tpi1b	ZDB-GENE-020416-4
Lyase		
Member of the fructose-bisphosphate aldolase, class-I	Aldocb	ZDB-GENE-030821-1
Member of the enolase	Eno1a	ZDB-GENE-030131-6048
Citric acid cycle related protein		
Belongs to the family of aconitase, mitochondrial-like	Aco2	ZDB-GENE-030131-1390
Member of the enolase	Eno2	ZDB-GENE-040704-27
Histone protein		
Core Histone		
Member of the histone H2A	H2ax	ZDB-GENE-040426-987
	Si:ch211-113a14.11	ZDB-GENE-121214-162
Member of the histone H4	Hist1h4l	ZDB-GENE-070927-10
Intracellular protein-Ependymin		
Member of the ependymin-related protein family (EPDRs)	Epd	ZDB-GENE-980526-111
Cytosolic protein		
Member of the complexin/synaphin family	Cplx2	ZDB-GENE-081113-1
ADF-H domain-containing protein		
Belongs to the family of ADF/Cofilin	Cfl1	ZDB-GENE-030131-215
Transporter protein-Primary active transporter		
Belongs to the cytochrome c oxidase subunit IV family and to the subfamily of cytochrome c oxidase subunit IV	Cox4i1	ZDB-GENE-030131-5175
Amidohydro-rel domain-containing protein		
Belongs to the hydantoinase/dihydropyrimidinase family and to the subfamily of dihydropyrimidinase-related protein 2	Dpysl2b	ZDB-GENE-031105-1

Remark: Protein Families and their respective functions were searched in the InterPro Classification of Protein Families and the ZFIN Database Information (https://www.ebi.ac.uk/interpro/protein/UniProt/ and www.zfin.org accessed on 17 February 2020).

50–1600 µg/kg of b.w. were tested in each assigned group. The zebrafish swimming pattern after exposure to 800 µg of OSLP did not show bottom-dwelling behavior. Diving to the bottom of tank can be a natural reflexive response of zebrafish. However, increased bottom-dwelling behavior has been linked to anxiety in the novel tank test [15,16]. The bottom dwelling frequency has been found reduced in zebrafish when treated with anxiolytic compounds [7,17]. These earlier findings thus lend support to the anxiolytic potential of OSLP in adult zebrafish, at least at a concentration greater than 800 µg/kg of body weight. Noteworthy however, OSLP at a concentration of 1600 µg is capable of causing lethal events in adult zebrafish. This finding has drawn a line to limit the maximum safe dose of OSLP achievable via intraperitoneal route to be not greater than 1600 µg/kg of body weight, at least in the case of zebrafish. This also lends support to the exclusion of 1600 µg OSLP for further analysis in this work. Building on the safety study outcomes and considering the maximum protective effects of OSLP at a safe concentration, 800 µg was chosen as the treatment dose in this study.

The OSLP safety study was crucial as there was no prior published scientific evidence on OSLP in both in vitro and in vivo models, let alone its neuroprotective potential. A prior literature search only yielded two studies on the ethanolic extracts of *Orthosiphon stamineus*; Choo et al. (2018) examined the anticonvulsive potential in adult zebrafish [9] and Ismail et al. (2017) reported on toxicity in zebrafish embryos [19]. As such, this work represents the first of its kind.

In this study, the PTZ-induced seizure model was established [7,12] to investigate the anticonvulsive potential of OSLP (800 µg/kg of b.w.) using adult zebrafish. Pre-treatment with OSLP 800 µg for 30 min brought about significant improvements in the PTZ-injected zebrafish, with a lower seizure score and a prolonged seizure onset time. Pre-treatment with OSLP 800 µg also produced a swimming pattern comparable to that of the untreated VC which received neither PTZ injection nor OSLP treatment (TC). It was seen that the O+P group managed to swim through the whole tank without showing an apparent preference for any spot or apparent bottom-dwelling behavior. Contradictorily, the representative zebrafish swimming pattern showed a bottom-dwelling behavior in the PTZ-injected group, which has been strongly linked to the anxious behavior in seizures [15,16]. A similar observation was also reported in two recent studies using PTZ-induced zebrafish [7,12]. Diazepam (DZP, 1.25 mg/kg) has been found in this study to efficaciously control seizures in the PTZ-injected zebrafish and thus, a swimming pattern comparable to that of the untreated VC was observed. Interestingly, the TC group which received neither PTZ injection nor DZP treatment, produced a swimming pattern comparable to that of the untreated VC group. This finding thus reaffirms that OSLP at 800 µg/kg of body weight does not produce lethal events and with that it could be potentially anticonvulsive. Nevertheless, one of the limitations in this study includes a considerably low yield of OSLP (approximately 0.3%) extracted from OS leaves and hence, based on the safety study (Section 3.1), only the maximal safe dose (800 µg/kg of b.w.) was used.

The PTZ-injected group had the highest mean total distance travelled and travelled about 60% longer distance than the untreated VC group. This uncontrolled movement has been strongly linked to burst neuronal firing in addition to the pass-out phenomenon in seizures [20,21]. A similar observation was also reported in two recent studies using PTZ-induced zebrafish [7,12]. A disruption occurred in the normal balance of excitation and inhibition following the injection of PTZ. Binding of PTZ to $GABA_A$ (γ-aminobutyric acid type A) receptors stimulated excitability in the brains and hence provoked uncontrolled seizures in the zebrafish. This explains the representative swim path of the PTZ-injected group which showed burst swimming activities (i.e., erratic movements, loss of direction) which taken together, contributed to the longest total distance travelled. Moreover, the PTZ-injected group spent a longer time in the lower half of tank, which could possibly be attributed to the bottom-dwelling behavior in seizures [15,16].

In contrast, pre-treatment with DZP significantly alleviated the manipulations of PTZ. A 57% reduction in the total distance travelled was seen in the DZP-treated group and it spent more time in the upper half of tank in a comparable manner to that of the untreated group. Interestingly however, it also spent a longer time in the bottom half of the tank, but the untreated group did not. This phenomenon could be attributed to the sedative effects of DZP. DZP is an anxiolytic benzodiazepine with fast-acting and long-lasting actions [22]. When administered intravenously, DZP has been shown to act within 1 to 3 min, while oral dosing onset ranges between 15 to 60 min; with a duration of action of more than 12 h. Similar to most benzodiazepines, DZP causes adverse effects including syncope (temporary loss of consciousness), sedation and confusion, to name a few [23]. A similar finding was also reported in three studies using DZP to treat zebrafish [7,12,24]. Pre-treatment with OSLP 800 µg also alleviated the manipulations of PTZ. A 20% reduction in the total distance travelled was seen in the OSLP-treated group and similarly, they spent more time in the upper half of tank compared to the DZP-treated group. Interestingly however, they did not spend a longer time in the bottom half of tank as the DZP-treated group did, but in a pattern more comparable to the untreated VC group. Hence, this outcome suggests that OSLP's anticonvulsive actions could be acting differently from DZP and with that, it might not produce the similar cognitive insults such as DZP. This similar outcome has been reported in Choo's study using *O. stamineus* ethanolic extracts to treat adult zebrafish [7]. On the market, DZP has since been one of the top selling AEDs of all time, well known for its fast onset of action and is often effective in adults [25,26]. However, DZP's high clinical efficacy in treating epilepsy and seizures comes with multiple adverse reactions such as suicidality, paradoxical CNS stimulation, syncope, sedation, depression and dystonia, to name a few [23]. These adverse effects are common in currently available AEDs. Worthy of mention, the TC group did not show any abnormal locomotion parameters and hence, reaffirming that this dose is considerably safe in the adult zebrafish.

Taken together, the outcomes of behavioral study suggest that OSLP at 800 µg/kg of body weight is potentially anticonvulsive. OSLP treatment produced milder anticonvulsant effects in comparison to DZP treatment, which is one of the standard AEDs available today.

In this study, two major neurotransmitters, namely GABA and Glu, were investigated. An interrupted GABA/Glu cycle was seen in the PTZ-injected zebrafish, with a drop in the mean GABA level but a surge in the mean Glu level. Distinctively, such anomalies were not found in the untreated zebrafish which did not receive PTZ injection. Additionally, the GABA/Glu ratio of PTZ-injected group remained the lowest. This thus shows a disruption in the normal balance of excitation and inhibition following the PTZ treatment. PTZ is a tetrazol derivative known to block $GABA_A$ receptor function [27]. PTZ suppresses GABA inhibitory activities which in turn potentiates the Glu excitatory activities in the brain and eventually results in an unbalanced GABA/Glu ratio. This finding has lent more support to the severe seizures seen in the PTZ-injected group. Pre-treatment with DZP, without surprise, significantly suppressed the excitatory neurotransmitter Glu, normalizing it to be comparable to the untreated VC group. Concurrently, the GABA levels in the DZP-treated group saw a slight elevation and this eventually improved the GABA/Glu ratio. A similar finding has been reported earlier [28]. DZP inhibits Glu release to suppress glutamatergic hyperactivity and hence, restores the balance between GABA and Glu to promptly arrest neuroexcitation [29,30]. Pre-treatment with OSLP has also improved the neurotransmitters profile, with significantly lower excitatory Glu levels. More interestingly, OSLP treatment brings the GABA/Glu ratio close to the DZP treatment. Although to a lesser degree than the pure drug control, taken together, these findings show that OSLP has GABA potentiating actions and antiglutamatergic effects. Moreover, the finding that TC group had a neurotransmitters profile comparable to the untreated VC group, has also buttressed the proposal of OSLP could be having neuroprotective potential.

The present protein expression study is useful in helping to predict the anticonvulsive mechanism of OSLP. The main findings are the following. First, mass spectrometry-based LFQ analysis compared the differentially expressed proteins in the seizure group (NC, induced by PTZ 170 mg/kg only) and the OSLP-treated seizure group (OSLP 800 µg/kg + PTZ 170 mg/kg). This identified a distinct protein expression profile of 29 differentially expressed proteins that had higher expressions in the O+P group than in the NC group. Second, functional annotation analysis found the protein bindings of SNARE (GO:149) and syntaxin (GO:19905) at intracellular localizations that were particularly interesting, given the fundamental role they play in the regulation of membrane fusion during presynaptic vesicle exocytosis. Third, KEGG pathway mapping proposed the synaptic vesicle cycle (04721) as the most probable pathway, in line with the strong association between SNARE and syntaxin proteins. These proteins are required in calcium (Ca^{2+})-dependent synaptic vesicle exocytosis. As shown, the trans-SNARE complex was assembled in the presence of SNARE proteins including complexin (Cplx), syntaxin (Stx), synaptotagmin (Syt), synaptosomal-associated protein of 25 kDa (Snap25) and vesicle-associated membrane protein (Vamp). According to ZFIN (https://zfin.org/ZDB-GENE-081113-1), gene cplx2 is predicted to orthologous to human gene CPLX2.

Complexin is an important regulator of synaptic vesicle exocytosis. Complexins, also called synaphins, are small cytosolic proteins. They form a small protein family with four isoforms, Cplx1–4 [31]. Cplx1 and Cplx2 are highly homologous. In particular, they bind to the SNARE complex which are expressed at presynaptic sites [32–35]. SNARE binding is a highly specialized regulation that is strictly regulated by synaptic fusion machinery. The basic components of a synaptic fusion machinery are the SNARE proteins namely Cplx, Stx, Syt, Snap25, Vamp, and two mammalian uncoordinated proteins (Munc13 and Munc18) [36]. The formation of the trans-SNARE complex is required in the vesicle priming phase. As the trans-SNARE complex forms, the vesicle is pulled close to the plasma membrane, where it is ready to fuse in response to the Ca^{2+} influx that is triggered by an action potential, usually in less than a millisecond. Complexin binds to the trans-SNARE complex and modulates the fusion process by either increasing or decreasing the height of the energy barrier for fusion. The height of the energy barrier for fusion is not only important for evoked release but also determines how likely vesicles are to fuse spontaneously in the absence of a Ca^{2+}-triggering signal. After fusion, the vesicle is retrieved by endocytosis and reloaded for another round of exocytosis [13,32,33,36]. Therefore, the binding of complexin to the SNARE complex is crucial for the normal priming and subsequent Ca^{2+}-evoked neurotransmitter release during presynaptic vesicle exocytosis.

The findings of protein expression study have suggested that synaptic vesicle cycle pathway could play a significant role in modulating the anticonvulsive mechanism of OSLP. OSLP could be regulating the release of GABA and Glu via calcium-dependent synaptic vesicle exocytosis. Similar findings have been reported by studies using samples from rats and patients [32,34,35]. Decreased expressions of complexin 2 have also been associated with neurodegenerative diseases including Alzheimer's, Huntington's, and Parkinson's; psychiatric disorders including schizophrenia and bipolar disorder [37–40], with seizures and epilepsy being common comorbidities [41–46].

OSLP could be a potential anticonvulsant. Found in OSLP, baicalein 7-O-glucuronosyltransferase and baicalin-beta-D-glucuronidase are responsible for the biosynthesis of baicalein and baicalin, respectively. Baicalein and baicalin have been reported to have anxiolytic activity and acting on GABA and glutamic acid in rat brains [47], binding to the benzodiazepine site of the $GABA_A$ receptor to potentiate GABA-mediated inhibition [48–50] and anticonvulsive action in the PTZ-induced seizure rat model [51]. Beta-mycrene synthase and R-linalool synthase are proteins responsible for the biosynthesis of myrcene and linalool respectively. Linalool has been reported to have antiepileptiform and antiseizure properties in PTZ-treated rats [52–54] whereas beta-mycrene has also been reported for sedative effects in human [55] and anticonvulsive effects in PTZ-treated rats [56]. Beta-mycrene synthase and R-linalool synthase might not directly act on cannabinoid receptors but could be producing synergic effects with future cannabinoid-based AEDs. The postulated synergistic contribution on both GABA and Glu neurotransmitters can increase the efficacy of future cannabinoid-based AEDs in managing epilepsy and seizures [57–60]. Rosmarinate synthase is involved in the biosynthesis of rosmarinic acid Choo, Kundap [7] suggested that rosmarinic acid (in an ethanolic extract of OS) is one of the probable antiepileptic components of the extract in adult zebrafish whereas similar findings in PTZ-induced seizures in mice have also been reported earlier [10,61].

5. Conclusions

The study suggests that OSLP could be a potential anticonvulsant. OSLP most likely regulates the release of the neurotransmitters, GABA and Glu, via calcium-dependent synaptic vesicle exocytosis mediated by the "synaptic vesicle cycle" pathway. To the best of our knowledge, this study is the first to show that OSLP can safely ameliorate epilepticeizures in adult zebrafish.

Author Contributions: Y.-S.C. designed, performed all the experiments and prepared the final manuscript; B.K.M.C. helped in the behavioral experiments and edited the final manuscript; P.K.A. aided in supervision and helped edit the final manuscript; M.F.S. and I.O. contributed to the design of research, supervised all aspects of the study and edited the final manuscript as submitted. All authors have read and agreed to the published version of the manuscript.

Funding: This research was funded by the NKEA EPP#1 Research Grant Scheme (NRGS) (NH1014D066), Ministry of Agriculture and Agro-based Industry, Malaysia and Global Asia in the 21st Century (GA21) Platform, Monash University Malaysia, Research Grant (GA-HW-18-L04).

Acknowledgments: The authors would like to thank Syafiq Asnawi Zainal Abidin and Nurziana Sharmilla Binti Nawawi for ESI-LCMS/MS technical support (LC-MS laboratory of Jeffrey Cheah School of Medicine and Health Sciences).

Conflicts of Interest: The authors declare no conflict of interest. The funders had no role in the design of the study; in the collection, analyses, or interpretation of data; in the writing of the manuscript, or in the decision to publish the results.

References

1. World Health Organisation. *Epilepsy: A Public Health Imperative: Summary*; World Health Organization: Geneva, Switzerland, 2019.
2. Jacob, S.; Nair, A.B. An updated overview on therapeutic drug monitoring of recent antiepileptic drugs. *Drugs R D* **2016**, *16*, 303–316. [CrossRef] [PubMed]
3. Luft, J.G.; Steffens, L.; Morás, A.M.; Da Rosa, M.S.; Leipnitz, G.; Regner, G.G.; Pflüger, P.F.; Gonçalves, D.; Moura, D.J.; Pereira, P. Rosmarinic acid improves oxidative stress parameters and mitochondrial respiratory chain activity following 4-aminopyridine and picrotoxin-induced seizure in mice. *Naunyn-Schmiedeberg's Arch. Pharmacol.* **2019**, *392*, 1347–1358. [CrossRef]
4. Chen, Z.; Brodie, M.J.; Liew, D.; Kwan, P. Treatment outcomes in patients with newly diagnosed epilepsy treated with established and new antiepileptic drugs: A 30-year longitudinal cohort study. *JAMA Neurol.* **2018**, *75*, 279–286. [CrossRef]
5. Helmstaedter, C.; Witt, J.-A. Chapter 28—Clinical neuropsychology in epilepsy: Theoretical and practical issues. In *Handbook of Clinical Neurology*; Stefan, H., Theodore, W.H., Eds.; Elsevier: Amsterdam, The Netherlands, 2012; Volume 107, pp. 437–459.
6. World Health Organisation. *WHO Traditional Medicine Strategy 2014–2023*; World Health Organisation: Geneva, Switzerland, 2013.
7. Zhu, H.-L.; Wan, J.-B.; Wang, Y.-T.; Li, B.-C.; Xiang, C.; He, J.; Li, P. Medicinal compounds with antiepileptic/anticonvulsant activities. *Epilepsia* **2014**, *55*, 3–16. [CrossRef] [PubMed]
8. Rabiei, Z. Anticonvulsant effects of medicinal plants with emphasis on mechanisms of action. *Asian Pac. J. Trop. Biomed.* **2017**, *7*, 166–172. [CrossRef]
9. Choo, B.K.M.; Kundap, U.P.; Kumari, Y.; Hue, S.-M.; Othman, I.; Shaikh, M.F. Orthosiphon stamineus leaf extract affects TNF-α and seizures in a zebrafish model. *Front. Pharmacol.* **2018**, *9*, 139. [CrossRef]
10. Coelho, V.R.; Vieira, C.G.; De Souza, L.P.; Moysés, F.; Basso, C.; Papke, D.K.M.; Pires, T.R.; Siqueira, I.R.; Picada, J.N.; Pereira, P. Antiepileptogenic, antioxidant and genotoxic evaluation of rosmarinic acid and its metabolite caffeic acid in mice. *Life Sci.* **2015**, *122*, 65–71. [CrossRef]
11. Howe, K.; Clark, M.D.; Torroja, C.F.; Torrance, J.; Berthelot, C.; Muffato, M.; Collins, J.E.; Humphray, S.; McLaren, K.; Matthews, L.; et al. The zebrafish reference genome sequence and its relationship to the human genome. *Nature* **2013**, *496*, 498–503. [CrossRef]
12. Norton, W.; Bally-Cuif, L. Adult zebrafish as a model organism for behavioural genetics. *BMC Neurosci.* **2010**, *11*, 90. [CrossRef]
13. Stewart, A.M.; Braubach, O.; Spitsbergen, J.; Gerlai, R.; Kalueff, A.V. Zebrafish models for translational neuroscience research: From tank to bedside. *Trends Neurosci.* **2014**, *37*, 264–278. [CrossRef]
14. OECD (Organisation for Economic Co-operation). *Development Test No. 203: Fish, Acute Toxicity Test*; OECD Publishing: Paris, France, 1992.

15. Blaser, R.E.; Rosemberg, D.B. Measures of anxiety in zebrafish (danio rerio): Dissociation of black/white preference and novel tank test. *PLoS ONE* **2012**, *7*, e36931. [CrossRef]
16. Kysil, E.V.; Meshalkina, D.A.; Frick, E.E.; Echevarria, D.J.; Rosemberg, D.B.; Maximino, C.; Lima, M.G.; Abreu, M.S.; Giacomini, A.C.; Barcellos, L.J. Comparative analyses of zebrafish anxiety-like behavior using conflict-based novelty tests. *Zebrafish* **2017**, *14*, 197–208. [CrossRef] [PubMed]
17. Gebauer, D.L.; Pagnussat, N.; Piato, Â.L.; Schaefer, I.C.; Bonan, C.D.; Lara, D.R. Effects of anxiolytics in zebrafish: Similarities and differences between benzodiazepines, buspirone and ethanol. *Pharmacol. Biochem. Behav.* **2011**, *99*, 480–486. [CrossRef]
18. OECD (Organisation for Economic Co-operation). *Development Test No. 203: Fish, Acute Toxicity Test*; OECD Publishing: Paris, France, 2018.
19. Ismail, H.F.; Hashim, Z.; Soon, W.T.; Ab Rahman, N.S.; Zainudin, A.N.; Majid, F.A.A. Comparative study of herbal plants on the phenolic and flavonoid content, antioxidant activities and toxicity on cells and zebrafish embryo. *J. Tradit. Complementary Med.* **2017**, *7*, 452–465. [CrossRef]
20. Kundap, U.P.; Kumari, Y.; Othman, I.; Shaikh, M.F. Zebrafish as a model for epilepsy-induced cognitive dysfunction: A pharmacological, biochemical and behavioral approach. *Front. Pharmacol.* **2017**, *8*, 515. [CrossRef] [PubMed]
21. Mormann, F.; Jefferys, J.G. Neuronal firing in human epileptic cortex: The ins and outs of synchrony during seizures: Dissociation of synchronization of neurons and field potentials. *Epilepsy Curr.* **2013**, *13*, 100–102. [CrossRef]
22. Scharfman, H.E. The neurobiology of epilepsy. *Curr. Neurol. Neurosci. Rep.* **2007**, *7*, 348–354. [CrossRef]
23. Griffin, C.E., 3rd; Kaye, A.M.; Bueno, F.R.; Kaye, A.D. Benzodiazepine pharmacology and central nervous system-mediated effects. *Ochsner J.* **2013**, *13*, 214–223. [PubMed]
24. Dhaliwal, J.S.; Saadabadi, A. Diazepam [Updated 2019 January 30]. In *StatPearls [Internet]*; StatPearls Publishing: Treasure Island, CA, USA, 2019.
25. Gupta, P.; Khobragade, S.B.; Shingatgeri, V.M.; Rajaram, S.M. Assessment of locomotion behavior in adult Zebrafish after acute exposure to different pharmacological reference compounds. *Drug Dev. Ther.* **2014**, *5*, 127–133. [CrossRef]
26. Calcaterra, N.E.; Barrow, J.C. Classics in chemical neuroscience: Diazepam (valium). *ACS Chem. Neurosci.* **2014**, *5*, 253–260. [CrossRef]
27. Kelly, T.H.; Delzer, T.A.; Martin, C.A.; Harrington, N.G.; Hays, L.R.; Bardo, M.T. Performance and subjective effects of diazepam and d-amphetamine in high and low sensation seekers. *Behav. Pharmacol.* **2009**, *20*, 505–517. [CrossRef] [PubMed]
28. Velíšek, L. Models of Generalized Seizures in Freely Moving Animals. In *Encyclopedia of Basic Epilepsy Research*; Philip, A.S., Ed.; Academic Press: Cambridge, MA, USA, 2009; pp. 775–780. [CrossRef]
29. Bernasconi, R.; Klein, M.; Martin, P.; Portet, C.; Maitre, L.; Jones, R.; Baltzer, V.; Schmutz, M. The specific protective effect of diazepam and valproate against isoniazid-induced seizures is not correlated with increased GABA levels. *J. Neural Transm.* **1985**, *63*, 169–189. [CrossRef] [PubMed]
30. Perks, A.; Cheema, S.; Mohanraj, R. Anaesthesia and epilepsy. *BJA Br. J. Anaesth.* **2012**, *108*, 562–571. [CrossRef] [PubMed]
31. Cao, L.; Bie, X.; Huo, S.; Du, J.; Liu, L.; Song, W. Effects of diazepam on glutamatergic synaptic transmission in the hippocampal CA1 area of rats with traumatic brain injury. *Neural Regen. Res.* **2014**, *9*, 1897–1901. [PubMed]
32. Trimbuch, T.; Rosenmund, C. Should I stop or should I go? The role of complexin in neurotransmitter release. *Nat. Rev. Neurosci.* **2016**, *17*, 118–125. [CrossRef] [PubMed]
33. Acuna, C.; Guo, Q.; Burré, J.; Sharma, M.; Sun, J.; Südhof, T.C. Microsecond Dissection of Neurotransmitter Release: SNARE-Complex Assembly Dictates Speed and Ca2+ Sensitivity. *Neuron* **2014**, *82*, 1088–1100. [CrossRef]
34. Li, Y.C.; Kavalali, E.T. Synaptic vesicle-recycling machinery components as potential therapeutic targets. *Pharm. Rev.* **2017**, *69*, 141–160. [CrossRef]
35. Snead, D.; Eliezer, D. Chapter Nine—Spectroscopic Characterization of Structure–Function Relationships in the Intrinsically Disordered Protein Complexin. In *Methods in Enzymology*; Rhoades, E., Ed.; Academic Press: Cambridge, MA, USA, 2018; Volume 611, pp. 227–286.

36. Tang, J. Complexins. In *Encyclopedia of Neuroscience*; Squire, L.R., Ed.; Academic Press: Oxford, UK, 2009; pp. 1–7.
37. Ungermann, C.; Langosch, D. Functions of SNAREs in intracellular membrane fusion and lipid bilayer mixing. *J. Cell Sci.* **2005**, *118*, 3819–3828. [CrossRef]
38. Moriya, Y.; Itoh, M.; Okuda, S.; Yoshizawa, A.C.; Kanehisa, M. KAAS: An automatic genome annotation and pathway reconstruction server. *Nucleic Acids Res.* **2007**, *35*, W182–W185. [CrossRef]
39. Roncon, P.; Soukupovà, M.; Binaschi, A.; Falciccia, C.; Zucchini, S.; Ferracin, M.; Langley, S.R.; Petretto, E.; Johnson, M.R.; Marucci, G. MicroRNA profiles in hippocampal granule cells and plasma of rats with pilocarpine-induced epilepsy–comparison with human epileptic samples. *Sci. Rep.* **2015**, *5*, 141–143. [CrossRef]
40. Chen, X.; Tomchick, D.R.; Kovrigin, E.; Araç, D.; Machius, M.; Südhof, T.C.; Rizo, J. Three-dimensional structure of the complexin/snare complex. *Neuron* **2002**, *33*, 397–409. [CrossRef]
41. Scarmeas, N.; Honig, L.S.; Choi, H.; Cantero, J.; Brandt, J.; Blacker, D.; Albert, M.; Amatniek, J.C.; Marder, K.; Bell, K.; et al. Seizures in alzheimer disease: Who, when, and how common? *Arch. Neurol.* **2009**, *66*, 992–997. [CrossRef] [PubMed]
42. Son, A.Y.; Biagioni, M.C.; Kaminski, D.; Gurevich, A.; Stone, B.; Di Rocco, A. Parkinson's disease and cryptogenic epilepsy. *Case Rep. Neurol Med.* **2016**, *2016*, 3745631. [CrossRef] [PubMed]
43. Sipilä, J.O.T.; Soilu-Hänninen, M.; Majamaa, K. Comorbid epilepsy in Finnish patients with adult-onset Huntington's disease. *BMC Neurol.* **2016**, *16*, 24. [CrossRef]
44. Mendez, M.F.; Grau, R.; Doss, R.C.; Taylor, J.L. Schizophrenia in epilepsy. *Seizure Psychos. Var.* **1993**, *43*, 1073.
45. Cascella, N.G.; Schretlen, D.J.; Sawa, A. Schizophrenia and epilepsy: Is there a shared susceptibility? *Neurosci. Res.* **2009**, *63*, 227–235. [CrossRef]
46. Knott, S.; Forty, L.; Craddock, N.; Thomas, R.H. Epilepsy and bipolar disorder. *Epilepsy Behav.* **2015**, *52*, 267–274. [CrossRef]
47. Awad, R.; Arnason, J.T.; Trudeau, V.; Bergeron, C.; Budzinski, J.W.; Foster, B.C.; Merali, Z. Phytochemical and biological analysis of skullcap (scutellaria lateriflora l.): A medicinal plant with anxiolytic properties. *Phytomedicine* **2003**, *10*, 640–649. [CrossRef]
48. Awad, R.; Levac, D.; Cybulska, P.; Merali, Z.; Trudeau, V.; Arnason, J. Effects of traditionally used anxiolytic botanicals on enzymes of the γ-aminobutyric acid (GABA). *Can. J. Physiol. Pharmacol.* **2007**, *85*, 933–942. [CrossRef]
49. Hanrahan, J.R.; Chebib, M.; Johnston, G.A.R. Flavonoid modulation of GABA(A) receptors. *Br. J. Pharmacol.* **2011**, *163*, 234–245. [CrossRef]
50. Wang, H.; Hui, K.-M.; Chen, Y.; Xu, S.; Wong, J.T.-F.; Xue, H. Structure-activity relationships of flavonoids, isolated from scutellaria baicalensis, binding to benzodiazepine site of GABAA receptor complex. *Planta Med.* **2002**, *68*, 1059–1062. [CrossRef] [PubMed]
51. Zhang, Z.; Lian, X.-y.; Li, S.; Stringer, J.L. Characterization of chemical ingredients and anticonvulsant activity of american skullcap (scutellaria lateriflora). *Phytomedicine* **2009**, *16*, 485–493. [CrossRef] [PubMed]
52. Jones, N.A.; Hill, A.J.; Smith, I.; Bevan, S.A.; Williams, C.M.; Whalley, B.J.; Stephens, G.J. Cannabidiol displays antiepileptiform and antiseizure properties in vitro and in vivo. *J. Pharm. Exp. Ther.* **2010**, *332*, 569–577. [CrossRef] [PubMed]
53. Hill, A.; Mercier, M.; Hill, T.; Glyn, S.; Jones, N.; Yamasaki, Y.; Futamura, T.; Duncan, M.; Stott, C.; Stephens, G. Cannabidivarin is anticonvulsant in mouse and rat. *Br. J. Pharm.* **2012**, *167*, 1629–1642. [CrossRef] [PubMed]
54. Hill, T.D.M.; Cascio, M.-G.; Romano, B.; Duncan, M.; Pertwee, R.G.; Williams, C.M.; Whalley, B.J.; Hill, A.J. Cannabidivarin-rich cannabis extracts are anticonvulsant in mouse and rat via a CB1 receptor-independent mechanism. *Br. J. Pharm.* **2013**, *170*, 679–692. [CrossRef] [PubMed]
55. Karniol, I.G.; Shirakawa, I.; Takahashi, R.N.; Knobel, E.; Musty, R.E. Effects of Δ^9-Tetrahydrocannabinol and Cannabinol in Man. *Pharmacology* **1975**, *13*, 502–512. [CrossRef] [PubMed]
56. De Barros, G.S.; Silva, C.M.M.; De Abreu Matos, F.J. Anticonvulsant activity of essential oils and active principles from chemotypes of Lippia alba (Mill.) NE Brown. *Biol. Pharm. Bull.* **2000**, *23*, 1314–1317.
57. Russo, E.B. Taming THC: Potential cannabis synergy and phytocannabinoid-terpenoid entourage effects. *Br. J. Pharmacol.* **2011**, *163*, 1344–1364. [CrossRef]
58. Reddy, D.S.; Golub, V.M. The pharmacological basis of cannabis therapy for epilepsy. *J. Pharmacol. Exp. Ther.* **2016**, *357*, 45–55. [CrossRef]

59. Perucca, E. Cannabinoids in the treatment of epilepsy: Hard evidence at last? *J. Epilepsy Res.* **2017**, *7*, 61–76. [CrossRef]
60. Katona, I. Cannabis and endocannabinoid signaling in epilepsy. In *Endocannabinoids*; Springer: Berlin/Heidelberg, Germany, 2015; pp. 285–316.
61. Grigoletto, J.; De Oliveira, C.V.; Grauncke, A.C.B.; De Souza, T.L.; Souto, N.S.; De Freitas, M.L.; Furian, A.F.; Santos, A.R.S.; Oliveira, M.S. Rosmarinic acid is anticonvulsant against seizures induced by pentylenetetrazol and pilocarpine in mice. *Epilepsy Behav.* **2016**, *62*, 27–34. [CrossRef] [PubMed]

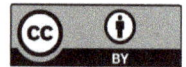

© 2020 by the authors. Licensee MDPI, Basel, Switzerland. This article is an open access article distributed under the terms and conditions of the Creative Commons Attribution (CC BY) license (http://creativecommons.org/licenses/by/4.0/).

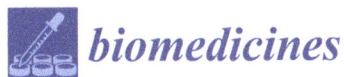

Review

Studying the Pathophysiology of Parkinson's Disease Using Zebrafish

Lisa M. Barnhill †, Hiromi Murata † and Jeff M. Bronstein *

David Geffen School of Medicine at UCLA, Department of Neurology and Molecular Toxicology Program, 710 Westwood Plaza, Los Angeles, CA 90095, USA; lbarnhill@ucla.edu (L.M.B.); muratahrm@gmail.com (H.M.)
* Correspondence: jbronste@mednet.ucla.edu; Tel.: +310-206-7999
† These authors contributed equally to this work.

Received: 18 June 2020; Accepted: 4 July 2020; Published: 7 July 2020

Abstract: Parkinson's disease is a common neurodegenerative disorder leading to severe disability. The clinical features reflect progressive neuronal loss, especially involving the dopaminergic system. The causes of Parkinson's disease are slowly being uncovered and include both genetic and environmental insults. Zebrafish have been a valuable tool in modeling various aspects of human disease. Here, we review studies utilizing zebrafish to investigate both genetic and toxin causes of Parkinson's disease. They have provided important insights into disease mechanisms and will be of great value in the search for disease-modifying therapies.

Keywords: Parkinson's disease; zebrafish; toxins; dopaminergic neuron

1. Introduction

Parkinson's disease (PD) is a neurodegenerative disorder leading to severe disability, affecting millions of people worldwide [1]. The clinical features of PD reflect the progressive loss of neurons throughout the nervous system. Dopaminergic neuron loss leads to many of the classic motor symptoms of PD, such as resting tremors and slowness of movement, but the pathology is much more widespread and results in many non-motor symptoms as well. Current treatments can improve the symptoms of PD but there are no therapies that alter the progression of the disease. It is essential to understand the pathophysiology of PD before developing disease-modifying therapies and zebrafish (ZF) offer unique qualities to add to this understanding.

2. What Is Known About the Pathophysiology of PD

The hallmark pathological finding in PD brains is the presence of intracytoplasmic inclusions called Lewy Bodies (LBs) [2]. Although the vast majority of cases of PD are sporadic, it was the discovery of a mutation in the α-synuclein (α-syn) gene in a family cluster that led to the identification of α-syn as the major component of LBs, both in this family but also in sporadic cases [3,4]. It is widely accepted that the aggregation and propagation of misfolded α-syn underlies the pathogenesis of PD [5,6]. When proteins misfold, they can form aggregates that lead to cell death. Several recently discovered lines of evidence support the self-propagation and spread of α-syn, leading to a predictable progression of PD [2,7]. α-Syn pathology appears to start in the gut and olfactory bulb, then spreading to the substantia nigra (SN) and other brain regions [2]. This process of templating was first described for prion disease but now has been proposed to underlie most neurodegenerative disorders [5,8].

Understanding the causes of protein misfolding and aggregation is essential for understanding the pathogenesis of the disease and are summarized in Figure 1. Increased expression of α-syn by gene duplication or promoter variations is sufficient to cause or increase the risk of developing PD [9–13]. α-Syn levels can also increase through disruption of its degradation. Both the ubiquitin proteasome system and autophagy degrade α-syn [14–19] and dysfunction of both of these processes have been implicated in PD. For example, mutations in genes that code for proteasome proteins (e.g., UCHL-1 and Parkin) and proteins involved in autophagy (e.g., GBA and LRRK2) markedly increase the risk of PD [20,21].

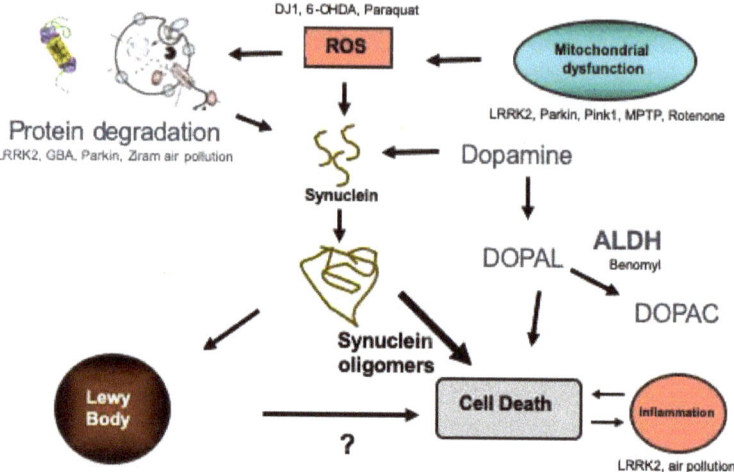

Figure 1. Summary of the proposed pathogenic pathways leading to Parkinson's disease. The genes and toxins that have been studied in zebrafish are listed in the pathways that they likely influence. Protein degradation refers to autophagy and the ubiquitin proteasome system. ROS refers to reactive oxygen species. ALDH refers to aldehyde dehydrogenase. DOPAL refers to 3,4-Dihydroxyphenylacetaldehyde and DOPAC is 3,4-Dihydroxyphenylacetic acid.

Mitochondrial dysfunction has also been implicated as a pathway leading to α-syn aggregation and PD [22–25]. The causes of mitochondrial dysfunction are diverse and can include both genetic (e.g., PINK1 and Parkin) and environmental (e.g., rotenone and TCE) insults [26–29]. There is also evidence that α-syn aggregates themselves lead to mitochondrial dysfunction, further propagating a prion-like cascade [30–34]. When mitochondria are damaged, they can be repaired or replaced. Mitophagy is the process by which mitochondria are targeted and degraded via macroautophagy, so dysfunction in autophagy may also lead to mitochondrial dysfunction.

Neuroinflammation (i.e., microglial and astrocyte activation) also appear to be a factor in the pathogenesis of PD [35–37]. Microglia are the resident immune cells of the CNS and play key roles in tissue repair and cellular homeostasis [38]. Inflammatory changes may cause injury, protect against it, or simply reflect neuronal injury [36,38–40]. Recent studies support a contributing role of inflammation to neuronal damage [37,40]. It is clear that inflammatory changes (microglial and astrocyte activation) are found in PD brains [40], and genetic alterations in several immune function-related genes (e.g., DJ-1, leucine-rich repeat protein kinase-2 (LRRK2), and HLA-DR) can alter the risk of developing PD [41,42].

3. Zebrafish as a Model Organism to Study PD

PD does not naturally occur in animals and since it can take decades to develop in humans, no model can accurately incorporate all aspects of the disease. With that said, different animal models can be utilized to study specific aspects of PD. For example, dopamine neurons can be selectively killed in rodents, resulting in some of the motor features of PD. These are excellent models for testing medicines that can relieve the symptoms of PD but may not prevent its pathogenesis. Other models focus on investigating the underlying molecular mechanisms that lead to PD, such as α-syn aggregation and dopaminergic cell loss. Measuring the perturbation of pathways leading to a disease has become a well-accepted approach in studying chronic disease (i.e., adverse outcome pathways (AOP) [43]). This is where ZF offer particular advantages over many other models [44]. Firstly, the transparent nature of the embryos and larvae allows for the use of non-invasive imaging techniques to study neuronal integrity, proteostasis, mitochondrial functions, and microglial activity in genetically modified fish using florescent reporters. Compared to rodents, ZF are also prolific external breeders. This allows researchers to easily genetically modify fertilized eggs without injury to the parent, minimize variation, and maximize experimental replicates. Furthermore, behavioral assays in ZF larvae can be performed in an automated and high-throughput manner, which can act as a powerful screening tool although the range of behaviors that can be measured is relatively limited [44].

Both genetic and toxin-induced ZF models have been used to study PD. A number of factors need to be considered when reviewing these studies. Most investigators utilize embryos and larvae to take advantage of their transparent nature but we must be cognizant that we are studying a degenerative disease in a developing organism [45]. Toxins can easily be added to the water but since the embryos are rapidly developing, the timing of exposure is very important. For example, some toxins affect notochord development during the first 24 h post fertilization (hpf), which would impair all subsequent behavioral assays. Embryos normally hatch approx. 3 days post fertilization (dpf), and the chorion can act as a barrier to toxins and other treatments added to the water. Some investigators choose to dechorionate the embryos prior to exposure, while others leave them intact [46]. Other considerations include the fact that the ZF blood brain barrier forms after 3 dpf, and the fish sexually differentiate at approx. 21 to 23 dpf [46,47]. When performing and reviewing ZF studies, it is important to consider factors such as these to maximize the benefit of using this model organism.

4. Genetic Models Used to Study PD

4.1. Synuclein

The first mutation found to cause a rare form of autosomal dominant (AD) PD was in the gene coding for α-syn [3]. This led to the finding that α-syn is the major component of LBs, both in the brains of this family but also in brains of sporadic cases [4]. Increased expression of α-syn by gene duplication is sufficient to cause PD [9–12] and the REP1 263 allele in the α-syn promoter, which confers a higher level of expression [48], is associated with an increased risk of developing PD [13] and faster progression in those that have it [49]. ZF express three syn genes: sncb, sncg1, and sncg2 (encoding β-, γ1-, and γ2-syn, respectively). They do not express an α-syn orthologue [50] although there is evidence that γ1-synuclein (γ1-syn) has a similar function as α-syn. γ1-Syn is highly expressed in the brain and is developmentally regulated in a similar manner as α-syn [51]. Knockdown of γ1-syn and ZF β-syn leads to hypokinesia and reduced dopamine levels, and expression of human α-syn can reverse these abnormalities [52].

We have transiently expressed γ1-syn in neurons using the *HuC* promoter and found it also forms thioflavin T binding to fibrils like α-syn, with similar kinetics [53]. Overexpression of γ1-syn in ZF neurons leads to the formation of aggregates in vivo and is neurotoxic in a similar manner as α-syn [53,54]. This model is limited by the inherent variability of transient expression and that the *HuC* promoter does not express well in dopaminergic neurons. We have made a stable transgenic line of fish using a Gal4/UAS expression system under the ZF HuC promoter (HuC:Gal4 x UAS:α-syn), but there is a much subtler phenotype (unpublished data). Despite these limitations, overexpression of α-syn in ZF neurons has proven to be useful in testing potential drugs that lower the neurotoxicity of α-syn aggregation [53,54].

4.2. LRRK2

Mutations in the leucine-rich repeat kinase 2 (LRRK2) gene are the most common cause of autosomal dominant PD and account for 1% of sporadic cases and 4% of familial cases [55]. The G2019S mutation is the most common, especially in Ashkenazi Jewish people or North African Berbers, but there are several other pathogenic variants. The penetrance is generally considered low (approx. 25%) but varies by the population studied [56]. Importantly, patients with LRRK2 mutations present with similar symptoms as idiopathic cases and most contain α-syn containing LBs [56].

LRRK2 is a protein with several domains, including both a serine/threonine kinase and a GTPase domain [21]. It is likely that all or most of the pathogenic mutations in the LRRK2 gene results in a toxic gain-of-function increase in kinase activity and kinase inhibition is considered a promising therapeutic drug target for both LRRK2-induced and idiopathic PD [21].

ZF contain a homologue of the human LRRK2 (hLRRK2) gene, and the protein contains all the functional domains of the human protein. The kinase domain is particularly conserved in ZF with a 71% homology [57]. Despite the fact that gain-of-function increase in kinase activity is considered the most likely mechanism whereby LRRK2 mutations lead to PD, ZF biologists have focused on knocking down the gene in ZF. Morpholino (MO) knockdown of the LRRK2 in ZF (zLRRK2) results in embryonic lethality with severe morphological and neuronal defects, including loss of tyrosine hydroxylase (TH)-positive neurons [57]. The effects of targeted deletion of the Trp-Asp-40 (WD) domain of zLRRK2 using MO is less clear. Sheng et al. [57] reported that this knockdown resulted in a Parkinson's phenotype including loss of TH+ neurons and locomotive dysfunction, while Ren et al. could not reproduce these findings despite using the same reagents [58].

More recently, Prabhudesai et al. knocked down a full length zLRRK2 in a dose-dependent manner and reported generalized morphological defects, loss of *HuC* and dopaminergic neurons, as well as increased levels of β-synuclein, PARK13, and SOD1. They also reported aggregation of β-synuclein; however, this is less clear since no staining for β-pleated sheets was performed and only low power images were shown [59]. These data confirm previous reports of the importance of LRRK2 in general development but also suggests it plays a role in proteostasis. No one yet has reported on the effects of increased kinase activity in ZF, which have a much more direct relevance to the etiology of PD in patients carrying a mutation in the LRRK2 gene.

The function of LRRK2 was further investigated by creating a mutation in the WD40 domain in zLRRK2 [60]. This mutation led to the fish being hyperactive and exhibiting a weakened antibacterial response. Transcriptome analysis revealed that this mutation in zLRRK2 altered the expression of the genes involved in infectious, immunological, and neurological diseases [60]. These studies add insight into why people with LRRK2 variants suffer from a higher incidence of Crohn's disease and leprosy.

4.3. GBA

Gaucher's disease (GD) is a relatively common autosomal recessive lysosomal storage disease caused by mutations in the glucocerebrosidase 1 (GBA) gene. GBA1 is a lysosomal enzyme required for the breakdown of glucosylceramide to ceramide and glucose and patients exhibit accumulation of glucocerebroside in the spleen, liver, and bone marrow. Clinically, GD presents in a very heterogenous manner. Patients can be asymptomatic or present with severe neurological decline with systemic problems. Several pathogenic mutations have been reported and heterozygote carriers are at an increased risk of developing PD [61]. Depending on the mutation, the risk of developing PD can increase from 2 to 19 fold [20]. GBA mutations result in loss of enzymatic activity of glucocerebrosidase, leading to lysosomal dysfunction that is believed to be responsible for the increased risk of PD. Patients with GBA mutations and PD have classic LBs, suggesting that the increased risk in these patients is due to a decreased degradation of α-syn through autophagy [20].

This concept that GBA mutations lead to an increased risk of PD by reducing α-syn degradation has been directly challenged by Keatinge et al. using their ZF GBA model [62]. They deleted 23 bp of the GBA orthologue that resulted in many of the characteristics of PD. Early on, they found sphingolipid accumulation, up regulation of miR-155 (a regulator of inflammation), and microglial activation. At 8 weeks post-fertilization (wpf), they reported decreased motor activity, dopaminergic cell loss, mitochondrial dysfunction, altered autophagy markers, and ubiquitin-positive intra-neuronal inclusions. Interestingly, all of these PD-like pathological changes occurred in the absence of α-syn and the ZF β- and γ1-synuclein levels were decreased. Furthermore, ablation of miR-155 expression did not alter microglial activation or the disease pathology [63]. Other features of GD were also apparent.

Uemura et al. knocked out GBA in medaka and reported some but not all of the findings of Keatinge et al. [64]. They reported infiltration of Gaucher-like cells into the brain, progressive aminergic neuronal loss, and microgliosis. Interestingly, they observed accumulation of α-syn in autophagosomes but knocking out α-syn in GBA-deficient medaka did not improve survival or the axonal swellings. Taken together, GBA deficiency results in dysfunction in autophagy as well as the accumulation of sphingolipids and proteins, such as α-syn; however, the α-syn is not necessary for neuronal loss.

4.4. Parkin

Mutations in the Parkin gene is the most common cause of autosomal recessive (AR) PD [55]. It is important to note that most PD patients with Parkin mutations do not have an LB pathology, even though they show fairly classic clinical signs of early onset PD [65]. For this reason, the pathological pathways leading to dopaminergic cell loss and clinical PD are likely different than the pathological pathways responsible for the majority of idiopathic or most other forms of genetic PD. The Parkin gene encodes for an E3 ligase that targets many proteins, including soluble α-syn, for degradation by the UPS or lysosomes. Parkin also plays an important role in targeting damaged mitochondria for clearance via mitophagy [65].

The ZF Parkin gene was cloned, and the protein was predicted to be 62% identical to the human Parkin protein and 78% identical in the most important functional regions [66]. MO knockdown of ZF Parkin led to reduced mitochondrial complex 1 activity and a 20% reduction in diencephalic dopaminergic neurons at 3 dpf. The authors reported that the Parkin knockdown ZF were more sensitive to MPP+ but the additional dopaminergic loss appeared to be additive. The fish swam normally at 5 dpf but had abnormal electron-dense material in the T tubules in muscle tissue [66].

Fett et al. also studied Parkin in ZF and described increased aggregation of Parkin under conditions of oxidative stress or in the presence of dopamine [67]. They used antisense technology to reduce the Parkin levels by 53%, but saw no morphological or behavioral alterations, and the dopamine neuron counts were normal at 3 dpf. Finally, they reported that overexpression of Parkin using a ubiquitous promoter reduced the number of apoptotic cell death while reduced levels of Parkin increased the death after heat shock determined by acridine orange.

4.5. (PTEN)-Induced Putative Kinase 1 (Pink1)

The 2nd most common cause of AR PD is mutations in the Pink1 gene, resulting in young onset disease [65]. LBs have been reported in two cases while they were absent in one report [68]. Pink 1 is a highly conserved 581 aa protein that is widely expressed in the CNS and associates with mitochondrial membranes. It is believed to play an important role, along with Parkin, to regulate mitochondrial quality, and the loss of function of Pink1 leads to disease [69].

MO knockdown of Pink1 has led to variable results in ZF. An early study reported severe developmental malformations, a reduction in dopaminergic neurons, and mitochondrial dysfunction [70]. Interestingly, Pink1 knockdown resulted in increased in GSK3β activity and GSK3β inhibitors partially rescued the malformations. In a study by Xi et al., MO knockdown of Pink1 did not lead to loss of dopamine neurons but altered patterning of their projections and altered locomotion [71]. Sallinen et al. reported that Pink1 protein was expressed in dopaminergic neurons and MO knockdown did not result in reduced dopaminergic neurons but did sensitize them to MPTP [72].

Flinn et al. took a different approach to study Pink1 [73]. They identified a fish line with mutant Pink1 from a mutagenized library. The knockout fish had a 25% reduction in dopaminergic neurons, which appeared to be relatively specific and not reflective of a more generalized developmental defect. They also observed microglial activation. The mitochondria in these fish had an abnormal morphology and reduced complex I and III activity. Taking a transcriptomic approach, they found that *TigarB* was highly upregulated and knockdown of *TigarB* reversed the mitochondrial defects caused by the loss of Pink1. Taken together, Pink1 appears to be important in maintaining dopaminergic neurons and mitochondrial function. The developmental malformations described by Anichtichik et al. were likely due to off-target effects.

4.6. DJ1

Mutations in the gene coding for DJ1 (PARK7) is another cause of AR PD, but LBs have yet to be described in brains of these patients [65]. The DJ1 protein is widely expressed and mostly localizes in the cytosol, as well as in the nucleus and mitochondria. Its function is not completely clear, but it appears to be able to sense oxidative stress and regulate anti-oxidant and anti-apoptotic gene expression [65].

The ZF orthologue of DJ1 is 83% identical to the human protein, and is expressed in the brain, muscle, and gut [74]. MO knockdown of DJ1 did not lead to loss of dopaminergic neurons, but did increase their sensitivity to H_2O_2 and proteasome inhibition [75]. Interestingly, overexpression of DJ1 in ZF astroglia led to increased expression of several genes related to oxidative stress in a similar pattern as nrf2 and was protective against MPTP toxicity [76].

5. Toxins and the Study of PD

There are a variety of reasons to study toxins in ZF with respect to PD. They can be used to create an anatomical model of PD by killing dopamine neurons. Others use them to study the biological plausibility of an association between exposure and disease. ZF are especially helpful in studying the mechanisms of action of toxins (i.e., adverse outcome pathways) and how they may alter the risk of PD. In particular, two different ZF lines, DAT-EGFP and VMAT2-EGFP, have been very useful in these studies to determine the effects of toxins on dopamine neurons [77,78]. Other studies utilized whole mount in situ hybridization or immunohistochemistry for labeling TH.

5.1. Toxins That Kill Dopamine Neurons

MPTP (1-methyl-4-phenyl-1,2,3,6-tetrahydropyridine) is one of the most commonly used toxins to kill dopamine neurons. It was discovered when addicted individuals injected the synthetic opioid MPPP that was contaminated with MPTP, and suddenly became Parkinsonian [79,80]. Its mechanism of toxicity is due to the enzymatic conversion of MPTP by MAO-B to MPP+, which is selectively taken up by the dopamine transporter (DAT) in dopamine neurons. This leads to the inhibition of mitochondrial complex I, which results in free radical formation, reduced ATP synthesis, and, ultimately, death of the neuron. MPTP-treated animals have been very useful as a model to test dopaminergic medications, but the mechanism of cell death is not necessarily related to that in PD [79].

Several groups have reported that MPTP treatment kills the dopamine neurons in ZF. The dose and timing of exposure likely accounts for the variability in reported effects. A single intraperitoneal injection of MPTP in adult ZF resulted in transient decreases in brain dopamine levels and locomotion, but not loss of dopamine neurons [81]. Embryonic and larval ZF are more sensitive to MPTP and exposure for 2–3 days beginning at 24 hpf results in loss of dopamine neurons and reduced locomotion [82–85]. The mechanism of toxicity of MPTP is the same in ZF as in mammals, since MAO-B and DAT inhibition block toxicity [83,84]. There were some morphological abnormalities when embryos were exposed to higher concentrations of MPTP [85].

6-Hydroxydopamine (6-OHDA) is another toxin used to kill dopamine neurons. It is taken up by DAT and kills neurons by a mechanism involving oxidative stress. Injection of 6-OHDA into adult ZF results in a small reduction in dopamine and locomotion, but no apparent loss of dopamine neurons [81]. Embryonic exposure to 6-OHDA resulted in a small reduction in dopaminergic neurons, but no change in locomotion [85].

5.2. Toxins Associated With the Pathogenesis of PD

Exposure to a number of environmental toxins, especially pesticides, have been associated with an increased risk of developing PD and ZF have been a valuable tool in determining if these associations represent causality.

5.2.1. Rotenone Is a Mitochondrial Complex I Inhibitor and Is Associated With an Increased Risk of PD

Systemic administration of rotenone in rats leads to α-syn accumulation, loss of dopamine neurons, and motor deficits. Systemic administration of rotenone in adult ZF had no effect of dopamine neurons or locomotion [82] but others have reported decreased dopamine, locomotion, and olfaction when put in the water [86,87]. Rotenone exposure to embryos results in a moderate loss of dopamine neurons, decreased locomotion, and occasional cardiac defects. There was no determination of the selectivity of the neuronal loss [85].

5.2.2. Paraquat Is Another Pesticide Associated With an Increased Risk of Developing PD

Paraquat is very similar to MPTP structurally, which is why it was initially studied. It has since been determined that, unlike MPTP, it is not a substrate for DAT or a complex I inhibitor but a redox cycler, and enhances oxidative stress in dopamine neurons [88]. In mammals, exposure to paraquat leads to an approximately 20% decrease in dopaminergic neurons and evidence of oxidative stress [89]. Dopamine neuron loss was greatly enhanced when used in combination with the fungicide maneb [90]. Interestingly, epidemiological studies have shown the risk of PD is also enhanced when exposed to maneb in addition to paraquat [91].

Treating ZF with paraquat has had mixed results. Bretaud et al. found no effect on embryos that were treated from 24 hpf to 5 dpf at concentrations up to 10 mg/L [82]. Nellore and Nandita reported decreased locomotion, dopamine, and serotonin, and evidence of oxidative stress when the embryos were treated with low dose paraquat from 18 to 96 hpf [92]. When ZF were treated with 1 mM paraquat from 3 to 7 dpf, Kalyn found a 16% decrease in dopamine neurons as well as decreased DAT and TH expression, but no change in behavior [85]. In adult ZF, IP injection every 3 days (total of six injections) of paraquat led to decreased locomotion but increased dopamine concentration, no change in TH expression, and decreased DAT expression [93]. When placed in the water for 4 weeks, paraquat had no effect on adult ZF [82].

5.2.3. Ziram Is a Dithiocarbamate Fungicide, and Is an E1 Ligase Inhibitor of the UPS

Exposure to ziram is associated with an increased risk of developing PD [91,94]. The biological plausibility of a causal association was tested using ZF embryos exposed to 50 nM of ziram at 24 hpf, resulting in selective loss of dopaminergic neurons and altered swimming in the dark in a similar manner to dopamine blockage [53]. Interestingly, the dopamine neuron loss was γ1-syn-dependent, since knockdown with MO was protective. Furthermore, CLR01, a drug that breaks apart γ1-synuclein fibrils, was also protective [53].

5.2.4. Benomyl Is Another Fungicide Found to Be Associated With an Increased Risk of Developing PD

Similar to ziram, it also killed dopamine neurons in a selective manner in ZF [95,96]. The mechanism of toxicity was found to be due to inhibition of aldehyde dehydrogenase that detoxifies the dopamine metabolite DOPAL [95,96].

5.2.5. Air Pollution Has Recently Been Found to Be Associated With an Increased Risk of PD and Alzheimer's Disease, Although the Mechanisms Remain Largely Unknown

Diesel exhaust particle extracts (DEPe), commonly used as a surrogate model of air pollution in health effects studies, was used to determine the biological plausibility and mechanisms of toxicity of this association. ZF embryos treated with DEPe for 24 h (24 to 48 hpf) and analyzed at 5 dpf resulted in loss of dopaminergic as well as non-dopaminergic neurons, and altered behavior [97,98]. Using a transgenic ZF line that measures neuronal autophagic flux [99], it was found that DEPe inhibited flux and that the enhancers of autophagy were protective of neuronal loss.

6. Conclusions

Animal models are essential for the study of disease mechanisms, as they allow us to determine the causes and lead us towards the discovery of better treatments. ZF offer several advantages over mammalian models in that that they are inexpensive, transparent, and easily manipulated genetically. Here, we reviewed many of the studies utilizing ZF that investigated genetic and environmental causes of PD. They have provided new insights into the pathogenesis of PD that have been extended into mammalian models. Future ZF studies will likely include high-throughput screens to discover the environmental toxins associated with PD as well as novel therapeutics to treat the disease.

Funding: This research was funded by grants from National Institute of Environmental Health Sciences, National Institutes of Health, T32ES015457 (LMB, HM), The Levine Foundation, and The Parkinson's Alliance.

Conflicts of Interest: The authors declare no conflict of interest.

References

1. Dorsey, E.R.; Constantinescu, R.; Thompson, J.P.; Biglan, K.M.; Holloway, R.G.; Kieburtz, K.; Marshall, F.J.; Ravina, B.M.; Schifitto, G.; Siderowf, A.; et al. Projected Number of People with Parkinson Disease in the Most Populous Nations, 2005 through 2030. *Neurology* **2007**, *68*, 384–386. [CrossRef] [PubMed]
2. Braak, H.; Del Tredici, K. Invited Article: Nervous System Pathology in Sporadic Parkinson Disease. *Neurology* **2008**, *70*, 1916–1925. [CrossRef] [PubMed]
3. Polymeropoulos, M.H.; Lavedan, C.; Leroy, E.; Ide, S.E.; Dehejia, A.; Dutra, A.; Pike, B.; Root, H.; Rubenstein, J.; Boyer, R.; et al. Mutation in the Alpha-Synuclein Gene Identified in Families with Parkinson's Disease [See Comments]. *Science* **1997**, *276*, 2045–2047. [CrossRef] [PubMed]
4. Spillantini, M.G.; Schmidt, M.L.; Lee, V.M.; Trojanowski, J.Q.; Jakes, R.; Goedert, M. Alpha-Synuclein in Lewy Bodies. *Nature* **1997**, *388*, 839–840. [CrossRef]
5. Jucker, M.; Walker, L.C. Self-Propagation of Pathogenic Protein Aggregates in Neurodegenerative Diseases. *Nature* **2013**, *501*, 45–51. [CrossRef]
6. Li, Q.; Liu, Y.; Sun, M. Autophagy and Alzheimer's Disease. *Cell. Mol. Neurobiol.* **2017**, *37*, 377–388. [CrossRef]
7. Luk, K.C.; Lee, V.M. Modeling Lewy Pathology Propagation in Parkinson's Disease. *Parkinsonism Relat. Disord.* **2014**, *20*, S85–S87. [CrossRef]
8. Prusiner, S.B.; Scott, M.R.; DeArmond, S.J.; Cohen, F.E. Prion Protein Biology. *Cell* **1998**, *93*, 337–348. [CrossRef]
9. Miller, D.W.; Hague, S.M.; Clarimon, J.; Baptista, M.; Gwinn-Hardy, K.; Cookson, M.R.; Singleton, A.B. Alpha-Synuclein in Blood and Brain from Familial Parkinson Disease with Snca Locus Triplication. *Neurology* **2004**, *62*, 1835–1838. [CrossRef]
10. Chartier-Harlin, M.C.; Kachergus, J.; Roumier, C.; Mouroux, V.; Douay, X.; Lincoln, S.; Levecque, C.; Larvor, L.; Andrieux, J.; Hulihan, M.; et al. Alpha-Synuclein Locus Duplication as a Cause of Familial Parkinson's Disease. *Lancet* **2004**, *364*, 1167–1169. [CrossRef]
11. Sibon, I.; Larrieu, D.; El Hadri, K.; Mercier, N.; Feve, B.; Lacolley, P.; Labat, C.; Daret, D.; Bonnet, J.; Lamaziere, J.M. Semicarbazide-Sensitive Amine Oxidase in Annulo-Aortic Ectasia Disease: Relation to Elastic Lamellae-Associated Proteins. *J. Histochem. Cytochem.* **2004**, *52*, 1459–1466. [CrossRef] [PubMed]
12. Ibanez, P.; Bonnet, A.M.; Debarges, B.; Lohmann, E.; Tison, F.; Pollak, P.; Agid, Y.; Durr, A.; Brice, A. Causal Relation between Alpha-Synuclein Gene Duplication and Familial Parkinson's Disease. *Lancet* **2004**, *364*, 1169–1171. [CrossRef]
13. Maraganore, D.M.; de Andrade, M.; Elbaz, A.; Farrer, M.J.; Ioannidis, J.P.; Kruger, R.; Rocca, W.A.; Schneider, N.K.; Lesnick, T.G.; Lincoln, S.J.; et al. Collaborative Analysis of Alpha-Synuclein Gene Promoter Variability and Parkinson Disease. *JAMA J. Am. Med Assoc.* **2006**, *296*, 661–670. [CrossRef]

14. Ebrahimi-Fakhari, D.; Cantuti-Castelvetri, I.; Fan, Z.; Rockenstein, E.; Masliah, E.; Hyman, B.T.; McLean, P.J.; Unni, V.K. Distinct Roles in Vivo for the Ubiquitin-Proteasome System and the Autophagy-Lysosomal Pathway in the Degradation of Alpha-Synuclein. *J. Neurosci. Off. J. Soc. Neurosci.* **2011**, *31*, 14508–14520. [CrossRef] [PubMed]
15. Cuervo, A.M.; Stefanis, L.; Fredenburg, R.; Lansbury, P.T.; Sulzer, D. Impaired Degradation of Mutant Alpha-Synuclein by Chaperone-Mediated Autophagy. *Science* **2004**, *305*, 1292–1295. [CrossRef] [PubMed]
16. Liu, C.W.; Giasson, B.I.; Lewis, K.A.; Lee, V.M.; Demartino, G.N.; Thomas, P.J. A Precipitating Role for Truncated Alpha-Synuclein and the Proteasome in Alpha-Synuclein Aggregation: Implications for Pathogenesis of Parkinson Disease. *J. Biol. Chem.* **2005**, *280*, 22670–22678. [CrossRef]
17. Mak, S.K.; McCormack, A.L.; Manning-Bog, A.B.; Cuervo, A.M.; Di Monte, D.A. Lysosomal Degradation of -Synuclein in Vivo. *J. Biol. Chem.* **2010**, *285*, 13621–13629. [CrossRef]
18. Zhang, N.Y.; Tang, Z.; Liu, C.W. Alpha-Synuclein Protofibrils Inhibit 26 S Proteasome-Mediated Protein Degradation: Understanding the Cytotoxicity of Protein Protofibrils in Neurodegenerative Disease Pathogenesis. *J. Biol. Chem.* **2008**, *283*, 20288–20298. [CrossRef]
19. Lee, H.J.; Khoshaghideh, F.; Patel, S.; Lee, S.J. Clearance of Alpha-Synuclein Oligomeric Intermediates Via the Lysosomal Degradation Pathway. *J. Neurosci. Off. J. Soc. Neurosci.* **2004**, *24*, 1888–1896. [CrossRef]
20. Pitcairn, C.; Wani, W.Y.; Mazzulli, J.R. Dysregulation of the Autophagic-Lysosomal Pathway in Gaucher and Parkinson's Disease. *Neurobiol. Dis.* **2019**, *122*, 72–82. [CrossRef]
21. Berwick, D.C.; Heaton, G.R.; Azeggagh, S.; Harvey, K. Lrrk2 Biology from Structure to Dysfunction: Research Progresses, but the Themes Remain the Same. *Mol. Neurodegener.* **2019**, *14*, 49. [CrossRef] [PubMed]
22. Dupuis, L. Mitochondrial Quality Control in Neurodegenerative Diseases. *Biochimie* **2013**, *100*, 177–183. [CrossRef] [PubMed]
23. Gautier, C.A.; Corti, O.; Brice, A. Mitochondrial Dysfunctions in Parkinson's Disease. *Revue Neurol.* **2013**, *170*, 339–343. [CrossRef] [PubMed]
24. Swerdlow, R.H.; Burns, J.M.; Khan, S.M. The Alzheimer's Disease Mitochondrial Cascade Hypothesis: Progress and Perspectives. *Biochim. Biophys. Acta* **2013**, *1842*, 1219–1231. [CrossRef] [PubMed]
25. Swomley, A.M.; Forster, S.; Keeney, J.T.; Triplett, J.; Zhang, Z.; Sultana, R.; Butterfield, D.A. Abeta, Oxidative Stress in Alzheimer Disease: Evidence Based on Proteomics Studies. *Biochim. Biophys. Acta* **2013**, *1842*, 1248–1257. [CrossRef] [PubMed]
26. Tanner, C.M.; Kamel, F.; Ross, G.W.; Hoppin, J.A.; Goldman, S.M.; Korell, M.; Marras, C.; Bhudhikanok, G.S.; Kasten, M.; Chade, A.R.; et al. Rotenone, Paraquat, and Parkinson's Disease. *Environ. Health Perspect.* **2011**, *119*, 866–872. [CrossRef] [PubMed]
27. Gash, D.M.; Rutland, K.; Hudson, N.L.; Sullivan, P.G.; Bing, G.; Cass, W.A.; Pandya, J.D.; Liu, M.; Choi, D.Y.; Hunter, R.L.; et al. Trichloroethylene: Parkinsonism and Complex 1 Mitochondrial Neurotoxicity. *Ann. Neurol.* **2008**, *63*, 184–192. [CrossRef]
28. Liu, M.; Choi, D.Y.; Hunter, R.L.; Pandya, J.D.; Cass, W.A.; Sullivan, P.G.; Kim, H.C.; Gash, D.M.; Bing, G. Trichloroethylene Induces Dopaminergic Neurodegeneration in Fisher 344 Rats. *J. Neurochem.* **2010**, *112*, 773–783. [CrossRef]
29. Goldman, S.M.; Quinlan, P.J.; Ross, G.W.; Marras, C.; Meng, C.; Bhudhikanok, G.S.; Comyns, K.; Korell, M.; Chade, A.R.; Kasten, M.; et al. Solvent Exposures and Parkinson Disease Risk in Twins. *Ann. Neurol.* **2011**, *71*, 776–784. [CrossRef]
30. Dryanovski, D.I.; Guzman, J.N.; Xie, Z.; Galteri, D.J.; Volpicelli-Daley, L.A.; Lee, V.M.; Miller, R.J.; Schumacker, P.T.; Surmeier, D.J. Calcium Entry and Alpha-Synuclein Inclusions Elevate Dendritic Mitochondrial Oxidant Stress in Dopaminergic Neurons. *J. Neurosci. Off. J. Soc. Neurosci.* **2013**, *33*, 10154–10164. [CrossRef]
31. Subramaniam, S.R.; Vergnes, L.; Franich, N.R.; Reue, K.; Chesselet, M.F. Region Specific Mitochondrial Impairment in Mice with Widespread Overexpression of Alpha-Synuclein. *Neurobiol. Dis.* **2014**, *70*, 204–213. [CrossRef] [PubMed]
32. Guardia-Laguarta, C.; Area-Gomez, E.; Rub, C.; Liu, Y.; Magrane, J.; Becker, D.; Voos, W.; Schon, E.A.; Przedborski, S. Alpha-Synuclein Is Localized to Mitochondria-Associated Er Membranes. *J. Neurosci.* **2014**, *34*, 249–259. [CrossRef] [PubMed]
33. Greenamyre, J.T.; Betarbet, R.; Sherer, T.B. The Rotenone Model of Parkinson's Disease: Genes, Environment and Mitochondria. *Parkinsonism Relat. Disord.* **2003**, *9*, S59–S64. [CrossRef]

34. Di Maio, R.; Barrett, P.J.; Hoffman, E.K.; Barrett, C.W.; Zharikov, A.; Borah, A.; Hu, X.; McCoy, J.; Chu, C.T.; Burton, E.A.; et al. Alpha-Synuclein Binds to Tom20 and Inhibits Mitochondrial Protein Import in Parkinson's Disease. *Sci. Transl. Med.* **2016**, *8*, 342ra78. [CrossRef]
35. Lull, M.E.; Block, M.L. Microglial Activation and Chronic Neurodegeneration. *Neurotherapeutics* **2010**, *7*, 354–365. [CrossRef] [PubMed]
36. Kannarkat, G.T.; Boss, J.M.; Tansey, M.G. The Role of Innate and Adaptive Immunity in Parkinson's Disease. *J. Parkinsons Dis.* **2013**, *3*, 493–514. [CrossRef] [PubMed]
37. Booth, H.D.E.; Hirst, W.D.; Wade-Martins, R. The Role of Astrocyte Dysfunction in Parkinson's Disease Pathogenesis. *Trends Neurosci.* **2017**, *40*, 358–370. [CrossRef]
38. Aguzzi, A.; Barres, B.A.; Bennett, M.L. Microglia: Scapegoat, Saboteur, or Something Else? *Science* **2013**, *339*, 156–161. [CrossRef]
39. Butchart, J.; Holmes, C. Systemic and Central Immunity in Alzheimer's Disease: Therapeutic Implications. *CNS Neurosci. Ther.* **2012**, *18*, 64–76. [CrossRef]
40. Deleidi, M.; Gasser, T. The Role of Inflammation in Sporadic and Familial Parkinson's Disease. *Cell. Mol. Life Sci. CMLS* **2013**, *70*, 4259–4273. [CrossRef]
41. Joshi, N.; Singh, S. Updates on Immunity and Inflammation in Parkinson Disease Pathology. *J. Neurosci. Res.* **2018**, *96*, 379–390. [CrossRef]
42. Mullett, S.J.; Di Maio, R.; Greenamyre, J.T.; Hinkle, D.A. Dj-1 Expression Modulates Astrocyte-Mediated Protection against Neuronal Oxidative Stress. *J. Mol. Neurosci.* **2013**, *49*, 507–511. [CrossRef] [PubMed]
43. Tan, Y.M.; Leonard, J.A.; Edwards, S.; Teeguarden, J.; Paini, A.; Egeghy, P. Aggregate Exposure Pathways in Support of Risk Assessment. *Curr. Opin. Toxicol.* **2018**, *9*, 8–13. [CrossRef] [PubMed]
44. Guo, S. Linking Genes to Brain, Behavior and Neurological Diseases: What Can We Learn from Zebrafish? *Genes Brain Behav.* **2004**, *3*, 63–74. [CrossRef] [PubMed]
45. Meyer, A. Phylogenetic Relationships and Evolutionary Processes in East African Cichlid Fishes. *Trends Ecol. Evol.* **1993**, *8*, 279–284. [CrossRef]
46. Westerfield, M. *The Zebrafish Book: A Guide for the Laboratory Use of Zebrafish (Danio Rerio)*, 4th ed.; University of Oregon Press: Eugene, Oregon, 2000.
47. Lee, S.L.J.; Horsfield, J.A.; Black, M.A.; Rutherford, K.; Gemmell, N.J. Identification of Sex Differences in Zebrafish (Danio Rerio) Brains During Early Sexual Differentiation and Masculinization Using 17alpha-Methyltestoterone. *Biol. Reprod.* **2018**, *99*, 446–460. [CrossRef] [PubMed]
48. Chiba-Falek, O.; Nussbaum, R.L. Effect of Allelic Variation at the Nacp-Rep1 Repeat Upstream of the Alpha-Synuclein Gene (Snca) on Transcription in a Cell Culture Luciferase Reporter System. *Hum. Mol. Genet.* **2001**, *10*, 3101–3109. [CrossRef] [PubMed]
49. Ritz, B.; Rhodes, S.L.; Bordelon, Y.; Bronstein, J. A-Synuclein Genetic Variants Predict Faster Motor Symptom Progression in Idiopathic Parkinson Disease. *PLoS ONE* **2012**, *7*, e36199. [CrossRef]
50. Sun, Z.; Gitler, A.D. Discovery and Characterization of Three Novel Synuclein Genes in Zebrafish. *Dev. Dyn. Off. Publ. Am. Assoc. Anat.* **2008**, *237*, 2490–2495.
51. Chen, Y.C.; Cheng, C.H.; Chen, G.D.; Hung, C.C.; Yang, C.H.; Hwang, S.P.; Kawakami, K.; Wu, B.K.; Huang, C.J. Recapitulation of Zebrafish Sncga Expression Pattern and Labeling the Habenular Complex in Transgenic Zebrafish Using Green Fluorescent Protein Reporter Gene. *Dev. Dyn. Off. Publ. Am. Assoc. Anat.* **2009**, *238*, 746–754.
52. Milanese, C.; Sager, J.J.; Bai, Q.; Farrell, T.C.; Cannon, J.R.; Greenamyre, J.T.; Burton, E.A. Hypokinesia and Reduced Dopamine Levels in Zebrafish Lacking Beta- and Gamma1-Synucleins. *J. Biol. Chem.* **2012**, *287*, 2971–2983. [CrossRef] [PubMed]
53. Lulla, A.; Barnhill, L.; Bitan, G.; Ivanova, M.I.; Nguyen, B.; O'Donnell, K.C.; Stahl, M.; Yamaashiro, C.; Klärner, F.G.; Schrader, T.; et al. Neurotoxicity of the Parkinson's Disease-Associated Pesticide Ziram Is Synuclein- Dependent in Zebrafish Embryos. *Environ. Health Perspect.* **2016**, *124*, 1766–1775. [CrossRef]
54. Prabhudesai, S.; Sinha, S.; Attar, A.; Kotagiri, A.; Fitzmaurice, A.G.; Lakshmanan, R.; Ivanova, M.I.; Loo, J.A.; Klarner, F.G.; Schrader, T.; et al. A Novel "Molecular Tweezer" Inhibitor of Alpha-Synuclein Neurotoxicity in Vitro and in Vivo. *Neurother. J. Am. Soc. Exp. Neurother.* **2012**, *9*, 464–476.
55. Trinh, J.; Farrer, M. Advances in the Genetics of Parkinson Disease. *Nat. Rev. Neurol.* **2013**, *9*, 445–454. [CrossRef] [PubMed]

56. Tolosa, E.; Vila, M.; Klein, C.; Rascol, O. Lrrk2 in Parkinson Disease: Challenges of Clinical Trials. *Nat. Rev. Neurol.* **2020**, *16*, 97–107. [CrossRef] [PubMed]
57. Sheng, D.; Qu, D.; Kwok, K.H.; Ng, S.S.; Lim, A.Y.; Aw, S.S.; Lee, C.W.; Sung, W.K.; Tan, E.K.; Lufkin, T.; et al. Deletion of the Wd40 Domain of Lrrk2 in Zebrafish Causes Parkinsonism-Like Loss of Neurons and Locomotive Defect. *PLoS Genet.* **2010**, *6*, e1000914. [CrossRef]
58. Ren, G.; Xin, S.; Li, S.; Zhong, H.; Lin, S. Disruption of Lrrk2 Does Not Cause Specific Loss of Dopaminergic Neurons in Zebrafish. *PLoS ONE* **2011**, *6*, e20630. [CrossRef]
59. Prabhudesai, S.; Bensabeur, F.Z.; Abdullah, R.; Basak, I.; Baez, S.; Alves, G.; Holtzman, N.G.; Larsen, J.P.; Moller, S.G. Lrrk2 Knockdown in Zebrafish Causes Developmental Defects, Neuronal Loss, and Synuclein Aggregation. *J. Neurosci. Res.* **2016**, *94*, 717–735. [CrossRef]
60. Sheng, D.; See, K.; Hu, X.; Yu, D.; Wang, Y.; Liu, Q.; Li, F.; Lu, M.; Zhao, J.; Liu, J. Disruption of Lrrk2 in Zebrafish Leads to Hyperactivity and Weakened Antibacterial Response. *Biochem. Biophys. Res. Commun.* **2018**, *497*, 1104–1109. [CrossRef]
61. Sidransky, E.; Lopez, G. The Link between the Gba Gene and Parkinsonism. *Lancet Neurol.* **2012**, *11*, 986–998. [CrossRef]
62. Keatinge, M.; Bui, H.; Menke, A.; Chen, Y.C.; Sokol, A.M.; Bai, Q.; Ellett, F.; Da Costa, M.; Burke, D.; Gegg, M.; et al. Glucocerebrosidase 1 Deficient Danio Rerio Mirror Key Pathological Aspects of Human Gaucher Disease and Provide Evidence of Early Microglial Activation Preceding Alpha-Synuclein-Independent Neuronal Cell Death. *Hum. Mol. Genet.* **2015**, *24*, 6640–6652. [CrossRef] [PubMed]
63. Watson, L.; Keatinge, M.; Gegg, M.; Bai, Q.; Sandulescu, M.C.; Vardi, A.; Futerman, A.H.; Schapira, A.H.V.; Burton, E.A.; Bandmann, O. Ablation of the Pro-Inflammatory Master Regulator Mir-155 Does Not Mitigate Neuroinflammation or Neurodegeneration in a Vertebrate Model of Gaucher's Disease. *Neurobiol. Dis.* **2019**, *127*, 563–569. [CrossRef] [PubMed]
64. Uemura, N.; Koike, M.; Ansai, S.; Kinoshita, M.; Ishikawa-Fujiwara, T.; Matsui, H.; Naruse, K.; Sakamoto, N.; Uchiyama, Y.; Todo, T.; et al. Viable Neuronopathic Gaucher Disease Model in Medaka (Oryzias Latipes) Displays Axonal Accumulation of Alpha-Synuclein. *PLoS Genet.* **2015**, *11*, e1005065. [CrossRef] [PubMed]
65. Hernandez, D.G.; Reed, X.; Singleton, A.B. Genetics in Parkinson Disease: Mendelian Versus Non-Mendelian Inheritance. *J. Neurochem.* **2016**, *139*, 59–74. [CrossRef]
66. Flinn, L.; Mortiboys, H.; Volkmann, K.; Koster, R.W.; Ingham, P.W.; Bandmann, O. Complex I Deficiency and Dopaminergic Neuronal Cell Loss in Parkin-Deficient Zebrafish (Danio Rerio). *Brain* **2009**, *132*, 1613–1623. [CrossRef]
67. Fett, M.E.; Pilsl, A.; Paquet, D.; van Bebber, F.; Haass, C.; Tatzelt, J.; Schmid, B.; Winklhofer, K.F. Parkin Is Protective against Proteotoxic Stress in a Transgenic Zebrafish Model. *PLoS ONE* **2010**, *5*, e11783. [CrossRef]
68. Samaranch, L.; Lorenzo-Betancor, O.; Arbelo, J.M.; Ferrer, I.; Lorenzo, E.; Irigoyen, J.; Pastor, M.A.; Marrero, C.; Isla, C.; Herrera-Henriquez, J.; et al. Pink1-Linked Parkinsonism Is Associated with Lewy Body Pathology. *Brain* **2010**, *133*, 1128–1142. [CrossRef]
69. Corti, O.; Brice, A. Mitochondrial Quality Control Turns out to Be the Principal Suspect in Parkin and Pink1-Related Autosomal Recessive Parkinson's Disease. *Curr. Opin. Neurobiol.* **2013**, *23*, 100–108. [CrossRef]
70. Anichtchik, O.; Diekmann, H.; Fleming, A.; Roach, A.; Goldsmith, P.; Rubinsztein, D.C. Loss of Pink1 Function Affects Development and Results in Neurodegeneration in Zebrafish. *J. Neurosci.* **2008**, *28*, 8199–8207. [CrossRef] [PubMed]
71. Xi, Y.; Ryan, J.; Noble, S.; Yu, M.; Yilbas, A.E.; Ekker, M. Impaired Dopaminergic Neuron Development and Locomotor Function in Zebrafish with Loss of Pink1 Function. *Eur. J. Neurosci.* **2010**, *31*, 623–633. [CrossRef]
72. Sallinen, V.; Kolehmainen, J.; Priyadarshini, M.; Toleikyte, G.; Chen, Y.C.; Panula, P. Dopaminergic Cell Damage and Vulnerability to Mptp in Pink1 Knockdown Zebrafish. *Neurobiol. Dis.* **2010**, *40*, 93–101. [CrossRef] [PubMed]
73. Flinn, L.J.; Keatinge, M.; Bretaud, S.; Mortiboys, H.; Matsui, H.; De Felice, E.; Woodroof, H.I.; Brown, L.; McTighe, A.; Soellner, R.; et al. Tigarb Causes Mitochondrial Dysfunction and Neuronal Loss in Pink1 Deficiency. *Ann. Neurol.* **2013**, *74*, 837–847. [CrossRef] [PubMed]
74. Bai, Q.; Mullett, S.J.; Garver, J.A.; Hinkle, D.A.; Burton, E.A. Zebrafish Dj-1 Is Evolutionarily Conserved and Expressed in Dopaminergic Neurons. *Brain Res.* **2006**, *1113*, 33–44. [CrossRef] [PubMed]
75. Bretaud, S.; Allen, C.; Ingham, P.W.; Bandmann, O. P53-Dependent Neuronal Cell Death in a Dj-1-Deficient Zebrafish Model of Parkinson's Disease. *J. Neurochem.* **2007**, *100*, 1626–1635. [CrossRef]

76. Froyset, A.K.; Edson, A.J.; Gharbi, N.; Khan, E.A.; Dondorp, D.; Bai, Q.; Tiraboschi, E.; Suster, M.L.; Connolly, J.B.; Burton, E.A.; et al. Astroglial Dj-1 over-Expression up-Regulates Proteins Involved in Redox Regulation and Is Neuroprotective in Vivo. *Redox Biol.* **2018**, *16*, 237–247. [CrossRef]
77. Xi, Y.; Yu, M.; Godoy, R.; Hatch, G.; Poitras, L.; Ekker, M. Transgenic Zebrafish Expressing Green Fluorescent Protein in Dopaminergic Neurons of the Ventral Diencephalon. *Dev. Dyn.* **2011**, *240*, 2539–2547. [CrossRef] [PubMed]
78. Wen, L.; Wei, W.; Wenchao, G.; Peng, H.; Xi, R.; Zheng, Z.; Zuoyan, Z.; Shuo, L.; Bo, Z. Visualization of Monoaminergic Neurons and Neurotoxicity of Mptp in Live Transgenic Zebrafish. *Dev. Biol.* **2008**, *314*, 84–92. [CrossRef]
79. Langston, J.W. The Etiology of Parkinson's Disease with Emphasis on the Mptp Story. *Neurology* **1996**, *47*, S153–S160. [CrossRef]
80. Langston, J.W.; Ballard, P.; Tetrud, J.W.; Irwin, I. Chronic Parkinsonism in Humans Due to a Product of Meperidine-Analog Synthesis. *Science* **1983**, *219*, 979–980. [CrossRef]
81. Anichtchik, O.V.; Kaslin, J.; Peitsaro, N.; Scheinin, M.; Panula, P. Neurochemical and Behavioural Changes in Zebrafish Danio Rerio after Systemic Administration of 6-Hydroxydopamine and 1-Methyl-4-Phenyl-1,2,3,6-Tetrahydropyridine. *J. Neurochem.* **2004**, *88*, 443–453. [CrossRef]
82. Bretaud, S.; Lee, S.; Guo, S. Sensitivity of Zebrafish to Environmental Toxins Implicated in Parkinson's Disease. *Neurotoxicol. Teratol.* **2004**, *26*, 857–864. [CrossRef] [PubMed]
83. Lam, C.S.; Korzh, V.; Strahle, U. Zebrafish Embryos Are Susceptible to the Dopaminergic Neurotoxin Mptp. *Eur. J. Neurosci.* **2005**, *21*, 1758–1762. [CrossRef] [PubMed]
84. McKinley, E.T.; Baranowski, T.C.; Blavo, D.O.; Cato, C.; Doan, T.N.; Rubinstein, A.L. Neuroprotection of Mptp-Induced Toxicity in Zebrafish Dopaminergic Neurons. *Brain Res. Mol. Brain Res.* **2005**, *141*, 128–137. [CrossRef] [PubMed]
85. Kalyn, M.; Hua, K.; Mohd Noor, S.; Wong, C.E.D.; Ekker, M. Comprehensive Analysis of Neurotoxin-Induced Ablation of Dopaminergic Neurons in Zebrafish Larvae. *Biomedicines* **2019**, *8*, 1. [CrossRef] [PubMed]
86. Wang, Y.; Liu, W.; Yang, J.; Wang, F.; Sima, Y.; Zhong, Z.M.; Wang, H.; Hu, L.F.; Liu, C.F. Parkinson's Disease-Like Motor and Non-Motor Symptoms in Rotenone-Treated Zebrafish. *NeuroToxicology* **2017**, *58*, 103–109. [CrossRef]
87. Unal, I.; Caliskan-Ak, E.; Ustundag, U.V.; Ates, P.S.; Alturfan, A.A.; Altinoz, M.A.; Elmaci, I.; Emekli-Alturfan, E. Neuroprotective Effects of Mitoquinone and Oleandrin on Parkinson's Disease Model in Zebrafish. *Int. J. Neurosci.* **2019**, *130*, 1–9.
88. Bus, J.S.; Gibson, J.E. Paraquat: Model for Oxidant-Initiated Toxicity. *Environ. Health Perspect.* **1984**, *55*, 37–46. [CrossRef] [PubMed]
89. Manning-Bog, A.B.; McCormack, A.L.; Li, J.; Uversky, V.N.; Fink, A.L.; Di Monte, D.A. The Herbicide Paraquat Causes up-Regulation and Aggregation of Alpha-Synuclein in Mice: Paraquat and Alpha-Synuclein. *J. Biol. Chem.* **2002**, *277*, 1641–1644. [CrossRef]
90. Thiruchelvam, M.; Richfield, E.K.; Baggs, R.B.; Tank, A.W.; Cory-Slechta, D.A. The Nigrostriatal Dopaminergic System as a Preferential Target of Repeated Exposures to Combined Paraquat and Maneb: Implications for Parkinson's Disease. *J. Neurosci. Off. J. Soc. Neurosci.* **2000**, *20*, 9207–9214. [CrossRef]
91. Wang, A.; Costello, S.; Cockburn, M.; Zhang, X.; Bronstein, J.; Ritz, B. Parkinson's Disease Risk from Ambient Exposure to Pesticides. *Eur. J. Epidemiol.* **2011**, *26*, 547–555. [CrossRef]
92. Nellore, J.; Nandita, P. Paraquat Exposure Induces Behavioral Deficits in Larval Zebrafish During the Window of Dopamine Neurogenesis. *Toxicol. Rep.* **2015**, *2*, 950–956. [CrossRef]
93. Bortolotto, J.W.; Cognato, G.P.; Christoff, R.R.; Roesler, L.N.; Leite, C.E.; Kist, L.W.; Bogo, M.R.; Vianna, M.R.; Bonan, C.D. Long-Term Exposure to Paraquat Alters Behavioral Parameters and Dopamine Levels in Adult Zebrafish (Danio Rerio). *Zebrafish* **2014**, *11*, 142–153. [CrossRef]
94. Chou, A.P.; Maidment, N.; Klintenberg, R.; Casida, J.E.; Li, S.; Fitzmaurice, A.G.; Fernagut, P.O.; Mortazavi, F.; Chesselet, M.F.; Bronstein, J.M. Ziram Causes Dopaminergic Cell Damage by Inhibiting E1 Ligase of the Proteasome. *J. Biol. Chem.* **2008**, *283*, 34696–34703. [CrossRef] [PubMed]
95. Fitzmaurice, A.G.; Rhodes, S.L.; Cockburn, M.; Ritz, B.; Bronstein, J.M. Aldehyde Dehydrogenase Variation Enhances Effect of Pesticides Associated with Parkinson Disease. *Neurology* **2014**, *82*, 419–426. [CrossRef]

96. Fitzmaurice, A.G.; Rhodes, S.L.; Lulla, A.; Murphy, N.; Lam, H.A.; O'Donnell, K.C.; Barnhill, L.; Casida, J.E.; Cockburn, M.; Sagasti, A.; et al. Aldehyde Dehydrogenase as a Potential Target for Toxicant-Induced Parkinson's Disease. *Proc. Natl. Acad. Sci. USA* **2013**, *110*, 636–641. [CrossRef] [PubMed]
97. Ritz, B.; P-Lee, C.; Hansen, J.; Lassen, C.F.; Ketzel, M.; Sorensen, M.; Raaschou-Nielsen, O. Traffic-Related Air Pollution Is a Risk Factor for Parkinson's Disease in Denmark. *Environ. Health Perspect.* **2016**, *124*, 351–356. [CrossRef] [PubMed]
98. Barnhill, L.M.; Khuansuwan, S.; Juarez, D.; Murata, H.; Araujo, J.A.; Bronstein, J.M. Diesel Exhaust Extract Exposure Induces Neuronal Toxicity by Disrupting Autophagy. *Toxicol. Sci. Off. J. Soc. Toxicol.* (in press). [CrossRef] [PubMed]
99. Khuansuwan, S.; Barnhill, L.M.; Cheng, S.; Bronstein, J.M. A Novel Transgenic Zebrafish Line Allows for in Vivo Quantification of Autophagic Activity in Neurons. *Autophagy* **2019**, *15*, 1–11. [CrossRef]

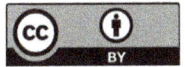

© 2020 by the authors. Licensee MDPI, Basel, Switzerland. This article is an open access article distributed under the terms and conditions of the Creative Commons Attribution (CC BY) license (http://creativecommons.org/licenses/by/4.0/).

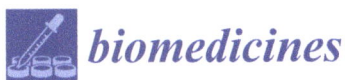

Article

Method Standardization for Conducting Innate Color Preference Studies in Different Zebrafish Strains

Petrus Siregar [1,†], Stevhen Juniardi [1,†], Gilbert Audira [1,2], Yu-Heng Lai [3], Jong-Chin Huang [4], Kelvin H.-C. Chen [4,*], Jung-Ren Chen [5,*] and Chung-Der Hsiao [1,2,6,*]

1 Department of Bioscience Technology, Chung Yuan Christian University, Chung-Li 320314, Taiwan; siregar.petrus27@gmail.com (P.S.); stvn.jun@gmail.com (S.J.); gilbertaudira@yahoo.com (G.A.)
2 Department of Chemistry, Chung Yuan Christian University, Chung-Li 320314, Taiwan
3 Department of Chemistry, Chinese Culture University, Taipei 11114, Taiwan; lyh21@ulive.pccu.edu.tw
4 Department of Biological Science & Technology, College of Medicine, I-Shou University, Kaohsiung 82445, Taiwan; hjc@mail.nptu.edu.tw
5 Department of Applied Chemistry, National Pingtung University, Pingtung 900391, Taiwan
6 Center for Nanotechnology, Chung Yuan Christian University, Chung-Li 320314, Taiwan
* Correspondence: kelvin@mail.nptu.edu.tw (K.H.-C.C.); jrchen@isu.edu.tw (J.-R.C.); cdhsiao@cycu.edu.tw (C.-D.H.)
† These authors contributed equally to this work.

Received: 22 June 2020; Accepted: 30 July 2020; Published: 3 August 2020

Abstract: The zebrafish has a tetrachromatic vision that is able to distinguish ultraviolet (UV) and visible wavelengths. Recently, zebrafish color preferences have gained much attention because of the easy setup of the instrument and its usefulness to screen behavior-linked stimuli. However, several published papers dealing with zebrafish color preferences have contradicting results that underscore the importance of method standardization in this field. Different laboratories may report different results because of variations in light source, color intensity, and other parameters such as age, gender, container size, and strain of fish. In this study, we aim to standardize the color preference test in zebrafish by measuring light source position, light intensity, gender, age, animal size to space ratio, and animal strain. Our results showed that color preferences for zebrafish are affected by light position, age, strain, and social interaction of the fish, but not affected by fish gender. We validated that ethanol can significantly induce color preference alteration in zebrafish which may be related to anxiety and depression. We also explored the potential use of the optimized method to examine color preference ranking and index differences in various zebrafish strains and species, such as the tiger barb and glass catfish. In conclusion, zebrafish color preference screening is a powerful tool for high-throughput neuropharmacological applications and the standardized protocol established in this study provides a useful reference for the zebrafish research community.

Keywords: zebrafish behavior; color preferences; toxicity assessment

1. Introduction

Color perception, an important trait that allows animals to recognize food, predators, shoaling, mating choices, and hiding places, has been reported to influence the learning behavior and memory formation of zebrafish [1,2]. Recent studies showed that zebrafish behavior could be used to evaluate the neurotoxicity of drugs [3,4]. Several transgenic zebrafish models [5,6] have been developed to assess behaviors based on various color cues and visual stimuli, such as T-maze [3,7], passive avoidance [8,9], Y-maze [10] and cross maze [6]. The pathway between the photoreceptor and the color spectrum recognition in animals and lower vertebrates are evolutionarily conserved [6]. Zebrafish have four different cones to distinguish UV and visible wavelengths. Specifically, the UV-cone has a peak sensitivity at 362 nm, the S-cone has a peak sensitivity at 417 nm, the M-cone peak sensitivity is at 480 nm, and the L-cone has a peak sensitivity at 556 nm [11]. Zebrafish larva responds to light at 3.5 day-post-fertilization (dpf), displays mobility from 5dpf onward, and is able to discern color from the early age of 5 dpf [6].

Several color preferences have been commonly demonstrated in zebrafish; however, the results were sometimes contradictory (summarized in Table A3). For example, either red [11,12] or blue [1,3,6,7,13,14] has been reported with the highest color preference ranking in zebrafish. Different color preference ranking results reported by different laboratories may be due to variations in the light source position (provided from the top or bottom positions), color intensity (different illumination lux), and/or physical parameters such as fish age and gender [1–3,6,7,11,13,14]. The variability of the assays can be overcome by standardizing the experimental conditions to ensure consistent results and ease in interpretation. In this study, we aim to standardize the innate color preference test condition in adult zebrafish by evaluating the potential effect of light source position and intensity, social interaction, gender, age, and strain of the tested fish. Furthermore, we applied the optimized protocol to evaluate the color preference difference in adult zebrafish exposed to ethanol to explore the potential uses of this setting for toxicity assessment.

2. Material and Methods

2.1. Animal Ethics and Animal Used in the Study

All the experimental protocols and procedures involving zebrafish were approved by the Committee for Animal Experimentation of the Chung Yuan Christian University (Number: CYCU104024, issued date 21 December 2015). All experiments were performed in accordance with the guidelines for laboratory animals. For intraspecies comparison, six zebrafish strains, AB, Tübingen long fin (TL), Wild Indian Karyotype (WIK), golden, absolute, and pet store-purchased (PET) were used. The TL zebrafish phenotype shows longer fins compared to the AB strain. The TL zebrafish are homozygous mutants for leo^{t1} and lof^{dt1}. leo^{t1} is a recessive mutation that causes spotting in adult zebrafish. The other mutation lof^{dt1} is a dominant homozygous viable mutation causing long fins [15,16]. The absolute mutant fish is a double mutant fish carrying the $ednrb1^{b140}$ and $mitfa^{b692}$. In zebrafish, $ednrb1$ is important in adult pigment pattern formation [17,18]. This fish is also carrying the $mitfa^{b692}$ mutation [19] which renders the skin transparent. The absolute mutant lacks melanophore, xanthophore, and most of the iridophore cells causing the transparent phenotype [20]. The golden zebrafish exhibited lightening of the pigmented stripes and golden phenotype. The golden phenotype is characterized by the mutation in $slc24a5$. This mutation causes a delayed and reduced development of melanin pigmentation in zebrafish. The mutation produced a lighter stripes in golden zebrafish [21]. The WIK strain was originally derived from a wild-caught line and is highly polymorphic compared to the AB strain. They are often used for genome mapping in zebrafish because of their characteristic of being highly polymorphic [22]. Meanwhile, the PET zebrafish were derived from a local aquarium in Taiwan, they represent the wild-type genetically and presumably have a heterogeneous genetic background [22]. For interspecies comparison, another two teleost species of tiger barb (*Puntigrus tetrazona*) and glass catfish (*Kryptopterus vitreolus*) were used. Four zebrafish strains, AB, TL, WIK, and absolute, were obtained from Taiwan Zebrafish Center at Academia Sinica (TZCAS), and the PET and the golden zebrafish strains, as well as the tiger barb and glass catfish, were purchased from a local pet store.

2.2. Color Preference Assay

The assay was conducted in a 21 × 21 × 10 cm acrylic tank and filled with 1.5 L of filtered water. Each half of the tank area with a size of 10.5 × 10.5 was covered with a color plate combination with lux intensity as listed in Table A1. All the color preference assays conducted in this study took place in the room temperature condition, which is around 26–28 °C. The temperature condition is the same with zebrafish maintenance conditions. Four 30W LED lights were positioned above (SerRickDon, Shenzhen, China) and one 60 × 60 cm 24W LED plate (Lumibox, Shenzhen, China) was positioned below the fish tanks to provide different combinations of illumination positions and intensities (Figures 1A and A1). A high-quality Couple-charged device (CCD) camera with a maximum resolution at 3264 × 2448 pixels and 30 frames per second (fps) frame rate (ONTOP, M2 module, Shenzhen, China) and an infrared (IR) camera (700–1000 nm detection window) with a maximum resolution at 1920 × 1080 pixels and 30 fps frame rate (3206_1080P module, Shenzhen, China) was used to record the fish locomotion activity. We also measured the reflectance of all color plates (Figure 1B and Table A2).

The high-quality CCD camera was used to record the blue–green color plate combination since the IR camera was not feasible in the tank with a blue–green color combination. The other color combinations (red–yellow, red–blue, red–green, yellow–blue, and yellow–green) were recorded by using the IR camera to increase the video signal-to-noise ratio (Figure 1C). The light intensity was measured by using a luminometer (Peakmeter Instruments Co., Ltd., Shenzhen, China). The luminometer's sensor was positioned facing the tank 5 cm above the water level to measure the light intensity (Figure 1B). The arrangement of four experimental tanks is shown in Figures 1A and A1 to increase the recording output. The wild-type AB strain zebrafish was used in this experiment. The zebrafish age used in this study is around 5–6 months old. Four experimental tanks were arranged side by side into a 2 × 2 array as shown in Figures 1A and A1 to increase the recording output. The experiments were divided into several different categories such as light position, tank size, social interaction, age, and gender to compare different variables that may affect the color preference result (summarized in Figure 1D). The light position, tank size, social interaction, and age were conducted in the color plate combination experiments. Social interaction and gender experiments were also conducted with half of the tank covered in color plate and the other half not covered (blank) (Figure 1E). All the experiments were conducted with a total of 24 fishes used in each category, except in ethanol-treated fish with a total of 12 fishes used in each ethanol-treated category.

The tank size comparison experiment was conducted to compare a 20 × 20 × 10 tank filled with 1.5 L and a 30 × 30 × 10 tank filled with 4.2 L which have the same height: the water-filled ratio. For comparing the effect of social interaction towards color preferences, the swimming activity of single zebrafish in one tank was compared with six zebrafishes shoaling in one tank. The gender effect was assessed by measuring the 5-month-old male and female zebrafish color preferences separately. The zebrafish age used for age-dependent color preference study was 3, 5, and 12 months old with a total of 24 fishes used in each age group. For all the color preference tests, the zebrafishes were placed into the water tank and immediately performed video recording by using IR or conventional camera for 30 min. No habituation time was performed in the experimental tank, and zebrafish movement was analyzed for 30 min in this study. Total Recorder software (High Criteria Inc., Richmond Hill, ON, Canada) was used to capture the video at a resolution of 1920 × 1080 pixel using the IR or conventional camera.

2.3. Data Analysis

The fish locomotion within 30 min of the recorded video was analyzed by using an open source idTracker software (Ver. 2.1, Cajal Institute, Madrid, Spain) [23]. The XY coordinates obtained by idTracker software was used to calculate the appearing times in different partitions of the zebrafish by using Microsoft Excel. The choice index equation was used to calculate the preferences of the zebrafish color preferences [24,25].

$$\text{Choice index} = \frac{\text{Time stay in color partition }(s) - \text{Time stay in a second color partition }(s)}{\text{Total video time }(s)} \quad (1)$$

2.4. Statistics

One-way ANOVA was used to analyze single group data for combined time point results with Tukey post hoc analysis. Non-parametric Kruskal–Wallis followed by Dunn's post hoc test was used to measure data that violated the normal distribution assumption. The statistical analysis was carried out by using GraphPad Prism 7.00 for Windows. The data shown were presented as mean ± SEM with $p < 0.05$ regarded as the statistically significant difference at 95% confidence.

3. Results

3.1. Overview of Experimental Design and Instrument Setting

To increase the test throughput, we set up four transparent acrylic containers with 20 cm (L) × 20 cm (W) × 10 cm (H) dimension and equipped them with four top lights and one bottom light (LED plate) sources to provide constant light intensity (Figures 1A and A1). A luminometer was used to measure the light intensity from either transmission light or reflection light (Figure 1B). The outlooking of fish images captured by using either conventional or infrared CCD is shown in Figure 1C. Seven experiments were conducted in order to understand the optimized color preference testing conditions (Figure 1D,E). For experiment 1, the potential light position effect on color preference was investigated to see whether the zebrafish exhibits distinct innate color preference when external light sources were provided from different positions. For experiment 2, the potential animal density effect was investigated to see whether the zebrafish exhibits distinct innate color preferences when they stay in different animal-to-space ratio conditions. For experiment 3, the potential social interaction (shoaling) effect was investigated by housing either single or six fishes in the same tank. For experiment 4, the potential gender effect was examined by conducting an innate color preference test using all male or female fishes. For experiment 5, the potential age effect was investigated by conducting a color preference test with zebrafish aged either 3-, 5- or 12-month-olds. For experiment 6, the potential strain effect was studied by conducting innate color preference tests with different strains of AB, TL, golden, absolute, and WIK. For experiment 7, the potential toxicological effect of ethanol on innate color preference was examined by exposing zebrafish (AB strain) to 1% ethanol for either 24 h or 96 h.

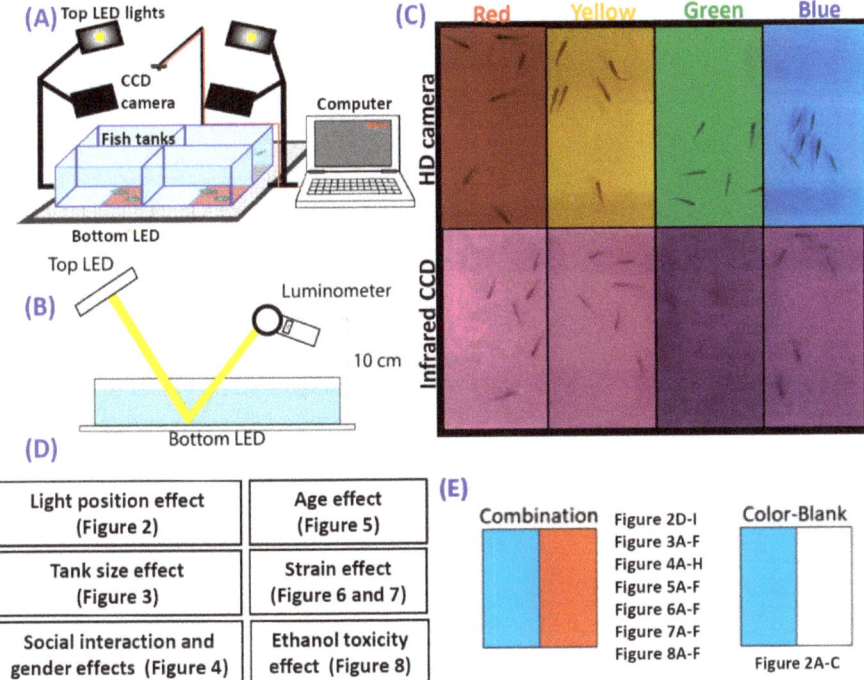

Figure 1. Experimental setup for color preference assay in zebrafish. (**A**) Schematic of the experimental setup and a picture of the experimental setup used for measuring zebrafish color preference in this study. (**B**) Schematic showing the position of the luminometer to measure the top and bottom light intensity. (**C**) Comparison of the images collected from regular Couple-charged device (CCD) (top) and infrared CCD cameras (bottom). (**D**) Experimental design and specific aims of this study. (**E**) Schematic illustrating tank area with color plate combination and color blank design.

3.2. Experiment 1: Light Source Position on Zebrafish Color Preferences

Various conditions of the zebrafish innate color preference tests used in separate laboratories sometimes lead to contradictory results in published studies (Table A3). We hypothesized that the light source position in the color preference test might affect zebrafish color preferences. To test the hypothesis, first, we compared the achromatic color plate with different light positions to determine whether different light sources affect zebrafish color preference. We found that the light source did not result in a significant difference with positions in achromatic plate comparison. In a white (0.000691 uWatt/nm) and grey (0.000207 uWatt/nm) combination, the zebrafish preferred to stay in the grey partition (Figure 2A). The white–grey combination ($F (3,92) = 1651, p = 0.9343$) showed no significant difference in effect whether the light source was placed at the bottom or on top (Figure 2A). In a white–black (0.0000342 uWatt/nm) combination, the zebrafish preferred the black partition (Figure 2B). The light source position also showed no significant effect on color preference in the white–black combination ($F (3,92) = 1249, p = 0.8649$) as seen in Figure 2B. In a grey and black comparison, the zebrafish preferred the black partition (Figure 2C). No significant effect on color preference was detected for top and bottom light position ($F (3,92) = 190.7, p = 0.9345$) in grey–black color combination (Figure 2C). This result showed zebrafish preferred to stay in a lower lux intensity partition regardless of different plate combinations and light positions.

Based on the above findings, we tested whether the innate color preference in adult zebrafish has an associated light position effect. We addressed this question by using a color plate combination and performed an innate color preference test with either a top (Figure 2K) or bottom (Figure 2J) light source. We subjected all four-color plates on two color combinations in each tank, so the total color combinations were six color combinations. Each color combination was tested either with a top light source or a bottom light source. Results showed that the bottom and top light sources have similar color preference ranking patterns (from most to least: red > blue > green > yellow). The green–blue (F (3,92) = 145.1, p = 0.0292) (Figure 2D), green–yellow (F (3,92) = 105.9, p = 0.2851) (Figure 2E), green–red (Figure 2G), red–yellow (F (3,92) = 394.6, p = 0.0195) (Figure 2H) and blue–yellow combinations (F (3,92) = 64.57, p = 0.0897) (Figure 2I) showed no significant differences in regard to color preference, regardless of whether the light source was placed at the bottom or on top. Interestingly, although the red–blue combination showed no difference in color preference ranking, it showed significant differences in color preference index (F (3,92) = 254.5, p = 0.0398). That is, the light source on top has a higher color preference index in red compared with the light source placed at the bottom (Figure 2F). Together, our results demonstrated the innate color preference ranking in zebrafish is red > blue > green > yellow, and this ranking is not associated with the light source provided either from the bottom (transmission light) or the top (reflection light) positions. Based on these results, using the top and bottom light sources makes the results much more stable and repeatable.

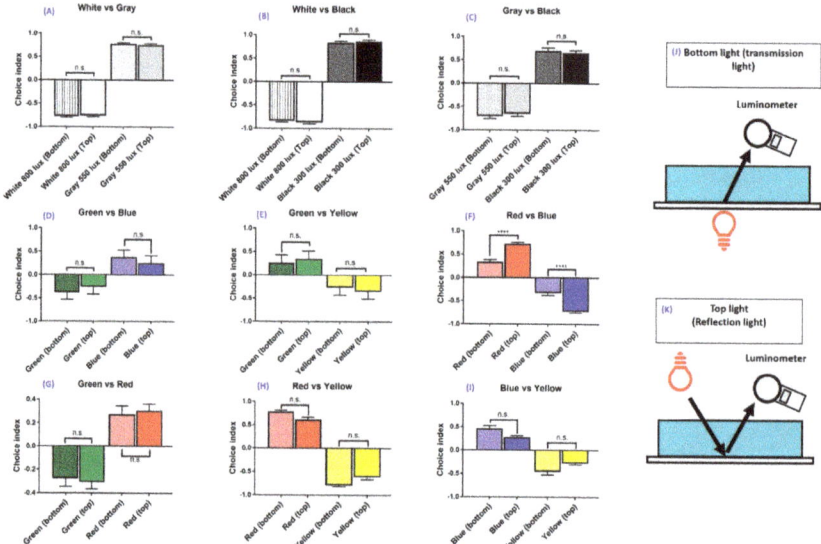

Figure 2. The effect of light intensity and light source position on the zebrafish swimming activity choice index. (**A–C**) The effect of different light intensity on the zebrafish swimming activity choice index. (**A**) White and grey combination, (**B**) white and black combination, (**C**) grey and black combination. (**D–I**) The effect of different color and light position on the zebrafish swimming activity choice index. (**D**) Green vs. blue combination, (**E**) green vs. yellow combination, (**F**) red vs. blue combination, (**G**) green vs. red combination, (**H**) red vs. yellow combination, (**I**) blue vs. yellow combination. (**J,K**) Schematic showing the light source positions either from the bottom or on top. The light intensity was measured by using a luminometer. The data are presented as mean ± SEM, n = 24 for each group. The difference was tested by one-way ANOVA and the significance level was set at, **** p < 0.0001. n.s. = non-significant.

3.3. Experiment 2: Tank Size (Animal Density) on Zebrafish Color Preferences

We also assessed whether the density of the tested animals plays a major role in color preferences which may cause the unrepeatability of the data. To reach this goal, zebrafishes were housed in different size containers at different fish-to-tank area ratios. The innate color preference for zebrafish housed in either a 20 × 20 × 10 cm tank (fish-to-tank ratio is 1:103, Figure 3G) or a 30 × 30 × 10 cm tank (fish-to-tank ratio is 1:224, Figure 3H) was measured and compared. Both the top light and bottom light sources were used simultaneously to get rid of any inconsistent factors in illumination. The fish-to-tank ratio was measured by using ImageJ software based on their relative pixel area. We found that there was no significant difference in either color preference ranking or index when using a 20 × 20 × 10 cm tank or a 30 × 30 × 10 cm tank in all color combinations tested (Figure 3A–F).

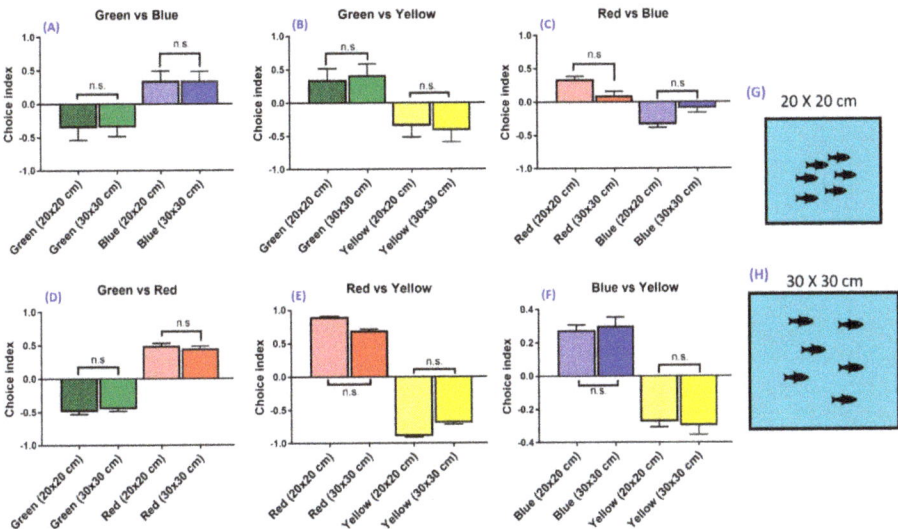

Figure 3. The effect of different tank sizes on the zebrafish swimming activity choice index. (**A**) Green vs. blue combination, (**B**) green vs. yellow combination, (**C**) red vs. blue combination, (**D**) green vs. red combination, (**E**) red vs. yellow combination, (**F**) blue vs. yellow combination. (**G**,**H**) Schematics showing two settings with different fish-to-tank ratios for assessment of the fish density effect. The data are presented as mean ± SEM, n = 24 for each group. The difference was tested by one-way ANOVA. n.s. = non-significant.

3.4. Experiment 3 and 4: Social Interaction and Gender on Zebrafish Color Preference

In order to maximize the assay throughput, we measured the locomotor activity of six fishes in the same container (Figure 4I). With the aid of locomotion tracking software, it is possible to perform multiple fish tracking in a single arena to increase the experimental throughputs. When multiple zebrafish swim together, they will display shoaling behavior to reduce anxiety and lower the risk of being captured by predators [12,26,27]. However, zebrafish color preference experiments in previous studies were often conducted with a single fish in a color preference chamber or maze [2,3]. Whether multiple fish and single fish display different color preferences is an interesting and unanswered question. By analyzing multiple fish, with the aid of idTracker software for individual identity recognition, our results showed that the single fish and multiple fish tested in a single arena showed a significant difference in color preference (Figure 4A). In a tank experiment with blank-color partition, the single fish showed avoidance of green, yellow and blue. Blank partition means a transparent partition or without a color plate. Thus, we obtained four color combinations: blank–red, blank–blue, blank–green, and blank–yellow combinations. On the contrary, when the test was given to a group of fish, green, yellow, blue and red were preferred, which showed an opposite preference between the color partitions.

We also used a color plate combination to investigate whether the multiple fish and single fish display different color preference rankings. We used four color plates, namely, red, blue, green and yellow, with a total of six color combinations in this social interaction experiment. The result showed that there was no significant difference between single and multiple fish color preference ranking in color combination, but the variances in the single fish were higher compared with the multiple fish experiment conditions (Figure 4C–H). Together, our results showed that the color preference data obtained from a test conducted with multiple fish are more reproducible and consistent compared to those in which a single fish was tested.

To date, the potential gender effect on color preference in zebrafish has not been adequately addressed [11]. To this end, we used sex-maturated males and females aged 6–8 months to investigate the potential gender-associated color preference difference (Figure 4J). The results showed that there was no significant difference in color preference between male and female zebrafishes tested in this study. The innate color preference ranking and index showed no significant difference between genders (Figure 4B). Therefore, in the subsequent experiments, zebrafishes with mixed gender were used to conduct color preference experiments.

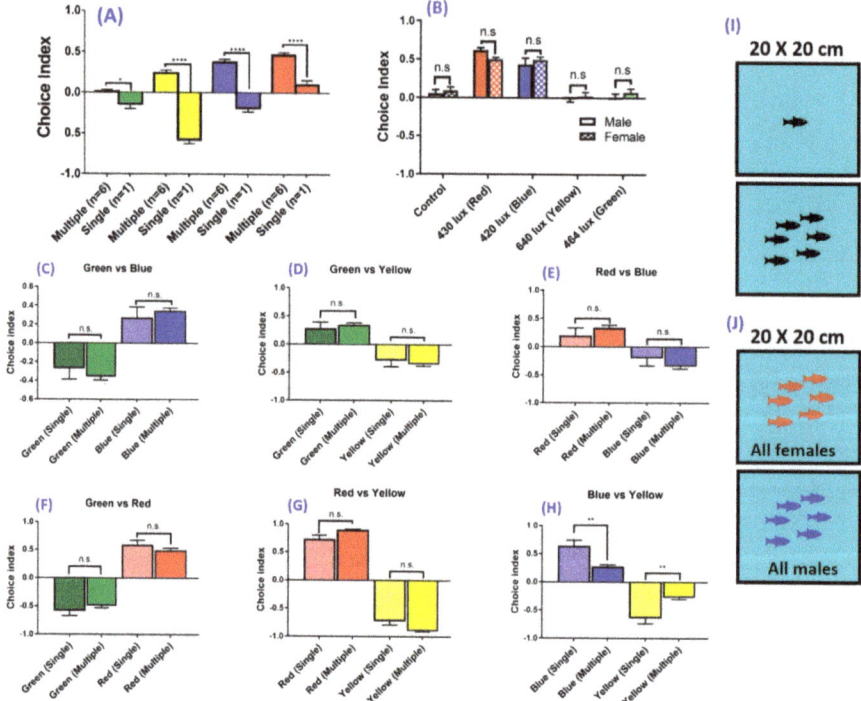

Figure 4. The effect of social interaction and gender on color preference using the top light source. (**A**) The effect of the single fish compared with multiple fish in a single tank on color preference using a blank-color partition. (**B**) The effect of gender on color preference using the light source on top. (**C–H**) The effect of social interaction on color preference using color combinations. (**C**) Green vs. blue combination, (**D**) green vs. yellow combination, (**E**) red vs. blue combination, (**F**) green vs. red combination, (**G**) red vs. yellow combination, (**H**) blue vs. yellow combination. (**I**) Schematics showing two settings in which either single or multiple fish were kept in a single tested tank. (**J**) Schematics showing two settings in which either six male or female fishes were kept in a single tested tank. The data are presented as mean ± SEM, n = 24 for each group. The difference was tested by one-way ANOVA and the significance level was set at * $p < 0.05$, ** $p < 0.01$, **** $p < 0.0001$. n.s. = non-significant.

3.5. Experiment 5: Age Effect on Zebrafish Color Preferences

A thorough review of the literature indicates that the potential effects of fish age on innate color preferences have not been carefully investigated in previous studies (Table A3). In this study, zebrafish with different ages from 3, 5 to 12 months old were subjected to color preference tests (Figure 5G). Results showed that their innate color preference ranking were the same (from most to least: red > blue > green > yellow) but the time they spent in the preferred color partition was different (Figure 5A–F). Notably, 12-month-old fish showed a relatively lower color preference index in blue–green (F (5,138) = 33.88, p = 0.4729) (Figure 5A) and red–green color combinations (F (5,138) = 61.39, p = 0.8010) (Figure 5D). However, the 3-month-old fish showed a relatively lower preference index compared with adult zebrafish in green–blue (F (5,138) = 33.88, p = 0.6579) (Figure 5A) and green–red (F (5,138) = 61.39, p = 0.0044) (Figure 5D) color combinations. It appears that the ability of the 3-month-old fish to discern color was higher compared with the 12-month-old fish because the time the 3-month-old fish chose their preferred colors was higher. There are also other possibilities to explain the differences that occurred in this experiment. Differences in the choice index may not be due to color preferences, but because of the fear or anxiety response. Old zebrafish could show fear or anxiety response to some colors and will likely show a freezing response and stay in the same color area. However, if the fish did not show a freezing response, then it could be interpreted as the color preference of the fish. In addition, the 5-month-old fish has the highest choice index in the green–blue combination (F (5,138) = 33.88, p = 0.0049) (Figure 5A) and green–red combination (F (5,138) = 61.39, p = 0.0163) (Figure 5D). Our result suggested that the optimal age for the color preference test in zebrafish is around 5 months old because they showed the highest choice index compared with other age groups.

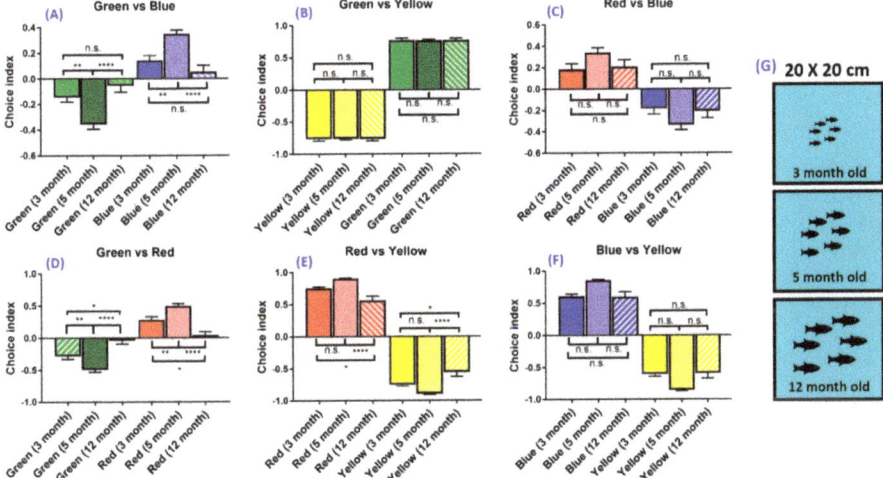

Figure 5. The effect of different ages on zebrafish color preference using the light source on top. (**A**) Green vs. blue combination, (**B**) green vs. yellow combination, (**C**) red vs. blue combination, (**D**) green vs. red combination, (**E**) red vs. yellow combination, (**F**) blue vs. yellow combination. (**G**) Schematics showing three settings with zebrafishes aged at either 3, 5 or 12 months old. The experiment was conducted with six zebrafishes inside one tank. The data are presented as mean ± SEM, n = 24 for each group. The difference was tested by one-way ANOVA and the significance level was set at * p < 0.05, ** p < 0.01, **** p < 0.0001. n.s. = non-significant.

3.6. Experiment 6: The Strain- and Species-Specific Effect on Zebrafish Color Preference

The most popular strain that has been used for color preference tests in previous studies is the AB strain (Table A3). Some previous reports used zebrafish from the local pet store and the variation in the fish genetic background might contribute to the inconsistent color preference test results seen in the literature. Here, we tested the hypothesis by examining the innate color preference among six different zebrafish strains, namely, AB, absolute, golden, TL, PET, and WIK for the first time. Using the optimized condition established in this study, we discovered that all six zebrafish strains display the same color preference, with the ranking from most to least as red > blue > green > yellow. However, the color preference index for each strain displayed a significant difference compared to their AB strain counterpart (Figure 6A–F).

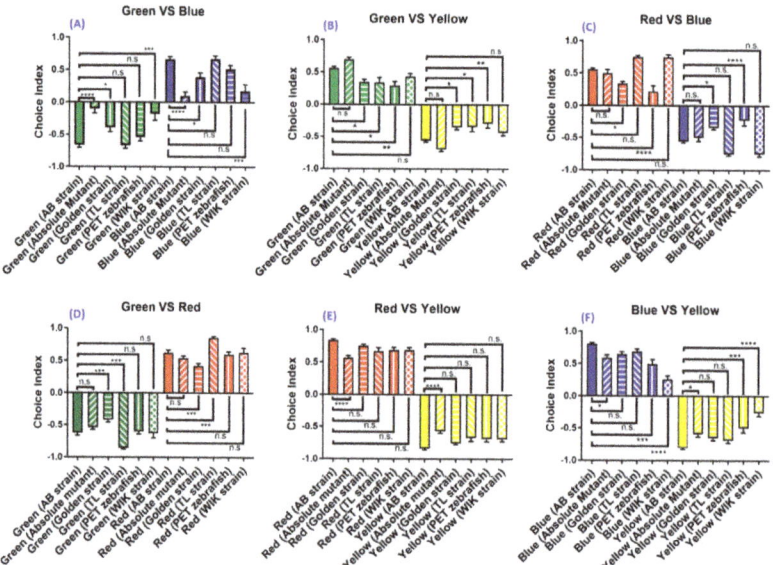

Figure 6. Color preference ranking and index difference between six different zebrafish strains. The color preference index for the (**A**) green vs. blue, (**B**) green vs. yellow, (**C**) red vs. blue, (**D**) green vs. red, (**E**) red vs. yellow, (**F**) and blue vs. yellow combinations. The data are presented as mean ± SEM, $n = 24$ for each strain, except for the Wild Indian Karyotype (WIK) strain ($n = 12$). The difference was tested by one-way ANOVA and the significance level was set at * $p < 0.05$, ** $p < 0.01$, *** $p < 0.001$, **** $p < 0.0001$. n.s. = non-significant.

Compared to the AB strain, the absolute mutant exhibited a lower choice index in green–blue (F (11,252) = 296.7, $p = 0.5117$) (Figure 6A), red–yellow (F (11,252) = 374.1, $p = 0.0181$) (Figure 6E), and blue–yellow color combinations (F (11,252) = 189.3, $p = 0.0457$), respectively (Figure 6F). The reduction in the choice index in green–blue combination suggests that the absolute mutant spent less time in the blue color compartment and more time in green compartments. A similar reduction in color choice indices can also be found in red–yellow and blue–yellow combinations (Figure 6A, E, F). Compared to AB, the golden strain manifests different choice indices in green–yellow (F (11,252) = 84.61, $p = 0.0273$) (Figure 6B), red–blue (F (11,252) = 111.4, $p = 0.0215$) (Figure 6C), and green–red (F (11,252) = 296.7, $p = 0.0009$) (Figure 6D) color combinations. Compared to the AB strain, the TL strain showed a reduced choice index in the green–yellow color combination (F (11,252) = 84.61, $p = 0.0208$) (Figure 6B). They also exhibit a higher choice index in the green–red color combination (F (11,252) = 296.7, $p = 0.0001$), which means that the TL strain prefers red and spent most of their time in the red area compared to the green area (Figure 6D). Different wild-type breeds such as the PET strain showed identical color preference rankings with the AB strain. However, the PET strain exhibited a lower choice index in the green–yellow color combination test (F (11,252) = 84.61, $p = 0.0020$), indicating that the PET strain zebrafish spent more time in the yellow compartment compared to the AB strain (Figure 6B). Similar results also were seen in the red–blue color combination (F (11,252) = 111.4, p = 0.0001) (Figure 6C) and the blue–yellow color combination (F (11,252) = 189.3, p = 0.0002) for the PET strain (Figure 6F). Finally, the WIK strain exhibited the same color preference ranking with their AB strain counterpart, but with reduced choice indices in some color combinations such as green–blue (F (11,252) = 74.17, p = <0.0001) and blue–yellow (F (11,252) = 189.3, p = <0.0001) (Figure 6A,F). In conclusion, by using the established protocol and conditions, we provided solid evidence to show that the color preference in six tested zebrafish strains (AB, absolute, golden, TL, PET, and WIK) display different color preference indices, however, the major color preference ranking does not appear to be associated with their genetic backgrounds.

Next, we asked whether the current optimized setting can be used to explore the color preference ranking and index for other small fish species. Two freshwater fishes, the tiger barb (*Puntigrus tetrazona*) and glass catfish (*Kryptopterus vitreolus*), with a similar body size to zebrafish were used in this study to explore the generality of the optimized experimental setting. Results showed that glass catfish display a similar color preference ranking with the AB strain zebrafish. It is intriguing to note that the tiger barb displays a distinct color preference ranking differing from that of the AB strain zebrafish. For the tiger barb, the innate color preference ranking is green > blue > red > yellow, while the AB strain zebrafish ranking is red > blue > green > yellow. The result in green–blue (F (5138) = 175.5, p = <0.0001), green–red (F (5138) = 49.2, p = <0.0001), and green–yellow color combinations (F (5138) = 358.3, p = <0.0001) indicate that green is the most preferred color for the tiger barb (Figure 7A,B,D). Similar to zebrafish, yellow is still the least preferred color for the tiger barb, which is corroborated by data collected from green–yellow, red–yellow, and blue–yellow color combinations (Figure 7B,E,F). In addition, the tiger barb exhibits lower choice indices in some color combinations, such as red–yellow (F (5138) = 429.1, p = <0.0001) and blue–yellow (F (5138) = 421.4, p = <0.0001) (Figure 7E,F).

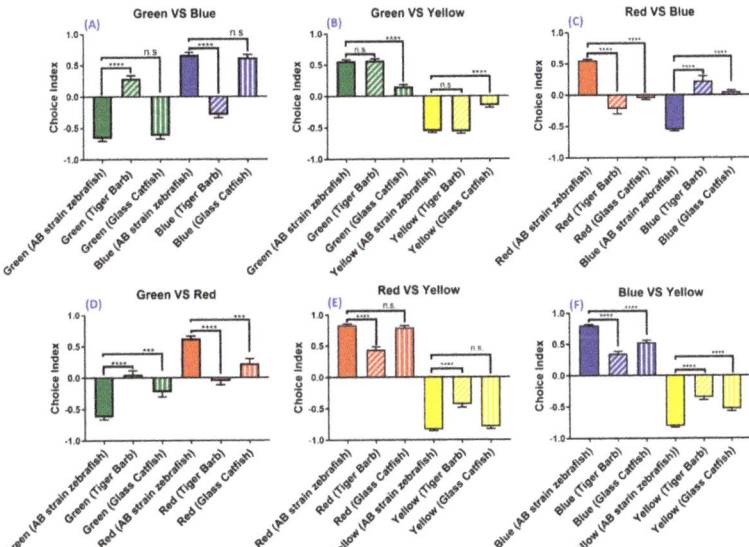

Figure 7. Color preference ranking and index difference for the tiger barb (*Puntigrus tetrazona*) and glass catfish (*Kryptopterus vitreolus*). The color preference index for the (**A**) green vs. blue, (**B**) green vs. yellow, (**C**) red vs. blue, (**D**) green vs. red, (**E**) red vs. yellow, (**F**) and blue vs. yellow combinations. The data are presented as mean ± SEM, n = 24 for each fish species. The difference was tested by one-way ANOVA and the significance level was set at *** p < 0.001, **** p < 0.0001. n.s. = non-significant.

For glass catfish, the innate color preference ranking is red >blue > green >yellow. The order is maintained as in zebrafish. This conclusion was supported by data collected from green–blue (F (5138) = 175.5, p = 0.9846), red–blue (F (5138) = 56.86, p = <0.0001), and blue–yellow color combinations (F (5138) = 421.4, p = <0.0001), where the blue choice index was higher than other colors (Figure 7A,C,F). Yellow is still the least favorite color of glass catfish, similar to the zebrafish and tiger barb (Figure 7). It can be seen that the yellow choice index in either green–yellow (F (5138) = 358.3, p = <0.0001), red–yellow (F (5138) = 429.1, p = 0.9604), or blue–yellow color combinations is the lowest compared to the other colors (Figure 7B,E,F). Together, our data clearly showed that the optimized experimental setting established in the present study can be applied to the innate color preference test conducted in other fish species.

3.7. Experiment 7: Effect of Ethanol on Zebrafish Color Preference

By using the optimized conditions described above, we aim to test the potential effect of environmental pollutants on color preference in zebrafish. In this experiment, we used ethanol as the potential pollutant to see their effects on color preference. Ethanol is extensively applied as a solvent in the industrial, research, and bioengineering process [28–30]. Excessive use of ethanol in industrial or research laboratories will likely become a new problem in the environment. Ethanol consumption has proved to have influence on the vestibulo-ocular system [31–34]. It also exhibits positional nystagmus and pursuit eye movements that further cause disturbed visual suppression [35–38]. Another experiment in zebrafish also proved that ethanol exposure to zebrafish embryos caused abnormalities of eye characteristics and affected the function of photoreceptors [39]. There is also a previous experiment that provides evidence that ethanol may affect visual systems, such as eye movements and fusion [40]. With all this evidence, we want to find out the effect of ethanol as an environmental pollutant on the color preference of zebrafish, as ethanol is known to affect the visual capabilities of animals and humans. Here, we took ethanol as an example to demonstrate chronological changes in the color preference of adult zebrafish after systematically being exposed to 1% ethanol. The AB strain zebrafish aged 5-month-old were exposed to 1% ethanol for either 24 h or 96 h. For most of the color combinations, the color preference ranking showed no significant change over time. This result suggests short-term ethanol exposure did not change the innate color preference ranking in zebrafish. However, it is intriguing to note that the color choice index in 1% ethanol-exposed zebrafish displayed a significant decrease in green–yellow (F (5,90) = 424.1, p = 0.0580) (Figure 8B) and blue–yellow combinations (F (5,90) = 307.6, p = <0.0001) over time (Figure 8F). In conclusion, the optimized protocol and settings for color preference ranking or index testing in zebrafish promises an applicable toxicity assessment for potential pollutants.

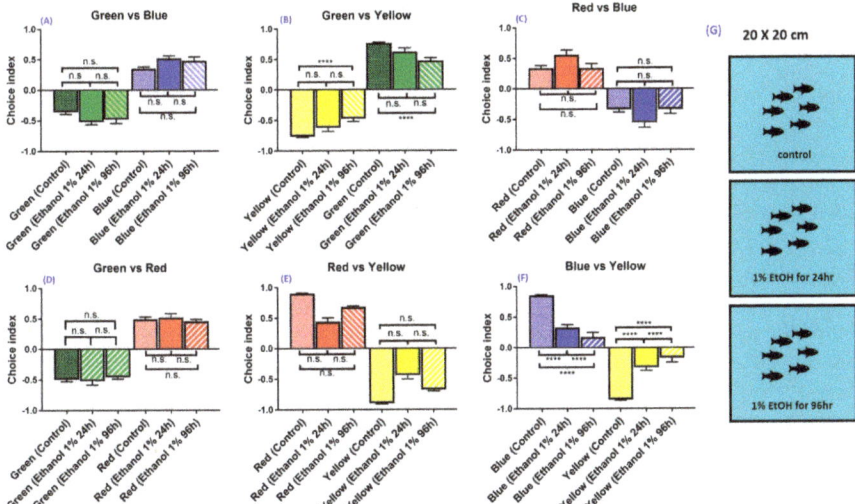

Figure 8. The effect of 1% ethanol on wild-type zebrafish with the light source on top. The ethanol at 1% concentration was systematically administered to zebrafish and their color preference changes were chronologically measured at 24 and 96 h. (**A**) Green vs. blue combination, (**B**) green vs. yellow combination, (**C**) red vs. blue combination, (**D**) green vs. red combination, (**E**) red vs. yellow combination, (**F**) blue vs. yellow combination. (**G**) Schematics showing three settings with either control or 1% ethanol exposure for 24 h or 96 h. The data are presented as mean ± SEM, control ($n = 24$); 1% ethanol, 24h ($n = 12$); 1% ethanol, 96h ($n = 12$). The difference was tested by one-way ANOVA and the significance level was set at **** $p < 0.0001$. n.s. = non-significant.

4. Discussion

Discrepancies in zebrafish color preference test results may have resulted from different factors that were not properly controlled and/or measured. The question of the potential influence of light intensity and light source position on color preference in zebrafish has not been adequately addressed. The zebrafish has been reported to prefer lower light intensity color, which is related to their strong preference towards blue [3]. Other parameters related to the living environment of the zebrafish may also affect color preferences.

In this study, carefully keeping the bottom light and top light at a similar light intensity, we found that the bottom light source and top light source gave similar results in both black–white and the color preference ranking and choice index (Figure 2). By careful control of the light position, intensity, and with a larger sample size, the zebrafish used in this study showed a preference for staying in the red and blue partitions, followed by staying in the green partition and avoiding the yellow partition. We concluded that the light intensity should be kept consistent in order to reduce bias for innate color preference in the zebrafish. However, the light source position did not affect zebrafish color preference.

Rhesus monkeys, chickens, turkeys, and mice have been reported to avoid red and yellow colors. These colors may be recognized as warning signals [41]. It has been reported that the color of feed may affect the behavior of zebrafish [12]. Avoidance of yellow discovered in the present study is in line with earlier studies showing that zebrafish tend to avoid yellow [1,7,14]. Yellow has a higher light intensity compared with the other colors, which may contribute to the avoidance behavior in the present study. Meanwhile, we found that red is the most preferred based on our zebrafish color preference test. Studies have shown that animals often prefer the color that is similar to or contrasts with the environment [42,43]. Animals tend to approach common colors that may help them find abundant food, while preference for a color that contrasts with the background may help animals to assess mate quality or to locate less common resources [44]. In addition, the preference towards red may be related to the color of the diet (red-colored pellet and artemia). Another study also showed that the zebrafish has an innate and relatively inflexible color preferences toward red [2].

We found that there is no significant effect of the tank size (animal density) used for the color preference test in the present study. This finding is in line with an experiment comparing differently sized tanks that had no significant effect in a novel tank test [45]. By using single fish in the single tank, we observed that the zebrafish had a different behavior compared to shoaling zebrafish. The single fish avoided going to color partitions even when the color partition had a lower light intensity compared to the blank partition, indicative of an altered behavior when the zebrafish were conditioned alone. A shoal of fish exhibited relaxed behavior when compared to the single fish scenario. We also observed that the freezing time for multiple fish was shorter as compared to that of a single fish. Such phenomenon may be affected by the social buffering effect of the zebrafish. Social interaction may ameliorate the anxiety level in zebrafish [46]. Animals' ability to distinguish objects and colors in the environment is helpful in finding food and communicating in groups [47]. Our results showed that social interaction influences the color preference choice index in zebrafish behavior (Figure 4A) and is consistent with such interpretation. In the color combination experiment, although the color preference ranking of the zebrafish did not change, the data variation in the single fish experiment was higher compared with the multiple fish experiment (Figure 4C–H). Moreover, in the present study, we found that sex difference did not have a significant effect on color preference ranking, suggesting that conducting color preference experiments using the mixed gender should be considered as a valid condition (Figure 4B).

Age plays an important role in the color preference of zebrafish (Figure 5A–F). The 12-month-old fish were incapable of differentiating the green color partition when compared to the 3-month-old and 5-month-old fish. The 3-month-old and 5-month-old fish showed similar patterns of color preference ranking and choice index. It has been reported that the zebrafish is able to recognize visual stimuli from the early age of 5 dpf, highlighting the importance of visual perception [48]. Furthermore, the zebrafish was reported to have different light preferences between their larval stage and adult stage. The larval stage showed light preference, while the adult fish showed light avoidance [24,49,50]. The previous experiments in zebrafish also proved that visual acuity of the normal fish will be improved with age [51]. In the blue and green color combination tests, the 12-month-old zebrafish prefer the blue partition over green partition, which may be caused by aging. In other color combinations, the color preference index in older fish was lowered, which may be due to reduced color sensitivity. One of the known aging symptoms in the zebrafish is retina degeneration, which affects color perception [52]. Besides aging, another factor also could cause abnormal zebrafish visual behavior, such as environmental conditions like abnormal lighting environments [51]. Different preferences between larval and adult stages also can be caused by different opsin expressions between both stages. The zebrafish has two different opsin genes: The middle/long wavelength sensitive (M/LW) and *Rhodopsin-like* (*RH2*) opsin genes [53]. Both of them are expressed in different times and areas in zebrafish. Expression of LWS-2 (sensitive to a shorter wavelength) in juvenile and larval zebrafish is more expressed than LWS-1 (longer-wavelength sensitive) in the retina. Meanwhile, in adult zebrafish, LWS-2 expressions are lower than LWS-1, indicating a spectral shift of opsin type from short to long [53,54]. Differences in the larval and adult stages also can be caused by dissimilar photoreceptor development and function. Larval zebrafish only have cones as the functional photoreceptor in the retina until 10 dpf [55]. In the larval stage, a light-responsive cone photoreceptor does not appear until 4 days post-fertilization. Cones that are sensitive to color in zebrafish larva also do not mature until 10 days post-fertilization [56–58]. In our study, zebrafish prefer red and blue and avoid green and yellow, which is similar to previous studies [6]. However, there are differences in the choice index between young and old zebrafish. This could be the anxiety or fear behavior toward some color and not because old zebrafish could not recognize the color like young zebrafish. Freezing has been suggested as a measurement of anxiety [59]. A previous study proved that longer freezing was observed in zones in which fish spent more time in a specific color area. Time spent in each area demonstrated a tendency as a stay time of preferred colors. However, there are two possibilities of inducing freezing by color. It can be a tendency to avoid a specific color that reflects an anxiety or fear response. Another possibility is the behavior of the appetitive quality of another color, which is the behavior of desire to satisfy bodily needs and more preferred by zebrafish [59,60]. Older zebrafish may show an anxiety or fear response to some colors and stay in a specific color area. This tendency could be misinterpreted as a preferred color behavior. Nevertheless, it could be a tendency for appetitive quality. With this fact in mind, it is better to also test the freezing movement or freezing time in zebrafish caused by color in the future. Meanwhile, our result showed that the sexually matured 5-month-old fish were favorable to perform the color preference-related study on because of the established ability of distinctive specific color preference.

The most important finding of this study is that we were able to provide solid evidence to show that different zebrafish strains gave similar innate color preference ranking when compared with the AB strain, which has been used as the wild-type control in most experiments. However, each strain seems to exhibit a different choice index. Previous studies have shown that zebrafish color preferences could be different depending on their source population [61]. Fish evolution and development may be reflected in color preferences [62], suggesting that source population, developmental, and evolutionary history may play a role in fish color preference, as seen in the fact that each strain showed a specific choice index. Another study also suggests that evolved and developed zebrafish in different physical environments could have a different color preference, and these preferences could impact their learning abilities [61]. In another species, color may be an important factor in the prey choice of predators [63]. Different species will have different color preferences depending on their favorite prey or food. A certain study manages to examine the reaction of various fish species to different models of foods. They found out that each strain preferred a different color depending on their choice of foods [64]. Our results are consistent with these studies, where the tiger barb and glass catfish exhibit different color preferences compared to zebrafish. Each has a different preferred color. Specifically, the zebrafish prefers red, the glass catfish prefers blue and red, and the tiger barb prefers green. Some studies in cichlid fish showed that different colored environments could induce a variety of changes to the retina, morphologically and physiologically, in support of our study that each species from different environments tends to have a specific color preference. Another study in the barramundi (*Lates calcarifer*) showed that different colored light environments could change fish color preference and shift their visual system. In line with our color preference results that different fish species from diverse environments could exhibit dissimilar color preference ranking or indices, the study also highlighted the relationship between organisms and their visual environment and suggested that color preference could influence animal growth [65].

Depression and anxiety have been linked with color preference changes in humans, and these changes have already been used to determine mental state in physiological studies [66]. Ethanol-treated fish showed a reduction in the choice index in the blue–yellow combination, similar to zebrafish depression behavior reported previously [14]. We also found that ethanol-treated fish exhibited a reduction in the choice index in the green–yellow combination. Ethanol has been known to cause anxiety and depression with long-term usage [67]. In this study, we demonstrated the potential application of the color preference assay for chemical toxicology in a behavioral study.

5. Conclusions

We have optimized the color preference test conditions to highlight the importance of keeping the light intensity constant and the advantage of using multiple shoaling settings to maximize the experimental throughput. We observed no significant effect due to different light positions or tank sizes in this study. We also showed that there was no gender effect on color preference in zebrafish. In addition, our results also highlight that the utilization of the color preference setting reported herein is suitable for performing toxicity assessment by analyzing their color choice indices in different color combinations. Together, we conclude that color preference is a sensitive marker that can be used to identify alteration caused by a compound or environmental change. Result in zebrafish strain tests showed that color preference ranking remains the same, and only the choice indices differ. However, different species such as the tiger barb and glass catfish could exhibit different color preference rankings. The optimized conditions established herein are thus generally applicable to evaluate potential toxicological or pharmaceutical effects of chemicals. A large number of the sample can be easily obtained by using this reported method ($n = 24$ for single videotaping), and we believe that the methodology proposed in the present study provides a robust tool for phenotypic screening for isolation of mutants with color preference deficiency in the future.

Author Contributions: Conceptualization, K.H.-C.C., J.-R.C. and C.-D.H.; methodology and software, P.S., S.J. and G.A.; validation, Y.-H.L. and J.-C.H.; formal analysis and investigation, P.S., S.J. and G.A.; writing—original draft preparation, P.S., S.J., K.H.-C.C., J.-R.C. and C.-D.H.; supervision, C.-D.H.; project administration, C.-D.H.; funding acquisition, K.H.-C.C. and C.-D.H. All authors have read and agreed to the published version of the manuscript.

Funding: This study was supported by the grants sponsored by the Ministry of Science Technology (MOST107-2622-B-033-001-CC2 and MOST108-2622-B-033-001-CC2) to C.-D.H. and MOST108-2113-M153-003 to K.H.-C.C. The funders have no role in study design, data collection and analysis, decision to publish, or preparation of the manuscript.

Acknowledgments: We thank Candy Chen for his assistance in fish care and Taiwan Zebrafish Core Facility at Academia Sinica (TZCAS) for the provision of zebrafish. We appreciate Marri Jmelou Roldan from University of Santo Tomas for providing English editing to enhance the quality of the paper.

Conflicts of Interest: The authors declare no conflicts of interest. The funders had no role in the design of the study; in the collection, analyses, or interpretation of data; in the writing of the manuscript, or in the decision to publish the results.

Appendix A

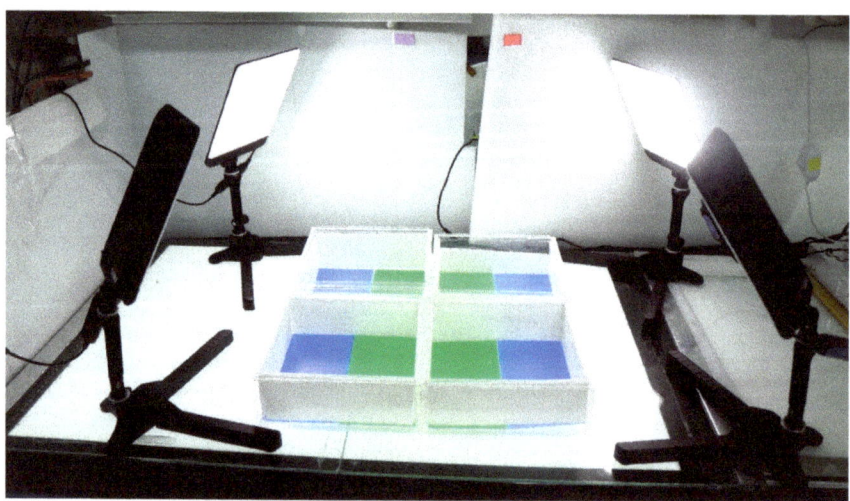

Figure A1. Instrument setting used to perform the color preference test in zebrafish.

Table A1. Illumination condition of the top and bottom light sources.

Color	Bottom Light Intensity (Lux)	Top Light Intensity (Lux)
Red	440	430
Yellow	450	533
Green	430	497
Blue	410	424

Table A2. Wavelength (spectrum), reflectance, and irradiance (emission intensity) of all color plates.

Color	Wavelength Spectrum (nm) and Maximum Wavelength	Reflectance (%)	Irradiance (uWatt/nm)
Red	625–740 (625)	97	0.000489
Yellow	565–590 (572)	99	0.000587
Green	500–565 (541)	100	0.000376
Blue	450–485 (456)	98	0.000358
White	380–700 (561)	100	0.000691
Gray	400–700 (564)	96	0.000207
Black	500–700 (588)	80	0.0000342

Table A3. Comparison of the conditions of the zebrafish innate color preference tests used in various laboratories.

Illumination Direction	Tank Type	Experimental Design	Fish Gender	Fish Strain	Color Preferences Ranking	References
Top	T-Maze with colored plastic sleeves	Single fish	N.D.	AB	Red = Green > Yellow = Blue = No color	[11]
	Two-chambered PP (23 × 15 × 15 cm)	n = 12				
Bottom (LED plate)	Transparent acrylic plastic sheeting with a thickness of 3 mm. The dimensions of the tank 230 × 150 × 150 mm	Single fish	N.D.	AB	Blue > White > Red	[13]
		n = 18				
Top	T-Maze	Single Fish	Male and Female	AB	Blue > Purple > Green > Yellow = Orange > Blank	[3]
		n = 7–10				
Bottom	T-maze setup (Noldus IT (Information Technology))	n = 12	N.D.	AB	Blue > Red > Green > Yellow	[7]
Bottom	Cross maze	Larvae	N.D.	Wild-type purchased from local pet stores	Blue > Red > Green	[6]
		n = 40				
Top (Colored Light)	20 l glass aquaria (40 × 25 × 30 cm)	Group of 10 fish	N.D.	Zebrafish obtained from a commercial supplier	Red > Green > White > Blue	[2]
Bottom	50 cm diameter transparent plastic tanks were divided into four laterals compartments of a similar size of 7 cm	n = 12	N.D.	Zebrafish obtained from a local fish farm	Blue = Green > Red = Yellow	[1]
Top	Cross-maze with sidearm covered in different colors	Single fish	N.D.	AB	Blue > Red = Green > Yellow	[14]
		n minimum = 8				

References

1. Oliveira, J.; Silveira, M.; Chacon, D.; Luchiari, A. The Zebrafish World of Colors and Shapes: Preference and Discrimination. *Zebrafish* **2015**, *12*, 166–173. [CrossRef] [PubMed]
2. Spence, R.; Smith, C. Innate and Learned Colour Preference in the Zebrafish, *Danio rerio*. *Ethology* **2008**, *114*, 582–588. [CrossRef]
3. Bault, Z.A.; Peterson, S.M.; Freeman, J.L. Directional and color preference in adult zebrafish: Implications in behavioral and learning assays in neurotoxicology studies. *J. Appl. Toxicol. JAT* **2015**, *35*, 1502–1510. [CrossRef]
4. Xu, X.; Weber, D.; Burge, R.; VanAmberg, K. Neurobehavioral impairments produced by developmental lead exposure persisted for generations in zebrafish (*Danio rerio*). *Neurotoxicology* **2016**, *52*, 176–185. [CrossRef] [PubMed]

5. Kim, O.H.; Cho, H.J.; Han, E.; Hong, T.I.; Ariyasiri, K.; Choi, J.H.; Hwang, K.S.; Jeong, Y.M.; Yang, S.Y.; Yu, K.; et al. Zebrafish knockout of Down syndrome gene, DYRK1A, shows social impairments relevant to autism. *Mol. Autism* **2017**, *8*. [CrossRef]
6. Park, J.S.; Ryu, J.H.; Choi, T.I.; Bae, Y.K.; Lee, S.; Kang, H.J.; Kim, C.H. Innate Color Preference of Zebrafish and Its Use in Behavioral Analyses. *Mol. Cells* **2016**, *39*, 750–755. [CrossRef]
7. Peeters, B.W.M.M.; Moeskops, M.; Veenvliet, A.R.J. Color Preference in *Danio rerio*: Effects of Age and Anxiolytic Treatments. *Zebrafish* **2016**, *13*, 330–334. [CrossRef]
8. Kim, Y.-H.; Lee, Y.; Kim, D.; Jung, M.W.; Lee, C.-J. Scopolamine-induced learning impairment reversed by physostigmine in zebrafish. *Neurosci. Res.* **2010**, *67*, 156–161. [CrossRef]
9. Yong-seok, C.; Chang-Joong, L.; Yeon-Hwa, K. MK-801-induced learning impairments reversed by physostigmine and nicotine in zebrafish. *Anim. Cells Syst.* **2011**, *15*, 115–121. [CrossRef]
10. Cognato Gde, P.; Bortolotto, J.W.; Blazina, A.R.; Christoff, R.R.; Lara, D.R.; Vianna, M.R.; Bonan, C.D. Y-Maze memory task in zebrafish (*Danio rerio*): The role of glutamatergic and cholinergic systems on the acquisition and consolidation periods. *Neurobiol. Learn. Mem.* **2012**, *98*, 321–328. [CrossRef]
11. Avdesh, A.; Martin-Iverson, M.T.; Mondal, A.; Chen, M.; Askraba, S.; Morgan, N.; Lardelli, M.; Groth, D.M.; Verdile, G.; Martins, R.N. Evaluation of color preference in zebrafish for learning and memory. *J. Alzheimer's Dis. JAD* **2012**, *28*, 459–469. [CrossRef] [PubMed]
12. Spence, R.; Gerlach, G.; Lawrence, C.; Smith, C. The behaviour and ecology of the zebrafish, *Danio rerio*. *Biol. Rev. Camb. Philos. Soc.* **2008**, *83*, 13–34. [CrossRef] [PubMed]
13. Jia, L.; Raghupathy, R.K.; Albalawi, A.; Zhao, Z.; Reilly, J.; Xiao, Q.; Shu, X. A colour preference technique to evaluate acrylamide-induced toxicity in zebrafish. *Comp. Biochem. Physiol. Toxicol. Pharmacol. CBP* **2017**, *199*, 11–19. [CrossRef] [PubMed]
14. Zhang, S.; Liu, X.; Sun, M.; Zhang, Q.; Li, T.; Li, X.; Xu, J.; Zhao, X.; Chen, D.; Feng, X. Reversal of reserpine-induced depression and cognitive disorder in zebrafish by sertraline and Traditional Chinese Medicine (TCM). *Behav. Brain Funct. BBF* **2018**, *14*. [CrossRef] [PubMed]
15. Iovine, M.K.; Johnson, S.L. Genetic analysis of isometric growth control mechanisms in the zebrafish caudal Fin. *Genetics* **2000**, *155*, 1321–1329. [PubMed]
16. Watanabe, M.; Iwashita, M.; Ishii, M.; Kurachi, Y.; Kawakami, A.; Kondo, S.; Okada, N. Spot pattern of leopard Danio is caused by mutation in the zebrafish connexin41. 8 gene. *EMBO Rep.* **2006**, *7*, 893–897. [CrossRef]
17. Trainor, P. *Neural Crest Cells: Evolution, Development and Disease*; Academic Press: Cambridge, MA, USA, 2013.
18. Parichy, D.M.; Mellgren, E.M.; Rawls, J.F.; Lopes, S.S.; Kelsh, R.N.; Johnson, S.L. Mutational analysis of endothelin receptor b1 (rose) during neural crest and pigment pattern development in the zebrafish *Danio rerio*. *Dev. Biol.* **2000**, *227*, 294–306. [CrossRef]
19. Sumbre, G.; De Polavieja, G.G. The world according to zebrafish: How neural circuits generate behavior. *Front. Neural Circuits* **2014**, *8*, 91.
20. Freeman, A.; Holland, R.; Hwang-Shum, J.-J.; Lains, D.; Matthews, J.; Murray, K.; Nasiadka, A.; Quinn, E.; Varga, Z.M.; Westerfield, M. 7 The Zebrafish International Resource Center. *Biol. Resour. Model Org. Collect. Charact. Appl.* **2019**, *1*, 113.
21. Lamason, R.L.; Mohideen, M.-A.P.; Mest, J.R.; Wong, A.C.; Norton, H.L.; Aros, M.C.; Jurynec, M.J.; Mao, X.; Humphreville, V.R.; Humbert, J.E. SLC24A5, a putative cation exchanger, affects pigmentation in zebrafish and humans. *Science* **2005**, *310*, 1782–1786. [CrossRef]
22. Meyer, B.M.; Froehlich, J.M.; Galt, N.J.; Biga, P.R. Inbred strains of zebrafish exhibit variation in growth performance and myostatin expression following fasting. *Comp. Biochem. Physiol. Part A Mol. Integr. Physiol.* **2013**, *164*, 1–9. [CrossRef] [PubMed]
23. Pérez-Escudero, A.; Vicente-Page, J.; Hinz, R.C.; Arganda, S.; de Polavieja, G.G. idTracker: Tracking individuals in a group by automatic identification of unmarked animals. *Nat. Methods* **2014**, *11*, 743. [CrossRef] [PubMed]
24. Lau, B.Y.B.; Mathur, P.; Gould, G.G.; Guo, S. Identification of a brain center whose activity discriminates a choice behavior in zebrafish. *Proc. Natl. Acad. Sci. USA* **2011**, *108*, 2581–2586. [CrossRef] [PubMed]
25. Zhang, B.; Yao, Y.; Zhang, H.; Kawakami, K.; Du, J. Left habenula mediates light-preference behavior in zebrafish via an asymmetrical visual pathway. *Neuron* **2017**, *93*, 914–928.e914. [CrossRef]

26. E Engeszer, R.; Alberici Da Barbiano, L.; Ryan, M.; M Parichy, D. Timing and Plasticity of Shoaling Behavior in the Zebrafish, *Danio rerio*. *Anim. Behav.* **2007**, *74*, 1269–1275. [CrossRef]
27. Norton, W.; Bally-Cuif, L. Adult zebrafish as a model organism for behavioural genetics. *BMC Neurosci.* **2010**, *11*, 90. [CrossRef]
28. Okiyama, D.C.; Soares, I.D.; Cuevas, M.S.; Crevelin, E.J.; Moraes, L.A.; Melo, M.P.; Oliveira, A.L.; Rodrigues, C.E. Pressurized liquid extraction of flavanols and alkaloids from cocoa bean shell using ethanol as solvent. *Food Res. Int.* **2018**, *114*, 20–29. [CrossRef]
29. Baümler, E.R.; Carrín, M.E.; Carelli, A.A. Extraction of sunflower oil using ethanol as solvent. *J. Food Eng.* **2016**, *178*, 190–197. [CrossRef]
30. Santamaria, R.; Reyes-Duarte, M.; Barzana, E.; Fernando, D.; Gama, F.; Mota, M.; Lopez-Munguia, A. Selective enzyme-mediated extraction of capsaicinoids and carotenoids from chili guajillo puya (*Capsicum annuum* L.) using ethanol as solvent. *J. Agric. Food Chem.* **2000**, *48*, 3063–3067. [CrossRef]
31. Barnes, G. The effects of ethyl alcohol on visual pursuit and suppression of the vestibulo-ocular reflex. *Acta Oto-Laryngol.* **1983**, *96*, 161–166. [CrossRef]
32. Barnes, G.; Crombie, J.; Edge, A. The effects of ethanol on visual–vestibular interaction during active and passive head movements. *Aviat. Space Environ. Med.* **1985**, *56*, 695–701. [PubMed]
33. Umeda, Y.; Sakata, E. Alcohol and the oculomotor system. *Ann. Otol. Rhinol. Laryngol.* **1978**, *87*, 392–398. [CrossRef] [PubMed]
34. Wilkinson, I. The influence of drugs and alcohol upon human eye movement. *Proc. R. Soc. Med.* **1976**, *69*, 479. [PubMed]
35. Aschan, G. Different types of alcohol nystagmus. *Acta Oto-Laryngol.* **1958**, *49*, 69–78. [CrossRef]
36. Baloh, R.; Sharma, S.; Moskowitz, H.; Griffith, R. Effect of alcohol and marihuana on eye movements. *Aviat. Space Environ. Med.* **1979**, *50*, 18–23.
37. Harder, T.; Reker, U. Influence of low dose alcohol on fixation suppression. *Acta Oto-Laryngol.* **1995**, *115*, 33–36. [CrossRef]
38. Takahashi, M.; Akiyama, I.; Tsujita, N.; Yoshida, A. The effect of alcohol on the vestibulo-ocular reflex and gaze regulation. *Arch. Oto-Rhino Laryngol.* **1989**, *246*, 195–199. [CrossRef]
39. Matsui, J.I.; Egana, A.L.; Sponholtz, T.R.; Adolph, A.R.; Dowling, J.E. Effects of ethanol on photoreceptors and visual function in developing zebrafish. *Investig. Ophthalmol. Vis. Sci.* **2006**, *47*, 4589–4597. [CrossRef]
40. Miller, R. The effect of ingested alcohol on fusion latency at various viewing distances. *Percept. Psychophys.* **1991**, *50*, 575–583. [CrossRef]
41. Sherwin, C.M.; Glen, E.F. Cage colour preferences and effects of home cage colour on anxiety in laboratory mice. *Anim. Behav.* **2003**, *66*, 1085–1092. [CrossRef]
42. Lunau, K.; Papiorek, S.; Eltz, T.; Sazima, M. Avoidance of achromatic colours by bees provides a private niche for hummingbirds. *J. Exp. Biol.* **2011**, *214*, 1607–1612. [CrossRef] [PubMed]
43. Endler, J.A.; Westcott, D.A.; Madden, J.R.; Robson, T. Animal visual systems and the evolution of color patterns: Sensory processing illuminates signal evolution. *Evolution* **2005**, *59*, 1795–1818. [CrossRef] [PubMed]
44. Dangles, O.; Irschick, D.; Chittka, L.; Casas, J. Variability in sensory ecology: Expanding the bridge between physiology and evolutionary biology. *Q. Rev. Biol.* **2009**, *84*, 51–74. [CrossRef] [PubMed]
45. Cachat, J.; Stewart, A.; Utterback, E.; Hart, P.; Gaikwad, S.; Wong, K.; Kyzar, E.; Wu, N.; Kalueff, A.V. Three-dimensional neurophenotyping of adult zebrafish behavior. *PLoS ONE* **2011**, *6*, e17597. [CrossRef] [PubMed]
46. Faustino, A.I.; Tacão-Monteiro, A.; Oliveira, R.F. Mechanisms of social buffering of fear in zebrafish. *Sci. Rep.* **2017**, *7*, 44329. [CrossRef]
47. Agrillo, C.; Piffer, L.; Bisazza, A. Number versus continuous quantity in numerosity judgments by fish. *Cognition* **2011**, *119*, 281–287. [CrossRef]
48. Morris, A.; Fadool, J. Studying rod photoreceptor development in zebrafish. *Physiol. Behav.* **2005**, *86*, 306–313. [CrossRef]
49. Bai, Y.; Liu, H.; Huang, B.; Wagle, M.; Guo, S. Identification of environmental stressors and validation of light preference as a measure of anxiety in larval zebrafish. *BMC Neurosci.* **2016**, *17*, 63. [CrossRef]
50. Maximino, C.; de Brito, T.M.; de Mattos Dias, C.A.G.; Gouveia, A.J.; Morato, S. Scototaxis as anxiety-like behavior in fish. *Nat. Protoc.* **2010**, *5*, 209. [CrossRef]

51. Bilotta, J. Effects of abnormal lighting on the development of zebrafish visual behavior. *Behav. Brain Res.* **2000**, *116*, 81–87. [CrossRef]
52. Anchelin, M.; Alcaraz-Pérez, F.; Martínez, C.M.; Bernabé-García, M.; Mulero, V.; Cayuela, M.L. Premature aging in telomerase-deficient zebrafish. *Dis. Models Mech.* **2013**, *6*, 1101–1112. [CrossRef]
53. Chinen, A.; Hamaoka, T.; Yamada, Y.; Kawamura, S. Gene duplication and spectral diversification of cone visual pigments of zebrafish. *Genetics* **2003**, *163*, 663–675. [PubMed]
54. Nawrocki, L.; Bremiller, R.; Streisinger, G.; Kaplan, M. Larval and adult visual pigments of the zebrafish, *Brachydanio rerio*. *Vis. Res.* **1985**, *25*, 1569–1576. [CrossRef]
55. Branchek, T. The development of photoreceptors in the zebrafish, *brachyDanio rerio*. II. Function. *J. Comp. Neurol.* **1984**, *224*, 116–122. [CrossRef] [PubMed]
56. Robinson, J.; Schmitt, E.A.; Dowling, J.E. Temporal and spatial patterns of opsin gene expression in zebrafish (*Danio rerio*). *Vis. Neurosci.* **1995**, *12*, 895–906. [CrossRef]
57. Saszik, S.; Bilotta, J.; Givin, C.M. ERG assessment of zebrafish retinal development. *Vis. Neurosci.* **1999**, *16*, 881–888. [CrossRef]
58. Korenbrot, J.I.; Mehta, M.; Tserentsoodol, N.; Postlethwait, J.H.; Rebrik, T.I. EML1 (CNG-modulin) controls light sensitivity in darkness and under continuous illumination in zebrafish retinal cone photoreceptors. *J. Neurosci.* **2013**, *33*, 17763–17776. [CrossRef]
59. Blaser, R.E.; Rosemberg, D.B. Measures of anxiety in zebrafish (*Danio rerio*): Dissociation of black/white preference and novel tank test. *PLoS ONE* **2012**, *7*, e36931. [CrossRef]
60. Pieróg, M.; Guz, L.; Doboszewska, U.; Poleszak, E.; Wlaź, P. Effects of alprazolam treatment on anxiety-like behavior induced by color stimulation in adult zebrafish. *Prog. Neuro Psychopharmacol. Biol. Psychiatry* **2018**, *82*, 297–306. [CrossRef]
61. Roy, T.; Suriyampola, P.S.; Flores, J.; López, M.; Hickey, C.; Bhat, A.; Martins, E.P. Color preferences affect learning in zebrafish, *Danio rerio*. *Sci. Rep.* **2019**, *9*, 14531. [CrossRef]
62. Fuller, R.C.; Noa, L.A.; Strellner, R.S. Teasing apart the many effects of lighting environment on opsin expression and foraging preference in bluefin killifish. *Am. Nat.* **2010**, *176*, 1–13. [CrossRef] [PubMed]
63. Johnsen, S. Cryptic and conspicuous coloration in the pelagic environment. *Proc. R. Soc. Lond. Ser. B Biol. Sci.* **2002**, *269*, 243–256. [CrossRef]
64. Protasov, V.R. *Vision and Near Orientation of Fish*; Israel Program for Scientific Translations: Jerusalem, Israel, 1970; Volume 5738.
65. Ullmann, J.F.; Gallagher, T.; Hart, N.S.; Barnes, A.C.; Smullen, R.P.; Collin, S.P.; Temple, S.E. Tank color increases growth, and alters color preference and spectral sensitivity, in barramundi (Lates calcarifer). *Aquaculture* **2011**, *322*, 235–240. [CrossRef]
66. Carruthers, H.R.; Morris, J.; Tarrier, N.; Whorwell, P.J. The Manchester Color Wheel: Development of a novel way of identifying color choice and its validation in healthy, anxious and depressed individuals. *BMC Med. Res. Methodol.* **2010**, *10*, 12. [CrossRef] [PubMed]
67. Langen, B.; Dietze, S.; Fink, H. Acute effect of ethanol on anxiety and 5-HT in the prefrontal cortex of rats. *Alcohol* **2002**, *27*, 135–141. [CrossRef]

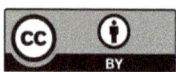

© 2020 by the authors. Licensee MDPI, Basel, Switzerland. This article is an open access article distributed under the terms and conditions of the Creative Commons Attribution (CC BY) license (http://creativecommons.org/licenses/by/4.0/).

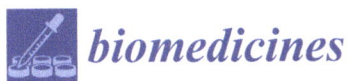

Review

Marijuana and Opioid Use during Pregnancy: Using Zebrafish to Gain Understanding of Congenital Anomalies Caused by Drug Exposure during Development

Swapnalee Sarmah [1],*, Marilia Ribeiro Sales Cadena [2], Pabyton Gonçalves Cadena [3] and James A. Marrs [1],*

1. Department of Biology, Indiana University Purdue University Indianapolis, 723 West Michigan St., Indianapolis, IN 46202, USA
2. Departamento de Biologia (DB), Universidade Federal Rural de Pernambuco. Av. Dom Manoel de Medeiros s/n, 52171-900 Dois Irmãos, Recife - PE, Brasil; marilia.sales@ufrpe.br
3. Departamento de Morfologia e Fisiologia Animal (DMFA), Universidade Federal Rural de Pernambuco. Av. Dom Manoel de Medeiros s/n, 52171-900 Dois Irmãos, Recife - PE, Brasil; pabyton.cadena@ufrpe.br
* Correspondence: ssarmah@iupui.edu (S.S.); jmarrs@iupui.edu (J.A.M.); Tel.: +1-317-274-7202 (S.S.); +1-317-278-0031 (J.A.M.)

Received: 4 July 2020; Accepted: 6 August 2020; Published: 8 August 2020

Abstract: Marijuana and opioid addictions have increased alarmingly in recent decades, especially in the United States, posing threats to society. When the drug user is a pregnant mother, there is a serious risk to the developing baby. Congenital anomalies are associated with prenatal exposure to marijuana and opioids. Here, we summarize the current data on the prevalence of marijuana and opioid use among the people of the United States, particularly pregnant mothers. We also summarize the current zebrafish studies used to model and understand the effects of these drug exposures during development and to understand the behavioral changes after exposure. Zebrafish experiments recapitulate the drug effects seen in human addicts and the birth defects seen in human babies prenatally exposed to marijuana and opioids. Zebrafish show great potential as an easy and inexpensive model for screening compounds for their ability to mitigate the drug effects, which could lead to new therapeutics.

Keywords: marijuana; opioid; congenital anomalies; THC; CBD; morphine; codeine; zebrafish; birth defects

1. Introduction

The status of marijuana legislation for medical and recreational purposes has changed in many states of the United States in recent years. As of 2020, 33 states and the District of Columbia of the United States passed laws that broadly legalized marijuana in some form. Out of those 33 states, 11 states and the District of Columbia have adopted the legalization of recreational marijuana [1]. This change has altered societal views on the use of marijuana, making the attitude more permissive. The benefit of medical marijuana for the treatment of many illnesses, including chronic pain, nausea, and various neurological symptoms has become increasingly clear. Importantly, the Food and Drug Administration (FDA) approved Epidiolex (plant-based prescription cannabidiol (CBD)) for the treatment of people aged 2 years and older to treat drug-resistant epilepsies like Dravet syndrome and Lennox–Gastaut syndrome (LGS). No matter how beneficial its therapeutic properties are, all marijuana products have side effects. The gaining popularity, the potential benefits, and easy access to marijuana are making people more reluctant to consider its adverse effects. The report from the 2017 National Survey on

Drug Use and Health (NSDUH) estimated 30.5 million people aged 12 or older used an illicit drug in the past 30 days (i.e., current use) [2]. Among these 30.5 million illicit drug users, 26.0 million were marijuana users, and 3.2 million misuse prescription pain relievers [2]. Notably, the potency of cannabis in marijuana products has shifted during the last two decades. A recent study has shown the overall increase in active ingredient content in the cannabis products, with greatly increased ∆9-tetrahydrocannabinol (THC: a psychoactive component from 3.4% in 1993 to 8.8% in 2008) relative to cannabidiol (a non-psychoactive component) [3,4]. These changes in use and potency of marijuana pose a high risk to the cannabis user [3].

Opioids are neuroactive drugs that are derived from the opium poppy (opiate) or synthesized in the laboratory (opioid). These drugs produce strong sedation, analgesia, and sleep. The use of opioids often begins with a prescription for acute pain treatment [5], but its long-term use can escalate to high doses, leading to addiction and overdose deaths [6]. Opioid overdoses have significantly increased in recent years. According to the World Health Organization, this increase is partly because of their frequent use as a pain medication to manage chronic non-cancer pain [7].

In the United States, opioid use either as prescription pain medications or as an illegal drug is widespread. There was an estimated 63,632 deaths due to drug overdose in the United States in 2016, out of which 19,413 deaths were associated with prescription opioids [7]. This was twice as high as the number in 2015 [7]. In 2018, ~67% of drug-related deaths (47,600 out of 70,237) involved opioid use [8]. The report from the 2017 NSDUH estimated that 11.4 million people aged 12 or older misused opioids in the past year, including 11.1 million pain reliever misusers and 886,000 heroin users. The majority of those people (62.6 percent) misused them to relieve physical pain [2].

2. Trends of Marijuana and Opioid Use during Pregnancy in Recent Decades

Increasingly, women of childbearing age use marijuana or opioids, which makes them very commonly used dependent substances during pregnancy in the United States after alcohol and tobacco [9,10]. Despite the fact that many states in the United States have adopted to legalize marijuana, none of the states have any regulation on its use during pregnancy. Cerdá M. et al. showed that the states with legal medical marijuana laws have significantly higher rates of marijuana use, abuse, and dependence compared to the states without such laws [11]. A nationwide study examining the prevalence of marijuana use among pregnant women using NSDUH data from 2007 to 2012 found out that 3.9% of pregnant women used marijuana in the previous month [12]. Another study used the NSDUH data from 2005 to 2014 and compared the marijuana use prevalence among married and unmarried pregnant women. This study showed that prenatal marijuana uses among unmarried women increased by 85% from 5.4% to 10% from 2005 to 2014, while the prevalence among married pregnant women remained mostly stable (1.5%) [13]. From 2009 through 2016, prenatal marijuana use in California increased from 4.2% to 7.1% [12,14]. Many women use marijuana to reduce morning sickness. This increasing trend of marijuana use by pregnant women is a great concern, especially when marijuana products contain high THC levels.

Opioid-containing medications are widely prescribed among reproductive-aged women with either private insurance or Medicaid [15]. In the United States, opioid overdose deaths among women increased more than five-fold between 1999 and 2010, and emergency department visits for misuse or abuse were even more frequent. For every opioid overdose death, there was about 30 emergency department visits [16]. Patrick et al. [17] found that 28% of around 112,000 pregnant women in the United States were prescribed opioid pain medication at least once during pregnancy, out of which 96.2% were short-acting opioid pain relievers. A study looking at the data from 2000 to 2007 with 1.1 million Medicaid-enrolled women from 46 U.S. states and Washington, DC found that one out of five women from that cohort of patients filled an opioid prescription during pregnancy [18]. The authors found that there was an increase in opioid prescriptions, especially codeine and hydrocodone, from 18.5% in 2000 to 22.8% in 2007 [18]. They also found a substantial regional variation in opioid prescription use during pregnancy ranging between 9.5% and 41.6% across the states. Another study of 534,500 women with completed pregnancies between 2005 and 2011 showed that 14.4% had an opioid prescription dispensed at some point during pregnancy. Of these, 2.2% had opioids dispensed three or more times during pregnancy [19]. This study, however, observed that there was a decline in opioid prescriptions to pregnant women from 14.9% to 12.9% between 2005 to 2011 [19]. A study done by the Centers for Disease Control and Prevention (CDC) estimated the proportion of privately insured and Medicaid-enrolled reproductive-aged women (15–44 years) who filled a prescription of opioid-containing medications from an outpatient pharmacy during 2008 to 2012, finding that approximately one in four privately insured and over one in three Medicaid-enrolled women filled a prescription for an opioid each year during that time. This study also found that an average of three opioids were prescribed for every four privately insured women and nearly two opioids were prescribed for each Medicaid-enrolled woman per year [15]. This increasing trend of opioid use by women of reproductive age is a great concern because 50% of pregnancies in the United States are unintended [15], and so, the exposure to the opioid during early prenatal development in unrecognized pregnancies is very likely.

These data on the marijuana and opioid use by reproductive-age women and pregnant mothers are alarming, which raises serious public health concerns as there is evidence of adverse pregnancy outcomes with prenatal marijuana or opioid exposure [20–24].

3. Patterns of Congenital Defects and Behavioral Changes Seen in Children Exposed to Marijuana in Utero

With the concern that legalization is making marijuana use more prevalent among pregnant women, Reece et. al. analyzed the overall patterns of birth defects in babies, without considering maternal age, in Colorado from 2000 to 2014 using data from the Colorado Responds to Children with Special Needs, the NSDUH, and the Drug Enforcement Agency [25]. This study identified multiple congenital defects that rose 5 to 37 times faster than the birth rate (3.3%) to generate in excess of 11,753 (22%) major anomalies. Those defects include cardiovascular (atrial septal defect, ventricular septal defect, patent ductus arteriosus, and others), spina bifida, microcephalus, Down's syndrome, central nervous system, genitourinary, respiratory, chromosomal, and musculoskeletal defects [25]. They also showed that cannabis was the only drug whose use grew during that period, while other drugs like pain relievers, cocaine, alcohol, and tobacco did not [25]. This study indicates a connection between congenital defects and marijuana use among Coloradans. However, in a previous study done by Marleen et. al. looking at the babies born with and without major congenital malformations between 1997 to 2003 compared with in utero illicit drug exposure, the investigators did not find associations between birth defects and mother's drug use (including marijuana) during pregnancy. They interviewed 15,208 mothers and examined 20 eligible categories of congenital malformations. Five percent of those mothers reported use of illicit drugs during pregnancy. However, they found the association between periconceptional cannabis use with an increased risk of anencephaly [26]. Other studies found links between in utero marijuana exposure to visual problem solving, visual-motor coordination, visual analysis, attention deficit, and behavioral problems [27,28]. Prenatal marijuana exposure was shown to be a significant predictor of marijuana use by adolescents [29].

4. Patterns of Congenital Defects and Behavioral Changes Seen after Prenatal Exposure to Opioid in Humans

The effect of prenatal exposure to opioids has been studied in recent years. Broussard et al. [30] described a correlation between opioid analgesic treatment in early pregnancy and certain birth defects, such as congenital heart disease, spina bifida, hydrocephaly, glaucoma, anterior chamber eye defects, and gastroschisis. Yazdy et al. [31] reported a two-fold increase risk of neural tube defects, including spina bifida, with maternal periconceptional opioid use. Minnes et al. [32] reviewed potential impacts on the development of the central nervous system and cognitive function associated with prenatal exposure to opiates and described less rhythmic swallowing, strabismus, possible cognitive delay, and defects in cognitive function. Moreover, autonomic dysregulation and nystagmus were associated with prenatal opiate exposed children [33]. Lind et al. [34] reported heart malformations as the most frequently reported malformations, followed by spina bifida and clubfoot in their systematic review of congenital defects related to maternal opioid use during pregnancy. However, the authors were concerned about the quality of the papers reviewed because of the lack of randomized control trials or other weaknesses found in the pregnancy literature on most medications. Maternal age was not taken into account in any of these studies.

Prenatal exposure to opiates leads to changes in behavior in babies. The prenatally opioid exposed neonate experiences opioid withdrawal symptoms because of the sudden discontinuation of the opioid after birth. Neonatal abstinence syndrome (NAS) is a postnatal drug abstinence syndrome characterized by a wide range of signs and symptoms including irritability, tremors, hypertonia, feeding intolerance, emesis, watery stools, seizures, and respiratory distress [17,23]. NAS-related withdrawal symptoms were recorded in 60 to 80 percent of newborns who were exposed to opioids such as heroin and methadone in utero [17]. The CDC reported diagnosis of seven NAS cases every 1000 newborn hospitalizations nationwide in 2016, which is three-fold higher than in 2008 (2.2 out of 1000 newborn) [35,36]. This is equivalent to 80 newborns with NAS every day [35,36]. In 1998, Bunikowski et al. reported NAS in the majority of drug-exposed infants during their first days of life. The researchers also found that children who are prenatally exposed to opiates had a mild developmental delay in the psychomotor system [37]. Minnes et al. [32] reviewed literature on potential impacts of prenatal opiate exposure and found a clear association between opiate exposure and anxiety, aggression, feelings of rejection, disruptive or inattentive behavior in babies. Recently, Conradt et al. reviewed the current literature to determine the short- and long-term neurodevelopmental outcomes of children with prenatal opioid exposure [38]. They also observed the symptoms in neonates as stated above. In addition, they showed that prenatal methadone or heroin exposure was associated with impaired mental, language, neuromotor, and psychomotor development. However, some of the studies they reviewed failed to account for important confounding variables or include a control group of unexposed children [38]. Lower IQ scores, differences in neurologic performance and language performance during elementary school education was also reported in the children exposed to opioids in utero. An increase in attention deficit hyperactivity disorder was observed in the children exposed to heroin in utero [33]. Children exposed to opioids prenatally also showed significantly lower visual–motor and perceptual performance scores [38].

These associations between in utero drug exposure and birth defects underscore the importance of understanding the mechanisms by which different opioids and marijuana ingredients cause birth defects. Different animal models are used to study the connections and mechanisms of opioid or marijuana use and specific birth defects [39].

5. Zebrafish: A Model System to Study the Effect of Marijuana and Opioid on Development and Behavior

Zebrafish is an outstanding model system to study vertebrate development. It is increasingly becoming a popular model to study the effects of exposure to different compounds during development because of its various advantages compared to the avian or mammalian systems [40–46]. It is easy to expose externally fertilized embryos to different drugs and to monitor their effects on development in transparent embryos. The developmental processes, genes, and regulatory networks are highly conserved between zebrafish and human. The zebrafish has been extensively used to study congenital defects including heart, eye, and neurodevelopmental defects caused by alcohol exposure [47–54] or the exposure to different environmental toxicants during development [43]. The zebrafish studies can dissect cellular and molecular changes during early embryogenesis (gastrulation) due to alcohol exposure [49,51]. Although the zebrafish brain is much simpler than a mammalian brain, it has a homologous organization, similar cellular morphology, and neurochemistry with mammals. Zebrafish larvae and adults have increasingly been used to study the nervous system, brain disorders, including disorders due to abuse of drugs seen in complex behaviors. Kalueff et al. wrote a comprehensive review showing striking similarities between zebrafish and mammalian brain biology and neurochemistry [55]. Zebrafish display anxiety, stress, and mood disorders, like other vertebrates [55,56]. Behaviors such as environment exploration, preference for light/dark environments, bottom-dwelling, peripheral preference, freezing/immobility, and irregular movements are used to measure anxiety, stress, and mood [57]. Behavioral phenotypes observed in zebrafish are strikingly similar to those observed in humans and rodents [55,57]. Thus, major brain disorders can be modeled in zebrafish in a cost-effective and simple way. As with any animal models in biomedicine, zebrafish have limitations and cannot fully recapitulate complex human brain disorders. Furthermore, some brain regions are less evolved than in mammals (e.g., the cerebral cortex) [57]. While some features, like neural physiology complexity, have been studied in less detail in zebrafish than mammalian models; the simplicity of the zebrafish model combined with genetic and genomic knowledge makes it attractive and useful [57].

5.1. Zebrafish Endocannabinoid Biology: A Gene-Level Comparison with Human

The human endocannabinoid system (eCBs) is composed of a set of cannabinoid receptors (mainly CNR1 and CNR2), endogenous cannabinoid ligands (2-arachidonoylglycerol, 2-AG; anandamide, AEA), different enzymes responsible for biosynthesis of cannabinoids (e.g., diacylglycerol lipase, DAGLa and DAGLb; ab-hydrolase domain containing 4, ABHD4; N-acyl phosphatidylethanolamine phospholipase D, NAPE-PLD; Glycerophosphodiester phosphodiesterase 1, GDE1) and degradation of cannabinoids (e.g., ab-hydrolase domain containing 6b, ABHD6B; fatty acid amide hydrolase families, FAAH and FAAH2A; monoglyceride lipase, MGLL) [58,59]. Unlike invertebrates, the eCB system is highly conserved between zebrafish and mammals, including humans. The zebrafish contain orthologs of all human cannabinoid signaling genes except N-acylethanolamine acid amidase gene [40,58,59]. Another difference is that zebrafish have two homologs for each of the four human genes FAAH2, PTGS2, TRPA1, and PPARA. Zebrafish Cnr1 and Cnr2 share 75% and 46% identity with their human counterparts [40,58].

An extensive body of research on the expression and the functions of zebrafish eCB genes are summarized in recent reviews [40,45,58,59]. During development, the expression of zebrafish cannabinoid receptor 1 (*cnr1*) was first detected in the pre-optic area as early as 1 day post fertilization (dpf). At the later larval stage, *cnr1* expression was detected in different parts of the brain, including the telencephalon, hypothalamus, tegmentum, and anterior hindbrain. Examining the expression in adult zebrafish brain showed a similar expression pattern [58,60–62]. Francesca et. al. detected high level cannabinoid receptor 2 (*cnr2*) mRNA expression as early as 4 hours post fertilization (hpf) [58]. The expression was reduced by 12 hpf and then went up again. In adults, *cnr2* mRNA was detected in gills, heart, intestine, muscle, spleen, and central nervous system [63].

The mRNAs encoding *dagla* and *daglb*, enzymes involved in the biosynthesis of the most abundant endocannabinoid 2-AG, were first detected during the early cleavage period suggesting that these mRNAs were maternally transmitted [58]. However, *dagla* and *daglb* were not detected during gastrulation and somitogenesis but detected again after 1 dpf [58]. In situ hybridization showed the expression of *dagla* throughout the anterior and posterior hindbrain at 2 dpf [62]. The mRNA expression of *nape-pld*, *abhd4*, and *gde1*, gene encoding enzymes involved in the synthesis of AEA, showed similar pattern as *dagl* genes. These genes also appeared to be maternally transmitted and were degraded during the pre-gastrulation period [58]. Francesca et. al. examined the expression until 4 dpf and showed that the zygotic expression begins around somitogenesis, which persisted at all time points that they examined [58].

The mRNAs encoding 2-AG degrading enzymes, *mgll*, and *abhd6a* were detected at low levels during early embryogenesis through organogenesis [58]. The 2-AG degrading enzyme *abhd12* was maternally transmitted, and its expression was high during early embryogenesis. The expression of *abhd12* was detected at all stages tested, until 4 dpf [58]. The mRNAs encoding proteins Faah and Faah2a, enzymes that degrade AEA, were detected at 1 hpf embryos, suggesting that those genes were maternally transmitted [58]. Zygotic transcripts were detected from 1 dpf until 4 dpf, the stages tested [58]. Table 1 summarizes the expression patterns of the zebrafish endocannabinoid signaling genes.

Table 1. Expression patterns of the zebrafish endocannabinoid signaling genes.

Gene Name	Maternal Deposition (Detected by RT-PCR)	First Zygotic Expression (Detected by RT-PCR)	Expressions in the Tissue (Detected by in situ Hybridization)
cannabinoid receptor 1 (cnr1)	yes [58]	1 dpf [58]	pre-optic area at 30 hpf; telencephalon, diencephalon, and midbrain at 50 hpf; olfactory bulb, midbrain, endoderm and liver at 72 and 96 hpf
cannabinoid receptor 2 (cnr2)	yes [58]	4 hpf * [58]	developing central nervous system at 24, and 48 hpf [64]; developing central nervous system, endoderm and liver at 72 and 96 hpf [64]
diacylglycerol lipase 1a (dagla)	yes (low expression) [58]	4 hpf * [58]	whole organism at 5–9 somite [65]; cranial ganglion, hindbrain, hypothalamus, midbrain, tegmentum, telencephalon at 48 hpf [62]
diacylglycerol lipase 1b (daglb)	yes (high expression) [58]	4 hpf * [58]	no in situ data at the embryo/larval stage
N-acyl phosphatidyl-ethanolamine phospholipase d (napepld)	yes (low expression) [58]	4 hpf * [58]	whole organism from 5 somite to 4 dpf [65]
ab-hydrolase domain containing 4 (abhd4)	yes (high expression) [58]	4 hpf * [58]	whole organism from 1 cell to 4 dpf [65,66],
Glycerophospho-diester phosphodiesterase 1 (gde1)	yes (high expression) [58]	4 hpf * [58]	basal level expression throughout the body at 1 cell to pec-fin stage [66].
ab-hydrolase domain containing 6a (abhd6a)	yes (low expression) [58]	24 hpf [58]	no in situ data available
ab-hydrolase domain containing 6b (abhd6b)	yes (moderate expression) [57]	72 hpf [58]	no in situ data available
ab-hydrolase domain containing 12 (abhd12)	yes (high expression) [57]	4 hpf [58]	brain, gill, neuromast at 5dpf [67]
fatty acid amide hydrolase family (faah)	yes [57]	24 hpf [58]	intestinal bulb, liver at long-pec to 4 dpf [68]
fatty acid amide hydrolase family 2a (faah2a)	yes [58]	24 hpf [58]	intestinal bulb, liver at long-pec to 4 dpf [66,68]
fatty acid amide hydrolase family 2a (faah2a)	yes [68]	3 hpf	intestinal bulb, liver at long-pec to 4 dpf [68]
monoglyceride lipase (mgll)	no [58]	4 hpf [58]	whole organism at 5–9 somite [65] brain, eye, pectoral fin, pronephric duct, pharynx at stages 26 somite to long-pec [65,69].

* the expression level varies at different developmental stages and peaks at different times.

Receptor-binding assays were done to examine if typical cannabinoid ligands for mammalian receptors can similarly bind to the zebrafish eCB receptors [70,71]. The study using the zebrafish brain homogenates and radiolabelled cannabinoid showed that a few typical cannabinoids did not fully recognize the cannabinoid-binding sites in zebrafish brain, but HU-210, WIN55212-2 and CP55940 bind to zebrafish eCB receptors very well. The affinity of the cannabinoids was determined as HU-210 > WIN55212-2 > CP55940 >anandamide [58,59,70]. Connors et al. showed that radiolabeled WIN55212-2 binds to the hypothalamus, optic tectum, and telencephalon targets in adult zebrafish brain sections [58,71].

The interactions of zebrafish receptors with those synthetic cannabinoids and the similarity in expression of zebrafish eCB genes with mammalian cannabinoid (CB) genes suggest that zebrafish CB signaling may serve the same function as mammalian CB signaling [59], and hence, zebrafish are a potentially useful model to study the effects of cannabinoid abuse on development and behavior.

5.2. Zebrafish Opioid Biology—Why the Zebrafish Is a Useful System to Study the Effects of Opioids

The human opioid signaling system consists of primarily three classical opioid receptors: the mu-opioid receptor (MORP), the kappa-opioid receptor (KORP), and the delta-opioid receptor (DORP). The fourth opioid receptor is nociception receptor (NOP). The NOP system is considered to be a part of the opioid system, although it produces antiopioid actions depending on the region in which it is expressed in the brain. These receptors are activated by endogenous ligands ß-endorphin (MORP ligand), dynorphin (KORP ligand), enkephalin and deltorphin (DORP ligand), nociceptin/orphanin FQ (N/OFQ) (NOP ligand) that result in physiological effects including analgesia, dysphoria, water diuresis, and antipruritic effects [40,45]. These ligands are derived from precursor compounds that are produced by the genes POMC, PENK, PDYN, and PNOC.

All four opioid receptors, the mu-opioid receptor, the kappa-opioid receptor, the delta-opioid receptor, and the nociception receptors are present in zebrafish [40,45]. Zebrafish have single homologs (*oprm1*, *oprk1*, *oprl1*) for three of the human opioid receptor genes, but the gene encoding delta-opioid receptor has a pair of homologs *oprd1a* and *oprd1b* [40,45]. Zebrafish and human opioid receptor genes and proteins share an average of 72% (range: 64%–77%) and of 87% (range: 77%–100%) identity, respectively [40,45]. Zebrafish has single homolog for *pdyn* but two copies of *pomc*, *penk*, and *pnoc* homologs [40,45]. The expression analyses of zebrafish opioid receptor genes showed that all opioid receptor genes are expressed during the first day of development, although *opkr1* expression is very low [45,72]. Robust expression of *oprm1* starts as early as 3 hpf, but high levels of *oprd1a* and *oprd1b* were detected first at 22 hpf [45,72]. The levels of expression for these receptors vary during different developmental stages, peaking at different times. The transcripts encoding NOP (*oprl1*) was detected at 0.5 hpf, which suggests that it is deposited maternally. Its expression was detected throughout embryonic development [73]. The expression of *oprk1* was first detected at 48 hpf [45].

In situ hybridization detected wide expressions of *opmr1* and *opd1b* in multiple CNS structures, including the telencephalon, epiphysis, diencephalon, midbrain, isthmus, cerebellum, pretectum, and hindbrain at 24 hpf, although the *opd1b* expression was weaker than *opmr1* [45,72]. Additional expression of *opd1b* was detected in the myotomes and spinal cord [72]. The expression patterns of these genes were more defined and at different CNS structures at 48 hpf [45,72]. The localization of *oprd1a* was detected in the telencephalon, epiphysis, pretectum, and cerebellum at 24 hpf and the hindbrain, spinal cord, and tegmentum at 30–36 hpf [45,72]. Table 2 summarizes the expression patterns of the zebrafish opioid signaling genes.

In general, the opioid receptors in zebrafish have analogous, conserved functions and pharmacological properties when compared to mammalian proteins, but there are differences in ligand selectivity between species caused by evolutionary changes of their receptor sequences [82].

Table 2. Expression patterns of the zebrafish opioid signaling genes.

Gene Name	Maternal Deposition (Detected by RT-PCR)	First Zygotic Expression (Detected by RT-PCR)	Expressions in the Tissue (Detected by in situ Hybridization)
mu-opioid receptor (oprm1)	yes [72]	3 hpf * [45,72]	telencephalon, epiphysis, diencephalon, midbrain, isthmus, cerebellum, pretectum, and hindbrain at 24 hpf; tegmentum, hypophysis, otic vesicle, and pectoral flipper at 48 hpf [45,72]
kappa-opioid receptor (oprk1)	yes (low expression) [65]	3 hpf [45,72]	no in situ data of the developing stages available
delta-opioid receptor (oprd1a)	yes (moderate expression) [65]	3 hpf [45,72]	whole organism at tail-bud stage [74]; telencephalon, epiphysis, pretectum, and cerebellum at 24 hpf; hindbrain, spinal cord, and tegmentum at 30–36 hpf [45,72]
delta-opioid receptor (oprd1b)	Yes (moderate expression) [65]	3 hpf [45,72]	whole organism at tail-bud stage [74]; telencephalon, epiphysis, diencephalon, midbrain, isthmus, cerebellum, pretectum, hindbrain, myotomes and spinal cord at 24 hpf [45,72]
nociception receptor (oprl1)	yes [73]	3 hpf [73]	diencephalon, hindbrain, midbrain, pretectum, telencephalon at 24 hpf [72]
prodynorphin (pdyn)	no data available	no data available	hypothalamus, lateral region at 2 dpf hindbrain, neuron at 5 dpf
proopiomelanocortin a (pomca)	yes [75]	shield [75]	whole organism at 64 cell [76]; Pituitary, hypothalamus at 2–5 dpf [77,78]
proopiomelanocortin b (pomcb)	no data available	no data available	preoptic area at 3 dpf [78]
proenkephalin a (penka)	no data available	no data available	diencephalon, epiphysis, dorsal telencephalon subpopulation of dorsal spinal cord neurons at 22–25 somite, 30–42 hpf [66]; central nervous system, retina at 5 dpf [66]
proenkephalin b (penkb)	no data available	no data available	dorsal posterior midbrain, diencephalon, spinal cord, posterior pronephric ducts at 22–25 somite, 30–42 hpf, and additionally hindbrain at 60 hpf [66]
prepronociceptin a (pnoca)	no data available	no data available	alpha pancreatic cells at 30 hpf [79], posterior pancreatic bud at 2 dpf [79]
prepronociceptin b (pnocb)	no data available	no data available	neurogenic field, preplacodal ectoderm at bud to 1–4 somites [80]; brain at 5 dpf [81]

* the expression level varies at different developmental stages and peaks at different times.

5.3. Zebrafish Studies on Effects of Embryonic Cannabinoid Exposure on Development

Given the embryonic expression of genes involved in eCB signaling including cannabinoid receptors, it is imperative to understand how modulation of the endocannabinoid system during embryonic development affects the morphology and the behavior of the fish. In the last three decades, several studies were done using zebrafish mutants and transgenic lines (deficient or overexpressed receptors), morpholinos, and the treatment of agonists or antagonists of the receptors. Those studies help decipher the roles of cannabinoid signaling in addiction, anxiety, immune system, energy homeostasis, food intake, learning and memory, and embryo development. The results of those studies were summarized in recent reviews [40,58]. Here we are emphasizing the most recent zebrafish studies that examined the effects of embryonic cannabinoid exposure on development, which shed light on the consequences of disrupting normal eCB signaling on the formation of different cell types, tissues, and organs. Endogenous cannabinoids (2-AG and AEA), synthetic cannabinoids, and cannabinoid antagonists were used in these studies (Table 3).

Table 3. Cannabinoid signaling modulators used in zebrafish studies and the treatment period during development.

Compound	Target	Concentration	Treatment Period
Δ9-Tetrahydro-cannabinol (THC)	CNR1/2 agonist	2–10 mg/L [83] 1–16 µM (0.3–5.0 mg/L) [84] 6 mg/L [85] 1 ppm–10 ppm [86]	5.25–10.75 hpf 2–96 hpf 5.25–10.75 hpf blastula-24 hpf
Cannabidiol (CBD)	CNR1/2 agonist	1–4 mg/L [83] 0.25–4 µM (0.07–1.25 mg/L) [84]	5.25–10.75 hpf 2–96 hpf
2-Arachidonoyl-glycerol (2-AG)	Endogenous CB	5 µM [87]	18–24, 30–36, or 30–96 hpf
Anandamide (AEA)	Endogenous CB	5 µM [87]	18–24, 30–36, or 30–96 hpf
O2545	CNR1/2 agonist	5 µM [87]	12–30 hpf
Arachidonyl-2′-chloroethylamide (ACEA)	CNR1 agonist	5 µM [87]	5.25–6.25, 8–10, 24–27 hpf
AM1241	CNR2 agonist	5–10 µM [87]	18–24, 30–36, 30–96 hpf
JWH015	CNR2 agonist	JW 5–10 µM [87]	12–30 hpf
WIN55,212-2	CNR1 agonist	1 nM–1 µM [88]	0–72, 0–96 hpf
AM251	CNR1 antagonist	100 nM–5 µM [88]; 10 nM, 20 nM [89]	0–72, 0–96 hpf
Rimonabant (SR141716A)	CNR1 antagonist	1 nM–1 µM [88]	0–72, 0–96 hpf
AM630	CNR2 antagonist	5–10 µM [87]	18–24, 30–38, 30–48, 30–96 hpf

Alteration of CB signaling during embryonic development has profound effects on the survival and hatching of zebrafish embryos. Ahmed et al. exposed the embryos to either psychoactive or non-psychoactive ingredients of marijuana (THC: 2–10 mg/L diluted from a stock solution of 1.0 mg/mL in methanol or CBD: 1–4 mg/L diluted from a stock solution of 1.0 mg/mL in methanol) during gastrulation between 5.25 hpf to 10.75 hpf [83]. Brief exposure to THC or CBD during gastrulation, only for a period of $5\frac{1}{2}$ h, significantly reduced the hatching rate of the larvae at 3 dpf. CBD was more potent in decreasing hatching than THC. CBD reduced the hatching to zero at the highest concentration tested [83]. The same treatment regimens of THC or CBD significantly reduced the survival rate of the larvae in a dose-dependent way. Like its effect on hatching, CBD exposure exerted more severe effects on survival, causing the death of more larvae [83]. Willett and her group employed waterborne exposure to CBD and THC by dissolving THC (0.3–5.0 mg/L) or CBD (0.07–1.25 mg/L) in 0.05% DMSO and validated their assay by measuring the water concentration and tissue bio-concentration of the drugs [84]. The actual THC concentrations in water at the start of exposure were between 64% and 88% of the expected concentrations, which declined to 16–32% of the initial concentration after 96 h of exposure, and actual CBD concentrations were only 33–40% of the expected concentrations that decreased to 0–3% of the initial concentration after 96 h of exposure [84]. At the end of the exposure, they measured the concentrations of the drugs in larvae and detected 0.28 mg/g of THC or 79 mg/g of CBD after a nominal 0.3 mg/mL of THC or CBD exposure. The embryos treated with higher concentrations of either THC or CBD from 2 to 96 hpf produced embryonic lethality [84]. The lethality by Δ9-THC exposure was observed and published as early as 1975, showing that exposure to 5 ppm or 10 ppm Δ9-THC from late blastula stage to 24 hpf led to the death of the larvae after 24 h [86].

The effects of specific CNR1 ligands showed different results to THC and CBD exposure. THC and CBD interact with both CNR1 and CNR2 receptors (THC binds to both types of receptors and CBD modifies the receptors' ability to bind to cannabinoids). Continuous exposure to different CNR1 receptor ligands WIN55,212-2 (1 nM-1 μM), AM251 (100 nM-5 μM) or rimonabant (SR141716A:1 nM-1 μM) at various concentrations from 0–72 hpf or 0–96 hpf, without the replacement of solution for the entire exposure period, did not impact hatching [88]. Although the highest concentration of WIN55,212-2 (1 μM; CNR1 agonist) caused complete embryonic lethality, lower concentrations had no impact on the survival of the embryos. Exposure to CNR1 antagonists AM251 or rimonabant also did not change the survival rate [88]. In another study, Migliarini et. al. showed that continuous exposure to AM251 at concentrations of 10 and 20 nM reduced hatching rates [89]. These studies suggest that modulating the cannabinoid system, specially CNR2 mediated cannabinoid signaling, even for a brief period during early development leads to lethality.

Short exposure to the THC (2–10 mg/L) or CBD (1–4 mg/L) during gastrulation causes many morphological changes in the embryos. The exposure caused deformities in the trunk including short body, curved tails, and blebbing at the tip of the tail. Higher exposure concentrations produced more severe deformities [83]. Waterborne exposure to THC (0.3–2.5 mg/L) or CBD (0.07–1.25 mg/L) from 2 to 96 hpf caused short and deformed body axis and bent distal trunk [84]. In fact, similar morphological anomalies were reported when embryos were exposed to 1–10 ppm Δ9-THC from the blastula stage until 24 hpf [86]. The morphology of the larvae was observed until 9 dpf. The lowest concentration of Δ9-THC (1 ppm) did not change the morphology of the larvae, but exposure to 2 ppm caused distal trunk anomalies that included a curved spine or bulbous-tipped tail [86]. On the other hand, continuous exposure to CNR1 antagonist AM251 (10 or 20 nM in ethanol) did not cause any distinguishable morphological changes [89]. These results indicate that cannabinoid signaling mediated by CNR2 receptor is active in the distal trunk during early development and blocking CNR1 receptor does not alter trunk morphology.

Early exposure to exogenous cannabinoids had negative effects on the heart rate. Exposure to THC (4–10 mg/L) during gastrulation from 5.25 to 10.75 hpf reduced the heart rate of larvae in a dose-dependent manner when examined at 2 dpf. The highest concentration of THC reduced the heart rate to 50% of the untreated control. Similar to THC, CBD exposure (1–4 mg/L CBD) for the same duration also reduced the heart rate of the larvae at 2 dpf, producing an even greater effect than that of THC [83]. Waterborne exposure to THC (0.3–2.5 mg/L) or CBD (0.07–1.25 mg/) from 2 to 96 hpf caused pericardial edema. This report also showed that CBD exposure was more potent in causing pericardial edema than THC, which exerted similar defects at a ten-times lower concentration than THC. The highest concentrations of both the drugs tested caused pericardial edema in all the embryos [84].

Chronic exposure to CNR1 agonist ACEA (6 mg/L suspended in ethanol) from 6 to 24 hpf induced microphthalmia, but a lower concentration of ACEA (3 mg/L) did not. However, when the embryos were treated with the combinations of 3 mg/L ACEA and 0.5% ethanol, the larvae had smaller eyes, suggesting a synergistic effect of CNR1 agonist and alcohol on interfering eye development [90]. Binge-like exposure of ACEA (3 and 12 mg/L) on eye development was examined by treating embryos during key developmental time points including the first hour of gastrulation (5.25–6.25 hpf), transition from gastrulation to neurulation (8–10 hpf) or during the formation of the five-vesicle brain (24–27 hpf). Higher concentrations of ACEA exposure at all the stages examined caused microphthalmia. Lower concentration (3 mg/L) of ACEA alone did not cause microphthalmia, but when treated with ethanol (1%), ACEA synergized with ethanol to induce microphthalmia. This study highlights the synergistic interaction of the CNR1 agonist and alcohol and shows how alcohol exposure exacerbates the defects caused by ACEA exposure [90]. Smaller eyes were also reported following waterborne exposure to CBD and THC [84]. These studies demonstrated the effect of prenatal cannabinoid exposure on eye development.

THC or CBD exposure during gastrulation from 5.25 to 10.75 hpf altered morphology and innervation patterns of primary and secondary motor neurons [83]. Exposure to CBD (3 mg/L) during gastrulation reduced the number of axonal branches of primary neurons in 2 dpf embryos, but THC exposure (6 mg/L) for a similar duration did not cause any change in primary neuron morphology. Both THC (6 mg/L) and CBD (3 mg/L) exposure exert severe effects on the secondary motor neurons compared with primary motor neurons. Dorsal, ventral, and lateral motor neuron branching patterns analyses using fluorescent labels showed undetectable dorsal branches and thinner ventral branches of secondary motor neurons in embryos treated with either 6 mg/L THC or 3 mg/L CBD. THC exposure did not alter lateral motor neuron branches, but CBD treatment significantly reduced those branches. Cannabinoid treatment altered synaptic activity at neuromuscular junctions (NMJs) and altered nicotinic acetylcholine receptor expression at NMJs [83]. Exposure to 6 mg/L THC during gastrulation, from 5.25 to 10.75 hpf slightly altered the axon diameter of Mauthner cells (M-cell), the neurons born during gastrulation and which are involved in escape response movements [85]. The muscle fibers of those larvae were slightly disorganized with subtle but significant changes in nicotinic acetylcholine receptor expression patterns [85].

A recent zebrafish study revealed the role of Cnr2 signaling on the production, expansion, and migration of embryonic hematopoietic stem cells [87]. By using different Cnr1 and Cnr2 signaling chemical modulators (Table 3) and genetic approaches, the investigators showed that Cnr2, but not Cnr1 regulates embryonic hematopoietic stem cell development. Cnr2-signaling optimizes the production, expansion, and migration of embryonic hematopoietic stem cells by modulating multiple downstream signaling pathways [87].

5.4. Zebrafish Studies Examining Effects of Embryonic Opioid Exposure on Development

Although the opioid system is active during early development and evidence shows the association of in utero opioid exposure and congenital defects in humans, there are only a handful of zebrafish studies aiming to understand the association between opioid exposure and birth defects. Sanchez-Simon et al. treated zebrafish embryos with 1, 10, and 100 nM of morphine during three different developmental periods: 5–24, 5–48 and 5–72 hpf to determine the effects of embryonic morphine exposure on neuronal fate [91]. They reported that 100 nM caused severe malformation and death in the embryos, while 1 nM did not produce measurable effects. Chronic exposure to 10 nM of morphine from 5–24 or 5–48 hpf enhanced cell proliferation and either induced or suppressed neuronal differentiation depending on neuronal populations. This study also showed that morphine protected motor and Pax-6-positive neurons against glutamate-induced damage. Interestingly, morphine exposure altered the expression of the opioid receptor genes [91]. The authors measured the concentration of morphine in the embryos after chronic exposure (5–24 or 5–48 hpf) and reported that only ~ 5% of the treatment concentration (10 nm) was present in the embryos [91]. In a later study, the group showed that morphine exposure caused nestin overexpression and delayed neural stem cell differentiation [92]. Microarray analyses after chronic exposure to 10 nM morphine from 5 to 24 hpf identified alteration of several genes associated with mu-opioid receptor expression and genes involved in neuronal development, CNS patterning processes, neuronal differentiation, dopaminergic neurotransmission, the serotonergic signaling pathway, and glutamatergic neurotransmission [93]. Rodriguez and her group showed that embryonic exposure to nociceptin altered the temporal and spatial expression pattern of NOP transcripts at 24 and 48 hpf [73]. Since the opioid system is active during zebrafish embryonic development, the advantages of the zebrafish model system can be exploited to understand prenatal opioid exposure effects.

5.5. Zebrafish Studies Examine Behavioral Defects Associated to Embryonic Exposure to Marijuana or Opioid

Many studies showed that the zebrafish behavioral repertoire changes after they have been exposed to psychoactive drugs, and those effects can be assayed using various techniques. Basnet et al. [56] nicely outlined the zebrafish behavior repertoire that can be used in neuropharmacology and reviewed the current literature on the utility of zebrafish larvae as a behavioral model in neuropharmacology. Zebrafish larvae show key behaviors like stress and anxiety. Zebrafish larvae are sensitive to different stimuli such as touch, olfaction, chemosensing, audition, heat, and vision. The zebrafish behavioral assay repertoire includes thigmotaxis, avoidance, startle response, optokinetic response, optomotor response, habituation, prey capture, response to predators, sleep/wake behavior, and locomotor response [56,94,95]. Zebrafish used as models of drug addiction (self-administration and conditioned place preference), withdrawal, anxiety-like behavior, pain, and cognition after cannabinoid and opioid exposure was recently reviewed [40], and those studies demonstrate the utility of zebrafish in studying human physiological conditions after drug exposure. Zebrafish could also be used to screen compounds with the potential to attenuate the drug effects, like opioid withdrawal syndrome symptoms. Khor et. al. modeled a morphine-withdrawal situation by treating adult fish continuously with 1.5 mg/L morphine for two weeks followed by withdrawal for 24 h, and the zebrafish displayed decreased exploratory behavior, increased erratic movement, elevated cortisol levels, indicating anxiety-related responses and stress [96]. Mitragynine is an alkaloid found in leaves of *Mitragyna speciosa*, a plant widely used by opiate addicts to mitigate the harshness of drug withdrawal. Exposure to mitragynine during the withdrawal phase attenuated majority of the stress-related swimming behaviors and lowered the whole-body cortisol level [96]. The authors also showed that mitragynine reduced the mRNA expression of corticotropin-releasing factor receptors and prodynorphin in zebrafish brain during the morphine withdrawal phase [96]. This study shows for the first time a possible link between mitragynine's ability to attenuate anxiety during opiate withdrawal and provided evidence for the utilization of the zebrafish to screen compounds for their ability to mitigate drug withdrawal effects. Together, these studies demonstrate the effectiveness of zebrafish as a model to study drug addiction and withdrawal.

6. Summary

Marijuana and opioid abuse are serious global health problems, which are more serious in the United States than most other countries, causing more than half a million deaths in the last two decades. The use of these drugs by pregnant and reproductive-age women has significantly increased in recent years. There is strong evidence for the association of prenatal drug exposure and congenital anomalies (Figure 1), which raises additional serious public health concerns. To combat the growing opioid overdose crisis, it was declared to be a public health emergency by the White House in 2017 [97]. The CDC outlined different focus areas to fight the drug abuse epidemic, and one of these is to advance research to better understand the epidemic and identify effective strategies to prevent it [8]. It will be important to better understand whether different cannabinoids and opioids exposure lead to adverse outcomes in babies, which would magnify the consequences of drug use in society. A challenge of evaluating drug exposure and birth defects is the potential contribution of other confounding factors such as maternal age, prenatal care, prenatal vitamins, diet, and exposure to other teratogens such as alcohol. For the studies related to developmental delay and cognitive function in babies, it is difficult to control for environment, nutrition, and socioeconomic factors. Using animal models, the direct effects of the drugs can be determined independent of other confounding factors.

Zebrafish provide a rapid and inexpensive platform to study the effects of drug exposure during development. Zebrafish studies showed various developmental defects caused by embryonic exposure to marijuana components (Figure 1). Those studies also indicated the differential sensitivity of the exogenous cannabinoids. Although the number of zebrafish studies examining the effects of different opioids on development is small, the existing evidence also showed developmental defects in fish. Zebrafish studies showed behavioral effects similar to human drug addiction and withdrawal symptoms. Although the human behavior response can never be completely replicated in the zebrafish, the fish experiments suggest that many drug-induced human and zebrafish phenotypes share common genetic and physiological factors. Recently, high-throughput zebrafish behavioral screens identified a novel group of antipsychotics, finazines, and their target, the sigma non-opioid intracellular receptor 1 [98–100]. These studies showed the utility of zebrafish in the discovery of new therapies for psychiatric disorders. Overall, zebrafish represents an exciting and emerging model to study the effects of drug exposure on development and could be a useful alternative vertebrate model for translational studies.

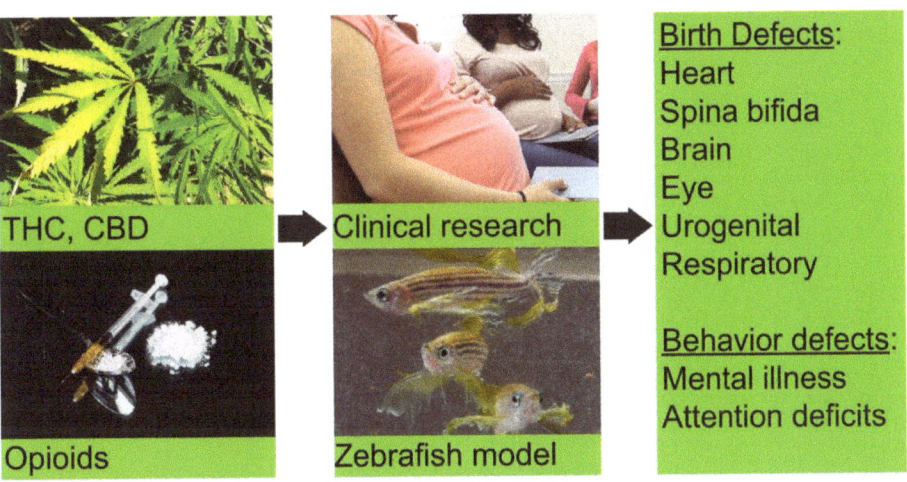

Figure 1. Schematic representations of drug use/abuse during pregnancy and birth outcomes. In utero exposure to Δ9-tetrahydrocannabinol (THC), cannabidiol (CBD) or opioids leads to congenital malformations and behavioral changes in babies. Exposure to cannabinoids or opioids during zebrafish development produced similar defects in embryos.

Funding: This work was supported by NIH/NIAAA 1 R21 AA026711.

Conflicts of Interest: The authors declare no conflict of interest.

References

1. State Marijuana Laws in 2019 Map. Governing-The future of states and localities. Available online: https://www.governing.com/gov-data/safety-justice/state-marijuana-laws-map-medical-recreational.html (accessed on 20 July 2020).
2. Bose, J.; Hedden, L.A.; Lipari, R.N.; Park-Lee, E. *Key Substance Use and Mental Health Indicators in the United States: Results from the 2017 National Survey on Drug Use and Health*; Substance Abuse and Mental Health Services Administration: Rockville, MD, USA, 2018.
3. Huestis, M.A. Human cannabinoid pharmacokinetics. *Chem. Biodivers.* **2007**, *4*, 1770–1804. [CrossRef] [PubMed]
4. Mehmedic, Z.; Chandra, S.; Slade, D.; Denham, H.; Foster, S.; Patel, A.S.; Ross, S.A.; Khan, I.A.; ElSohly, M.A. Potency trends of Delta9-THC and other cannabinoids in confiscated cannabis preparations from 1993 to 2008. *J. Forensic Sci.* **2010**, *55*, 1209–1217. [CrossRef] [PubMed]
5. Shah, A.; Hayes, C.J.; Martin, B.C. Characteristics of Initial Prescription Episodes and Likelihood of Long-Term Opioid Use—United States, 2006–2015. *Morb. Mortal. Wkly. Rep.* **2017**, *66*, 265–269. [CrossRef] [PubMed]
6. Mattson, C.L.; O'Donnell, J.; Kariisa, M.; Seth, P.; Scholl, L.; Gladden, R.M. Opportunities to Prevent Overdose Deaths Involving Prescription and Illicit Opioids, 11 States, July 2016–June 2017. *MMWR Morb. Mortal. Wkly. Rep.* **2018**, *67*, 945–951. [CrossRef]

7. Information Sheet on Opioid Overdose. Available online: https://www.who.int/substance_abuse/information-sheet/en/ (accessed on 30 June 2020).
8. Opioid Overdose. Centers for Disease Control and Prevention. Available online: https://www.cdc.gov/drugoverdose/index.html (accessed on 20 July 2020).
9. McHugh, R.K.; Wigderson, S.; Greenfield, S.F. Epidemiology of substance use in reproductive-age women. *Obstet. Gynecol. Clin. North Am.* **2014**, *41*, 177–189. [CrossRef]
10. Forray, A. Substance use during pregnancy. *F1000Research* **2016**, *5*. [CrossRef]
11. Cerda, M.; Wall, M.; Keyes, K.M.; Galea, S.; Hasin, D. Medical marijuana laws in 50 states: Investigating the relationship between state legalization of medical marijuana and marijuana use, abuse and dependence. *Drug Alcohol Depend.* **2012**, *120*, 22–27. [CrossRef]
12. Ko, J.Y.; Farr, S.L.; Tong, V.T.; Creanga, A.A.; Callaghan, W.M. Prevalence and patterns of marijuana use among pregnant and nonpregnant women of reproductive age. *Am. J. Obstet. Gynecol.* **2015**, *213*, 201.e1–201e.10. [CrossRef]
13. Oh, S.; Salas-Wright, C.P.; Vaughn, M.G.; DiNitto, D.M. Marijuana use during pregnancy: A comparison of trends and correlates among married and unmarried pregnant women. *Drug Alcohol Depend.* **2017**, *181*, 229–233. [CrossRef]
14. Young-Wolff, K.C.; Tucker, L.Y.; Alexeeff, S.; Armstrong, M.A.; Conway, A.; Weisner, C.; Goler, N. Trends in Self-reported and Biochemically Tested Marijuana Use Among Pregnant Females in California From 2009–2016. *JAMA* **2017**, *318*, 2490–2491. [CrossRef]
15. Ailes, E.C.; Dawson, A.L.; Lind, J.N.; Gilboa, S.M.; Frey, M.T.; Broussard, C.S.; Honein, M.A. Opioid Prescription Claims Among Women of Reproductive Age – United States, 2008–2012. In *Morbidity and Mortality Weekly Report (MMWR)*; Centers for Disease Control and Prevention: Atlanta, GA, USA, 2015; Volume 64, pp. 37–41.
16. Mack, K.A.; Jones, C.M.; Paulozzi, L.J. Vital signs: Overdoses of prescription opioid pain relievers and other drugs among women—United States, 1999–2010. *MMWR Morb. Mortal. Wkly. Rep.* **2013**, *62*, 537–542.
17. Patrick, S.W.; Schumacher, R.E.; Benneyworth, B.D.; Krans, E.E.; McAllister, J.M.; Davis, M.M. Neonatal Abstinence Syndrome and Associated Health Care Expenditures: United States, 2000–2009. *JAMA* **2012**, *307*, 1934–1940. [CrossRef] [PubMed]
18. Desai, R.J.; Hernandez-Diaz, S.; Bateman, B.T.; Huybrechts, K.F. Increase in prescription opioid use during pregnancy among Medicaid-enrolled women. *Obstet. Gynecol.* **2014**, *123*, 997–1002. [CrossRef] [PubMed]
19. Bateman, B.T.; Hernandez-Diaz, S.; Rathmell, J.P.; Seeger, J.D.; Doherty, M.; Fischer, M.A.; Huybrechts, K.F. Patterns of opioid utilization in pregnancy in a large cohort of commercial insurance beneficiaries in the United States. *Anesthesiology* **2014**, *120*, 1216–1224. [CrossRef] [PubMed]
20. Volkow, N.D.; Han, B.; Compton, W.M.; Blanco, C. Marijuana Use During Stages of Pregnancy in the United States. *Ann. Intern. Med.* **2017**, *166*, 763–764. [CrossRef] [PubMed]
21. Yazdy, M.M.; Desai, R.J.; Brogly, S.B. Prescription Opioids in Pregnancy and Birth Outcomes: A Review of the Literature. *J. Pediatr. Genet.* **2015**, *4*, 56–70. [CrossRef]
22. Martins, F.; Oppolzer, D.; Santos, C.; Barroso, M.; Gallardo, E. Opioid Use in Pregnant Women and Neonatal Abstinence Syndrome-A Review of the Literature. *Toxics* **2019**, *7*, 9. [CrossRef]
23. Desai, R.J.; Huybrechts, K.F.; Hernandez-Diaz, S.; Mogun, H.; Patorno, E.; Kaltenbach, K.; Kerzner, L.S.; Bateman, B.T. Exposure to prescription opioid analgesics in utero and risk of neonatal abstinence syndrome: Population based cohort study. *BMJ* **2015**, *350*, h2102. [CrossRef]
24. Volkow, N.D.; Compton, W.M.; Wargo, E.M. The Risks of Marijuana Use During Pregnancy. *JAMA* **2017**, *317*, 129–130. [CrossRef]
25. Reece, A.S.; Hulse, G.K. Cannabis Teratology Explains Current Patterns of Coloradan Congenital Defects: The Contribution of Increased Cannabinoid Exposure to Rising Teratological Trends. *Clin. Pediatr.* **2019**, *58*, 1085–1123. [CrossRef]
26. van Gelder, M.M.; Reefhuis, J.; Caton, A.R.; Werler, M.M.; Druschel, C.M.; Roeleveld, N.; National Birth Defects Prevention, S. Maternal periconceptional illicit drug use and the risk of congenital malformations. *Epidemiology* **2009**, *20*, 60–66. [CrossRef] [PubMed]
27. Willford, J.A.; Chandler, L.S.; Goldschmidt, L.; Day, N.L. Effects of prenatal tobacco, alcohol and marijuana exposure on processing speed, visual-motor coordination, and interhemispheric transfer. *Neurotoxicol. Teratol.* **2010**, *32*, 580–588. [CrossRef] [PubMed]

28. Fried, P.A.; Watkinson, B. Visuoperceptual functioning differs in 9- to 12-year olds prenatally exposed to cigarettes and marihuana. *Neurotoxicol. Teratol.* **2000**, *22*, 11–20. [CrossRef]
29. Day, N.L.; Goldschmidt, L.; Thomas, C.A. Prenatal marijuana exposure contributes to the prediction of marijuana use at age 14. *Addiction* **2006**, *101*, 1313–1322. [CrossRef]
30. Broussard, C.S.; Rasmussen, S.A.; Reefhuis, J.; Friedman, J.M.; Jann, M.W.; Riehle-Colarusso, T.; Honein, M.A. Maternal treatment with opioid analgesics and risk for birth defects. *Am. J. Obstet. Gynecol.* **2011**, *204*, 314-e1. [CrossRef]
31. Yazdy, M.M.; Mitchell, A.A.; Tinker, S.C.; Parker, S.E.; Werler, M.M. Periconceptional use of opioids and the risk of neural tube defects. *Obstet. Gynecol.* **2013**, *122*, 838–844. [CrossRef]
32. Minnes, S.; Lang, A.; Singer, L. Prenatal tobacco, marijuana, stimulant, and opiate exposure: Outcomes and practice implications. *Addict. Sci. Clin. Pract.* **2011**, *6*, 57–70.
33. Ross, E.J.; Graham, D.L.; Money, K.M.; Stanwood, G.D. Developmental Consequences of Fetal Exposure to Drugs: What We Know and What We Still Must Learn. *Neuropsychopharmacology* **2015**, *40*, 61–87. [CrossRef]
34. Lind, J.N.; Interrante, J.D.; Ailes, E.C.; Gilboa, S.M.; Khan, S.; Frey, M.T.; Dawson, A.L.; Honein, M.A.; Dowling, N.F.; Razzaghi, H.; et al. Maternal Use of Opioids During Pregnancy and Congenital Malformations: A Systematic Review. *Pediatrics* **2017**, *139*, e20164131. [CrossRef]
35. Neonatal Abstinence Syndrome (NAS) Among Newborn Hospitalizations. 2019. Available online: www.hcup-us.ahrq.gov/faststats/nas/nasmap.jsp (accessed on 20 July 2020).
36. Data and Statistics About Opioid Use During Pregnancy. Available online: https://www.cdc.gov/mmwr/preview/mmwrhtml/mm6402a1.htm (accessed on 20 July 2020).
37. Bunikowski, R.; Grimmer, I.; Heiser, A.; Metze, B.; Schäfer, A.; Obladen, M. Neurodevelopmental outcome after prenatal exposure to opiates. *Eur. J. Pediatrics* **1998**, *157*, 724–730. [CrossRef]
38. Conradt, E.; Flannery, T.; Aschner, J.L.; Annett, R.D.; Croen, L.A.; Duarte, C.S.; Friedman, A.M.; Guille, C.; Hedderson, M.M.; Hofheimer, J.A.; et al. Prenatal Opioid Exposure: Neurodevelopmental Consequences and Future Research Priorities. *Pediatrics* **2019**, *144*. [CrossRef] [PubMed]
39. Reddy, U.M.; Davis, J.M.; Ren, Z.; Greene, M.F.; Opioid Use in Pregnancy, N.A.S.; Childhood Outcomes Workshop Invited, S. Opioid Use in Pregnancy, Neonatal Abstinence Syndrome, and Childhood Outcomes: Executive Summary of a Joint Workshop by the Eunice Kennedy Shriver National Institute of Child Health and Human Development, American College of Obstetricians and Gynecologists, American Academy of Pediatrics, Society for Maternal-Fetal Medicine, Centers for Disease Control and Prevention, and the March of Dimes Foundation. *Obstet. Gynecol.* **2017**, *130*, 10–28. [CrossRef] [PubMed]
40. Demin, K.A.; Meshalkina, D.A.; Kysil, E.V.; Antonova, K.A.; Volgin, A.D.; Yakovlev, O.A.; Alekseeva, P.A.; Firuleva, M.M.; Lakstygal, A.M.; de Abreu, M.S.; et al. Zebrafish models relevant to studying central opioid and endocannabinoid systems. *Prog. Neuro-Psychopharmacol. Biol. Psychiatry* **2018**, *86*, 301–312. [CrossRef] [PubMed]
41. Bailey, J.; Oliveri, A.; Levin, E.D. Zebrafish model systems for developmental neurobehavioral toxicology. *Birth Defects Res. Part C Embryo Today Rev.* **2013**, *99*, 14–23. [CrossRef] [PubMed]
42. Duncan, K.M.; Mukherjee, K.; Cornell, R.A.; Liao, E.C. Zebrafish models of orofacial clefts. *Dev. Dyn. Off. Publ. Am. Assoc. Anat.* **2017**, *246*, 897–914. [CrossRef]
43. Sarmah, S.; Marrs, J.A. Zebrafish as a Vertebrate Model System to Evaluate Effects of Environmental Toxicants on Cardiac Development and Function. *Int. J. Mol. Sci.* **2016**, *17*, 2123. [CrossRef]
44. Gerlai, R. Using zebrafish to unravel the genetics of complex brain disorders. *Curr. Top. Behav. Neurosci.* **2012**, *12*, 3–24. [CrossRef]
45. Klee, E.W.; Schneider, H.; Clark, K.J.; Cousin, M.A.; Ebbert, J.O.; Hooten, W.M.; Karpyak, V.M.; Warner, D.O.; Ekker, S.C. Zebrafish: A model for the study of addiction genetics. *Hum. Genet.* **2012**, *131*, 977–1008. [CrossRef]
46. Marrs, J.A.; Clendenon, S.G.; Ratcliffe, D.R.; Fielding, S.M.; Liu, Q.; Bosron, W.F. Zebrafish fetal alcohol syndrome model: Effects of ethanol are rescued by retinoic acid supplement. *Alcohol* **2010**, *44*, 707–715. [CrossRef]
47. Sarmah, S.; Marrs, J.A. Complex cardiac defects after ethanol exposure during discrete cardiogenic events in zebrafish: Prevention with folic acid. *Dev. Dyn. Off. Publ. Am. Assoc. Anat.* **2013**, *242*, 1184–1201. [CrossRef]
48. Sarmah, S.; Marrs, J.A. Embryonic Ethanol Exposure Affects Early- and Late-Added Cardiac Precursors and Produces Long-Lasting Heart Chamber Defects in Zebrafish. *Toxics* **2017**, *5*. [CrossRef]

49. Sarmah, S.; Muralidharan, P.; Curtis, C.L.; McClintick, J.N.; Buente, B.B.; Holdgrafer, D.J.; Ogbeifun, O.; Olorungbounmi, O.C.; Patino, L.; Lucas, R.; et al. Ethanol exposure disrupts extraembryonic microtubule cytoskeleton and embryonic blastomere cell adhesion, producing epiboly and gastrulation defects. *Biol. Open* **2013**, *2*, 1013–1021. [CrossRef] [PubMed]
50. Sarmah, S.; Muralidharan, P.; Marrs, J.A. Embryonic Ethanol Exposure Dysregulates BMP and Notch Signaling, Leading to Persistent Atrio-Ventricular Valve Defects in Zebrafish. *PLoS ONE* **2016**, *11*, e0161205. [CrossRef] [PubMed]
51. Sarmah, S.; Srivastava, R.; McClintick, J.N.; Janga, S.C.; Edenberg, H.J.; Marrs, J.A. Embryonic ethanol exposure alters expression of sox2 and other early transcripts in zebrafish, producing gastrulation defects. *Sci. Rep.* **2020**, *10*, 3951. [CrossRef]
52. Muralidharan, P.; Sarmah, S.; Marrs, J.A. Zebrafish retinal defects induced by ethanol exposure are rescued by retinoic acid and folic acid supplement. *Alcohol* **2015**, *49*, 149–163. [CrossRef]
53. Muralidharan, P.; Sarmah, S.; Marrs, J.A. Retinal Wnt signaling defect in a zebrafish fetal alcohol spectrum disorder model. *PLoS ONE* **2018**, *13*, e0201659. [CrossRef]
54. Muralidharan, P.; Sarmah, S.; Zhou, F.C.; Marrs, J.A. Fetal Alcohol Spectrum Disorder (FASD) Associated Neural Defects: Complex Mechanisms and Potential Therapeutic Targets. *Brain Sci.* **2013**, *3*, 964–991. [CrossRef]
55. Kalueff, A.V.; Stewart, A.M.; Gerlai, R. Zebrafish as an emerging model for studying complex brain disorders. *Trends Pharmacol. Sci.* **2014**, *35*, 63–75. [CrossRef]
56. Basnet, R.M.; Zizioli, D.; Taweedet, S.; Finazzi, D.; Memo, M. Zebrafish Larvae as a Behavioral Model in Neuropharmacology. *Biomedicines* **2019**, *7*, 23. [CrossRef]
57. Kalueff, A.V.; Echevarria, D.J.; Stewart, A.M. Gaining translational momentum: More zebrafish models for neuroscience research. *Prog. Neuro-Psychopharmacol. Biol. Psychiatry* **2014**, *55*, 1–6. [CrossRef]
58. Oltrabella, F.; Melgoza, A.; Nguyen, B.; Guo, S. Role of the endocannabinoid system in vertebrates: Emphasis on the zebrafish model. *Dev. Growth Differ.* **2017**, *59*, 194–210. [CrossRef] [PubMed]
59. Krug, R.G., II; Clark, K.J. Elucidating cannabinoid biology in zebrafish (Danio rerio). *Gene* **2015**, *570*, 168–179. [CrossRef] [PubMed]
60. Lam, C.S.; Rastegar, S.; Strahle, U. Distribution of cannabinoid receptor 1 in the CNS of zebrafish. *Neuroscience* **2006**, *138*, 83–95. [CrossRef] [PubMed]
61. Nishio, S.; Gibert, Y.; Berekelya, L.; Bernard, L.; Brunet, F.; Guillot, E.; Le Bail, J.C.; Sanchez, J.A.; Galzin, A.M.; Triqueneaux, G.; et al. Fasting induces CART down-regulation in the zebrafish nervous system in a cannabinoid receptor 1-dependent manner. *Mol. Endocrinol.* **2012**, *26*, 1316–1326. [CrossRef] [PubMed]
62. Watson, S.; Chambers, D.; Hobbs, C.; Doherty, P.; Graham, A. The endocannabinoid receptor, CB1, is required for normal axonal growth and fasciculation. *Mol. Cell Neurosci.* **2008**, *38*, 89–97. [CrossRef] [PubMed]
63. Rodriguez-Martin, I.; Herrero-Turrion, M.J.; Marron Fdez de Velasco, E.; Gonzalez-Sarmiento, R.; Rodriguez, R.E. Characterization of two duplicate zebrafish Cb2-like cannabinoid receptors. *Gene* **2007**, *389*, 36–44. [CrossRef] [PubMed]
64. Liu, L.Y.; Alexa, K.; Cortes, M.; Schatzman-Bone, S.; Kim, A.J.; Mukhopadhyay, B.; Cinar, R.; Kunos, G.; North, T.E.; Goessling, W. Cannabinoid receptor signaling regulates liver development and metabolism. *Development* **2016**, *143*, 609–622. [CrossRef]
65. Martella, A.; Sepe, R.M.; Silvestri, C.; Zang, J.; Fasano, G.; Carnevali, O.; De Girolamo, P.; Neuhauss, S.C.; Sordino, P.; Di Marzo, V. Important role of endocannabinoid signaling in the development of functional vision and locomotion in zebrafish. *FASEB J.* **2016**, *30*, 4275–4288. [CrossRef]
66. Thisse, B.; Thisse, C. Fast Release Clones: A High Throughput Expression Analysis. Available online: https://zfin.org/ (accessed on 20 July 2020).
67. Tingaud-Sequeira, A.; Raldua, D.; Lavie, J.; Mathieu, G.; Bordier, M.; Knoll-Gellida, A.; Rambeau, P.; Coupry, I.; Andre, M.; Malm, E.; et al. Functional validation of ABHD12 mutations in the neurodegenerative disease PHARC. *Neurobiol. Dis.* **2017**, *98*, 36–51. [CrossRef]
68. Krug, R.G., II; Lee, H.B.; El Khoury, L.Y.; Sigafoos, A.N.; Petersen, M.O.; Clark, K.J. The endocannabinoid gene faah2a modulates stress-associated behavior in zebrafish. *PLoS ONE* **2018**, *13*, e0190897. [CrossRef]
69. Thisse, B.; Pflumio, S.; Fürthauer, M.; Loppin, B.; Heyer, V.; Degrave, A.; Woehl, R.; Lux, A.; Steffan, T.; Charbonnier, X.Q.; et al. Expression of the Zebrafish Genome During Embryogenesis. Available online: https://zfin.org/ (accessed on 20 July 2020).

70. Rodriguez-Martin, I.; Marron Fernandez de Velasco, E.; Rodriguez, R.E. Characterization of cannabinoid-binding sites in zebrafish brain. *Neurosci. Lett.* **2007**, *413*, 249–254. [CrossRef] [PubMed]
71. Connors, K.A.; Valenti, T.W.; Lawless, K.; Sackerman, J.; Onaivi, E.S.; Brooks, B.W.; Gould, G.G. Similar anxiolytic effects of agonists targeting serotonin 5-HT1A or cannabinoid CB receptors on zebrafish behavior in novel environments. *Aquat. Toxicol.* **2014**, *151*, 105–113. [CrossRef] [PubMed]
72. Sanchez-Simon, F.M.; Rodriguez, R.E. Developmental expression and distribution of opioid receptors in zebrafish. *Neuroscience* **2008**, *151*, 129–137. [CrossRef] [PubMed]
73. Macho Sanchez-Simon, F.; Rodriguez, R.E. Expression of the nociceptin receptor during zebrafish development: Influence of morphine and nociceptin. *Int. J. Dev. Neurosci.* **2009**, *27*, 315–320. [CrossRef] [PubMed]
74. Lopez-Bellido, R.; Barreto-Valer, K.; Sanchez-Simon, F.M.; Rodriguez, R.E. Cocaine modulates the expression of opioid receptors and miR-let-7d in zebrafish embryos. *PLoS ONE* **2012**, *7*, e50885. [CrossRef] [PubMed]
75. Hansen, I.A.; To, T.T.; Wortmann, S.; Burmester, T.; Winkler, C.; Meyer, S.R.; Neuner, C.; Fassnacht, M.; Allolio, B. The pro-opiomelanocortin gene of the zebrafish (Danio rerio). *Biochem. Biophys. Res. Commun.* **2003**, *303*, 1121–1128. [CrossRef]
76. Faught, E.; Vijayan, M.M. The mineralocorticoid receptor is essential for stress axis regulation in zebrafish larvae. *Sci. Rep.* **2018**, *8*, 18081. [CrossRef]
77. Eachus, H.; Bright, C.; Cunliffe, V.T.; Placzek, M.; Wood, J.D.; Watt, P.J. Disrupted-in-Schizophrenia-1 is essential for normal hypothalamic-pituitary-interrenal (HPI) axis function. *Hum. Mol. Genet.* **2017**, *26*, 1992–2005. [CrossRef]
78. Nasif, S.; de Souza, F.S.; Gonzalez, L.E.; Yamashita, M.; Orquera, D.P.; Low, M.J.; Rubinstein, M. Islet 1 specifies the identity of hypothalamic melanocortin neurons and is critical for normal food intake and adiposity in adulthood. *Proc. Natl. Acad. Sci. USA* **2015**, *112*, E1861–E1870. [CrossRef]
79. Tarifeno-Saldivia, E.; Lavergne, A.; Bernard, A.; Padamata, K.; Bergemann, D.; Voz, M.L.; Manfroid, I.; Peers, B. Transcriptome analysis of pancreatic cells across distant species highlights novel important regulator genes. *BMC Biol.* **2017**, *15*, 21. [CrossRef]
80. Lleras-Forero, L.; Tambalo, M.; Christophorou, N.; Chambers, D.; Houart, C.; Streit, A. Neuropeptides: Developmental signals in placode progenitor formation. *Dev. Cell* **2013**, *26*, 195–203. [CrossRef] [PubMed]
81. Woods, I.G.; Schoppik, D.; Shi, V.J.; Zimmerman, S.; Coleman, H.A.; Greenwood, J.; Soucy, E.R.; Schier, A.F. Neuropeptidergic signaling partitions arousal behaviors in zebrafish. *J. Neurosci.* **2014**, *34*, 3142–3160. [CrossRef] [PubMed]
82. Bao, W.; Volgin, A.D.; Alpyshov, E.T.; Friend, A.J.; Strekalova, T.V.; de Abreu, M.S.; Collins, C.; Amstislavskaya, T.G.; Demin, K.A.; Kalueff, A.V. Opioid Neurobiology, Neurogenetics and Neuropharmacology in Zebrafish. *Neuroscience* **2019**, *404*, 218–232. [CrossRef] [PubMed]
83. Ahmed, K.T.; Amin, M.R.; Shah, P.; Ali, D.W. Motor neuron development in zebrafish is altered by brief (5-hr) exposures to THC ((9)-tetrahydrocannabinol) or CBD (cannabidiol) during gastrulation. *Sci. Rep.* **2018**, *8*, 10518. [CrossRef]
84. Carty, D.R.; Thornton, C.; Gledhill, J.H.; Willett, K.L. Developmental Effects of Cannabidiol and Delta9-Tetrahydrocannabinol in Zebrafish. *Toxicol. Sci.* **2018**, *162*, 137–145. [CrossRef]
85. Amin, M.R.; Ahmed, K.T.; Ali, D.W. Early Exposure to THC Alters M-Cell Development in Zebrafish Embryos. *Biomedicines* **2020**, *8*, 5. [CrossRef]
86. Thomas, R.J. The toxicologic and teratologic effects of delta-9-tetrahydrocannabinol in the zebrafish embryo. *Toxicol. Appl. Pharmacol.* **1975**, *32*, 184–190. [CrossRef]
87. Esain, V.; Kwan, W.; Carroll, K.J.; Cortes, M.; Liu, S.Y.; Frechette, G.M.; Sheward, L.M.; Nissim, S.; Goessling, W.; North, T.E. Cannabinoid Receptor-2 Regulates Embryonic Hematopoietic Stem Cell Development via Prostaglandin E2 and P-Selectin Activity. *Stem Cells* **2015**, *33*, 2596–2612. [CrossRef]
88. Zuccarini, G.; D'Atri, I.; Cottone, E.; Mackie, K.; Shainer, I.; Gothilf, Y.; Provero, P.; Bovolin, P.; Merlo, G.R. Interference with the Cannabinoid Receptor CB1R Results in Miswiring of GnRH3 and AgRP1 Axons in Zebrafish Embryos. *Int. J. Mol. Sci.* **2019**, *21*, 168. [CrossRef]
89. Migliarini, B.; Carnevali, O. A novel role for the endocannabinoid system during zebrafish development. *Mol. Cell Endocrinol.* **2009**, *299*, 172–177. [CrossRef]

90. Boa-Amponsem, O.; Zhang, C.; Mukhopadhyay, S.; Ardrey, I.; Cole, G.J. Ethanol and cannabinoids interact to alter behavior in a zebrafish fetal alcohol spectrum disorder model. *Birth Defects Res.* **2019**, *111*, 775–788. [CrossRef] [PubMed]
91. Sanchez-Simon, F.M.; Arenzana, F.J.; Rodriguez, R.E. In vivo effects of morphine on neuronal fate and opioid receptor expression in zebrafish embryos. *Eur. J. Neurosci.* **2010**, *32*, 550–559. [CrossRef] [PubMed]
92. Jimenez-Gonzalez, A.; Garcia-Concejo, A.; Leon-Lobera, F.; Rodriguez, R.E. Morphine delays neural stem cells differentiation by facilitating Nestin overexpression. *Biochim. Biophys. Acta Gen. Subj.* **2018**, *1862*, 474–484. [CrossRef] [PubMed]
93. Herrero-Turrion, M.J.; Rodriguez-Martin, I.; Lopez-Bellido, R.; Rodriguez, R.E. Whole-genome expression profile in zebrafish embryos after chronic exposure to morphine: Identification of new genes associated with neuronal function and mu opioid receptor expression. *BMC Genom.* **2014**, *15*, 874. [CrossRef]
94. Muniandy, Y. The Use of Larval Zebrafish (Danio rerio) Model for Identifying New Anxiolytic Drugs from Herbal Medicine. *Zebrafish* **2018**, *15*, 321–339. [CrossRef]
95. Maximino, C.; de Brito, T.M.; da Silva Batista, A.W.; Herculano, A.M.; Morato, S.; Gouveia, A. Measuring anxiety in zebrafish: A critical review. *Behav. Brain Res.* **2010**, *214*, 157–171. [CrossRef]
96. Khor, B.-S.; Amar Jamil, M.F.; Adenan, M.I.; Chong Shu-Chien, A. Mitragynine Attenuates Withdrawal Syndrome in Morphine-Withdrawn Zebrafish. *PLOS ONE* **2011**, *6*, e28340. [CrossRef]
97. Ongoing Emergencies & Disasters. Available online: https://www.cms.gov/About-CMS/Agency-Information/Emergency/EPRO/Current-Emergencies/Ongoing-emergencies (accessed on 20 July 2020).
98. Rennekamp, A.J.; Huang, X.P.; Wang, Y.; Patel, S.; Lorello, P.J.; Cade, L.; Gonzales, A.P.; Yeh, J.R.; Caldarone, B.J.; Roth, B.L.; et al. sigma1 receptor ligands control a switch between passive and active threat responses. *Nat. Chem. Biol.* **2016**, *12*, 552–558. [CrossRef]
99. Leung, L.C.; Mourrain, P. Drug discovery: Zebrafish uncover novel antipsychotics. *Nat. Chem. Biol.* **2016**, *12*, 468–469. [CrossRef]
100. Bruni, G.; Rennekamp, A.J.; Velenich, A.; McCarroll, M.; Gendelev, L.; Fertsch, E.; Taylor, J.; Lakhani, P.; Lensen, D.; Evron, T.; et al. Zebrafish behavioral profiling identifies multitarget antipsychotic-like compounds. *Nat. Chem. Biol.* **2016**, *12*, 559–566. [CrossRef]

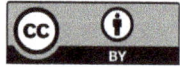

© 2020 by the authors. Licensee MDPI, Basel, Switzerland. This article is an open access article distributed under the terms and conditions of the Creative Commons Attribution (CC BY) license (http://creativecommons.org/licenses/by/4.0/).

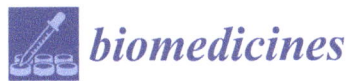

Review

An Overview of Methods for Cardiac Rhythm Detection in Zebrafish

Fiorency Santoso [1,2,†], Ali Farhan [3,†], Agnes L. Castillo [4], Nemi Malhotra [5], Ferry Saputra [2], Kevin Adi Kurnia [2], Kelvin H.-C. Chen [6], Jong-Chin Huang [6,*], Jung-Ren Chen [7,*] and Chung-Der Hsiao [1,2,8,*]

1. Master Program in Nanotechnology, Chung Yuan Christian University, Chung-Li 320314, Taiwan; fiorency_santoso@yahoo.co.id
2. Department of Bioscience Technology, Chung Yuan Christian University, Chung-Li 320314, Taiwan; ferrysaputratj@gmail.com (F.S.); kevinadik-adi@hotmail.com (K.A.K.)
3. Department of Bioinformatics and Biotechnology, Government College University Faisalabad, Punjab 38000, Pakistan; smalifarhan@gmail.com
4. Faculty of Pharmacy, The Graduate School and Research Center for the Natural and Applied Sciences, University of Santo Tomas, Manila 1008, Philippines; alcastillo@ust.edu.ph
5. Department of Biomedical Engineering, Chung Yuan Christian University, Chung-Li 320314, Taiwan; nemi.malhotra@gmail.com
6. Department of Applied Chemistry, National Pingtung University, Pingtung 900391, Taiwan; kelvin@mail.nptu.edu.tw
7. Department of Biological Science & Technology College of Medicine, I-Shou University, Kaohsiung 82445, Taiwan
8. Center of Nanotechnology, Chung Yuan Christian University, Chung-Li 320314, Taiwan
* Correspondence: hjc@mail.nptu.edu.tw (J.-C.H.); jrchen@isu.edu.tw (J.-R.C.); cdhsiao@cycu.edu.tw (C.-D.H.)
† These authors contributed equally to this work.

Received: 12 July 2020; Accepted: 1 September 2020; Published: 4 September 2020

Abstract: The heart is the most important muscular organ of the cardiovascular system, which pumps blood and circulates, supplying oxygen and nutrients to peripheral tissues. Zebrafish have been widely explored in cardiotoxicity research. For example, the zebrafish embryo has been used as a human heart model due to its body transparency, surviving several days without circulation, and facilitating mutant identification to recapitulate human diseases. On the other hand, adult zebrafish can exhibit the amazing regenerative heart muscle capacity, while adult mammalian hearts lack this potential. This review paper offers a brief description of the major methodologies used to detect zebrafish cardiac rhythm at both embryonic and adult stages. The dynamic pixel change method was mostly performed for the embryonic stage. Other techniques, such as kymography, laser confocal microscopy, artificial intelligence, and electrocardiography (ECG) have also been applied to study heartbeat in zebrafish embryos. Nevertheless, ECG is widely used for heartbeat detection in adult zebrafish since ECG waveforms' similarity between zebrafish and humans is prominent. High-frequency ultrasound imaging (echocardiography) and modern electronic sensor tag also have been proposed. Despite the fact that each method has its benefits and limitations, it is proved that zebrafish have become a promising animal model for human cardiovascular disease, drug pharmaceutical, and toxicological research. Using those tools, we conclude that zebrafish behaviors as an excellent small animal model to perform real-time monitoring for the developmental heart process with transparent body appearance, to conduct the in vivo cardiovascular performance and gene function assays, as well as to perform high-throughput/high content drug screening.

Keywords: zebrafish; cardiac physiology; heart rate; detection method

1. Why Zebrafish Behavior Is a Good in vivo Model to Address Cardiac Physiology and Toxicology?

Zebrafish have been widely used as an in vivo model for toxicology evaluation. Toxicity screening may include information on the potential off-target effects of target compounds on the cardiac system, central nervous system, intestinal tract, auditory and visual functions, and bone formation. Cardiotoxicity is one of the major concerns in toxicological studies. It is associated with potential QT interval prolongation, an indicator of fatal cardiac side effects in the heart's electric cycle [1]. The use of zebrafish has been reported to be very reliable, describing the potential toxicity of drugs to the human cardiovascular system [2]. Human cardiovascular disorders have been recapitulated in zebrafish genetic models [3]. Moreover, numerous human cardiovascular drugs have demonstrated similar effects on zebrafish physiology. It is reported that humans' cardiac electrophysiology is more similar to that in zebrafish than in rodents [4]. A previous study has shown that more than 95% of drugs that induce QT prolongation in humans have similar effects in zebrafish [5]. Effects of chemicals on zebrafish cardiac development have been reported in a study by Incardona et al. [6], Transient changes in zebrafish cardiac conduction have been observed after exposure to Polycyclic Aromatic Hydrocarbons (PAHs), which are pollutants in the aquatic environment. The result shows no effect on the initial stages of cardiac loop formation. However, significant changes occur after loop formation, including the development of cardiac valves, formation of trabeculae, and the thickening of the ventricular myocardium. Additionally, biological characteristics, ease of genetic manipulation, facilitation of chemical screening, and genetic similarity to humans are features that contributed to zebrafish as a versatile animal model for cardiovascular research. Previously, zebrafish have been generated to study lipid metabolism and hypercholesteremia, major risk factors for cardiovascular disease [3]. Furthermore, Chen et al. reported mutations in zebrafish, useful for in-depth cardiac development research [7]. These advantages make zebrafish a suitable animal model for cardiac physiology and toxicity studies.

Zebrafish's hearts consists of two chambers, an atrium, and a ventricle, which has a similar pumping mechanism to mammals' hearts in cellular and molecular levels [8]. These similarities include the flow of the blood from sinus venosus into an atrium; the blood moves through the ventricle to the aorta as controlled and directed by the heart valves; has specialized endocardium musculature that drives a high-pressure system; the regulation of heart rhythm controlled by electrical current that flows through the heart, causing the muscles to contract and blood pumped out; and a pacemaker that discharged the electrical current determines the heart rate [9]. Moreover, the zebrafish heart rate was reported at 140–180 bpm, where it is much closer to the human fetal heart rate (130–170 bpm), which is far slower compared to mouse heart rate (300–600 bpm) [10].

As a human cardiovascular disease model, adult zebrafish can be applied to study damage of myocardial tissue caused by prolonged ischemia and hypoxia, which is typical of myocardial infarction and a leading cause of heart failure. Adult zebrafish hearts regenerate, while adult mammalian hearts do not. Adult zebrafish are reported to have the robust regenerative ability in the heart muscle [11]. They can regenerate their ventricles without having a visible scar when surgical amputated or cryo-injured. Moreover, both atrium and ventricle can regenerate in response to genetic cardiomyocyte ablation, even if the ablation is widespread enough to initially cause clinical heart failure [12]. The cardiovascular system is also linked to the zebrafish swimming stamina. Generally, there are a 20 to 50 beats per minute increase in heart rate associated with swimming activity as early as day 5, suggesting that neural or hormonal mechanisms required for heart rate acceleration are functional in early development. Alteration in the heart rate is closely related to the cardiac output. A lower heart rate could reflect lower cardiac output for any given swimming speed in the high stamina group, where this phenomenon could be comparable to athletes [13].

2. Overview of Embryo Cardiac Rhythm Detection

Zebrafish embryos have been widely used to understand heart development and physiology, due to their body transparency, small body size, high fecundity, rapid developmental process, and similar heart structures as humans. These are some features that help scientists to understand the mechanisms in mammals [14]. In addition to transparency, small body size and high fecundity make embryonic zebrafish a fitting animal model in a high throughput heart rate assay. The assay scored 229 (95%) heart rates out of 240 arrayed embryos per 96-well plates, and the heart rates were scored accurately [15]. Other advantages of using zebrafish embryo are the ease of genetic manipulation which can also facilitate identification of the function of human mutations [16] and its ability to survive for several days (4–5 days) without active circulation, providing enough time to study the defects and to dissect cellular and molecular mechanisms [10]. Zebrafish heart development can be traced back to 5 h post-fertilization (hpf) during which cardiac progenitor cells were originated. These cells will migrate to reside in the posterior half of the anterior lateral plate mesoderm (ALPM) during the gastrulation process at 15 hpf. At 24 hpf, heart tube will form and initiate cardiac contraction [17]. Finally, the heart loop from the right-sided ventricle and left-sided atrium can be observed at 48 hpf, although major heart structures have been formed, the heart is still immature and lacking functions for supporting future growth [16]. Regarding this information, zebrafish embryo at 48 hpf can be used to see the whole heartbeat frequency and early-stage chemical treatment as early as 3 hpf can be performed to observe developmental effects [10].

There are several methods to assess cardiac functions in zebrafish embryos, including the manual counting from slow-motion replay in the video, micro pressure systems, microscope techniques, and electrocardiogram devices. However, using electrocardiographic signals in a zebrafish embryo requires precise positioning of the electrodes to obtain reproducible signals [18]. Kang et al. found outthat counting heartbeats manually was more unreliable as there is a high possibility of biased results due to individual error, which measures the variation between repeated experiments by an individual, and from the crowd error, which measures the variation between different operators, even when the counting was done by trained individuals [19]. Gaur et al. [20] also reported the manual counting method. Three independent researchers counted the heartbeat from 10-second length video and, validation was also performed by exposing the zebrafish embryo to Isoproterenol, a well-known beta-adrenergic agonist, which increases heart rate. Their results showed that manual counting is unreliable and may lead to inaccurate data due to the variably experienced researchers.

In overcoming the drawback of manual analysis, several approaches have been developed to monitor cardiac function in zebrafish, such as automated and semi-automated based on computer-controlled, image-based heartbeat detection techniques. Fink et al. [21] and Ocorr et al. [22] outlined a semi-automatic technique of analyzing heartbeats based on the variation of intensity changes over a set of pixels selected by a manually provided threshold, and by stacking a manually selected vertical slice containing the ventricular wall. Other research manually selected the Region of Interest (ROI) before performing an automatic method of characterizing the cardiac function in zebrafish embryos [23]. On the other hand, for the sake of time efficiency, automatic counting was then developed [18,21,24–26]. The development of automated algorithms for estimating heart rate in zebrafish larvae begins with the automatic determination of a suitable ROI and heart rate calculation [25]. Comparison of previously published method to detect cardiac rhythm in zebrafish larvae can be found in Table 1.

Table 1. Comparison of the methods for cardiac rhythm detection in zebrafish embryos.

Author and Published Year	Require a Transgenic Fish Line?	Require a Special Script to Run the Software?	Major Platform to Calculate Heartbeat Regularity	Major Facility to Capture Heartbeat Images	Region of Interests (ROI)	What Kind of Message Can Be Obtained?	Automated Calculation?	References
ImageJ-Based Methods								
(Santoso, Sampurna et al., 2019)	No	No	ImageJ (dynamic pixel changes method)	Inverted microscope mounted with high-speed CCD camera	Dorsal Aorta	Atrium rhythm and heartbeat frequency	No	[27]
(Sampurna, Audira et al., 2018)	No	No	ImageJ (dynamic pixel changes method)	CCD mount onto dissecting microscope	Heart	Atrium and ventricle rhythm, whole heartbeat frequency	No	[28]
(Gaur, Pullaguri et al., 2018)	No	No	ImageJ (pixel intensity changes method)	An inverted microscope (Olympus IX73 series) equipped with a 10-MP camera (ProCAM HS-10 MP)	Heart	Whole heartbeat frequency	No	[20]
(van Opbergen, Koopman et al., 2018)	Yes	Not mentioned	ImageJ and MATLAB (method not mentioned)	Upright widefield microscope (Cairn research, Kent, UK) with a high-speed camera (AndorZyla 4.2 plus sCMOS)	Heart	Whole heartbeat frequency	Yes	[29]
Matlab-Based Methods								
(Gierten, Pylatiuk et al., 2019)	Yes	Yes	MATLAB (dynamic pixel changes method)	An ACQUIFER wide-field high content screening microscope equipped with a white LED array	Heart	Whole heartbeat frequency	Yes	[24]
(Akerberg, Burns, et al., 2019)	No	Yes	Matlab (deep learning platform)	ZEISS Lightsheet Z.1 microscope and optical microscope	Heart	Whole heartbeat frequency, Cardiac Function Parameters	Yes	[30]
(Xing, Huynh, et al., 2018)	No	Yes	Matlab	Electrophysiological recordings by an Opticam attached to the microscope	Heart	Whole heartbeat frequency	Yes	[31]
(Krishna, Chatti, et al., 2017)	No	Yes	Matlab	Zeiss Stereo Discovery V8 zoom stereo microscope with a ProRes color camera C3 (3 Megapixels)	Heart	Whole heartbeat frequency	Yes	[25]
(De Luca, Zaccaria et al., 2014)	Yes	Yes	MATLAB (threshold value method)	Leica TCS SP5X II confocal laser-scanning inverted microscope equipped with a tandem scanning system	Heart	Atrium and ventricle rhythm, whole heartbeat frequency	Yes	[18]
(Pylatiuk, Sanchez, et al., 2014)	Yes	Yes	MATLAB (threshold value method)	An inverted microscope (Leica DMIL LED) with a digital camera (Leica DFC 400)	Heart	Whole heartbeat frequency	Yes	[26]
(Fink, Callol-Massot et al., 2009)	No	Yes	MATLAB	Hamamatsu EM-CCD digital camera mounted on Leica DM-LFSA microscope	Heart	Atrium and ventricle rhythm, whole heartbeat frequency	Yes	[21]

Table 1. Cont.

Author and Published Year	Require a Transgenic Fish Line?	Require a Special Script to Run the Software?	Major Platform to Calculate Heartbeat Regularity	Major Facility to Capture Heartbeat Images	Region of Interests (ROI)	What Kind of Message Can Be Obtained?	Automated Calculation?	References
Commercial Software-Based Methods								
(Martin, Tennant, et al., 2019)	No	Yes	FishRateZ software (commercial) (pixel intensity changes method)	AndorZyla 4.2 sCMOS (Andor Technologies, Belfast, NI, UK) camera mounted to a Nikon Ti microscope (Nikon Instruments, Melville, NY, USA)	Heart	Whole heartbeat frequency	Yes	[32]
(Yozzo, Isales, et al., 2013)	Yes	Yes	MetaXpress 4.0.0.24 software (commercial)	ImageXpress Micro (IXM) Widefield High-Content Screening	Heart	Whole heartbeat frequency	Yes	[33]
(Chan, Lin, et al., 2009)	No	Yes	A custom-made program which developed in C# language was used for digital motion analysis	Stereo-microscope (Olympus) equipped with a 3-color CCD camera	Caudal blood vessel	Whole heartbeat frequency	Yes	[34]
(Lin, S.J. 2016)	No	Yes	SoftEdge™ (IonOptix Corporation)	Light microscope (Axiovert 100 V microscope, Carl Zeiss, Jena, Germany)	Heart	Whole heartbeat frequency	Yes	[35]
(Ocorr, Fink, et al., 2009)	No	Yes	Semi-automatic Optical Heartbeat Analysis (SOHA)	Not mentioned	Heart	Whole heartbeat frequency, heart diameter measurements	Yes	[2]
Zgenebio and RasVector Technology	No	No	Rv Visual Pulse Analysis	CCD mount onto dissecting microscope	Heart	Atrium and ventricle rhythm	Yes	(https://www.zgenebio.com.tw)
Viewpoint Company	No	No	MicroZebraLab	Not mentioned	Heart	Whole heartbeat frequency	Yes	(http://www.viewpoint.fr/en/home)
Noldus Company	No	No	Danioscope Software	ZEISS SteREO Discovery.V8 microscope	Heart	Whole heartbeat frequency	Yes	(https://www.noldus.com/danioscope)

3. Commercial or Third-Party Software

Normally, heart rate assays in zebrafish embryo are performed on one embryo per video/imaging field [9,27]. The high-throughput method from multiple zebrafish embryos per imaging field was established [32]. FisHRateZ, a LabVIEW-based program, can measure the heart rate of multiple zebrafish embryo per imaging field. By utilizing an algorithm to locate the heart automatically and derive average pixel intensity vs. time, data were generated from each embryo's cardiac cycle. FisHRateZ increases the throughput and reliability of the cardiotoxicity screening method. This method is the first approach to detect and place ROI on multiple zebrafish up to five embryones/well. However, the algorithm is unable to assign precise ROIs on overlapping embryos. Therefore, this study suggests that analysis might provide better results with two embryones/well [32]. Another commercial software is MetaXpress. It is a high content image analysis software that uses interactive semi-automated journal scripts to isolate the region of interest and quantify heart rate, circulation, pericardial area, and intersegmental vessel area. Moreover, a fully automated journal script has been used to quantify body length. The main principle of MetaXpress is to detect the heart rate based on intensity variation [33]. SoftEdge Myocyte Cell Length Acquisition Module, developed by IonOptix Corporation (https://www.ionoptix.com/), provides an edge-detection system to evaluate systolic and diastolic by using automatic video. The edge detection is based on either image intensity or the derivative of image intensity. The software analyzes each video image and treats the crossing of the threshold values as the edge location [35]. RvVisualPulse software developed by Zgenebio and RasVector Technology in Taiwan (https://www.zgenebio.com.tw), can simultaneously track the cardiac rhythm in both atrium and ventricle. This software's basic principle is also based on dynamic pixel change and very convenient for potential arrhythmia detection in zebrafish. Another two third-party software called MicroZebraLab from Viewpoint company (http://www.viewpoint.fr/en/home) and DanioScope from Nodules company (https://www.noldus.com/danioscope) also can be used for cardiac rhythm measurement with the advantages of easy operation.

4. Dynamic Pixel Changes Method

Matlab is one of the software commonly used to measure heart rate in zebrafish embryo [18,21,24–26]. Detection and quantification of movement can be performed by algorithms written in Matlab. The Frame Brightness Algorithm tracks changes in average light intensity of each frame combined with a Changing Pixel Intensity Algorithm to detect movement by comparing the intensity changes in individual pixels from one frame to the next. During heart contraction, frame brightness decreases in correspondence to darker pixels. As the heart muscle contracts, the cell membrane becomes more concentrated and obscures more of the transmitted light [21]. A similar approach also has been taken by other researchers [24–26]. However, the Matlab programs were too complicated for researchers who did not have a computer programing language background.

To overcome the scriptwriting requirement, the open-source software of ImageJ, initially developed by the National Institutes of Health (USA), is a public domain, Java-based image processing program [36]. The ImageJ platform is adaptable with no requirement of scriptwriting to execute the program. Similar to Matlab's approach, the cardiac rhythm measurement method is based on the dynamic pixel changes in the heart region. Sampurna et al. [9] proposed an image-based method that did not require transgenic fish or expensive instruments to detect heart rate. Only a conventional dissecting microscope and a less expensive charged-coupled device (CCD) were needed. The highest peak rhythm represented the greatest abundance of red blood cells pumped out of the heart chamber is defined as a contraction (systolic phase). On the other hand, the lowest peak rhythm represented the greatest abundance of red blood cells, which filled the heart chamber and was defined as relaxation (diastolic phase). In previous studies, zebrafish heartbeat calculations mainly focused on the whole heartbeat. The atrium and ventricle beating rhythm was not studied in detail. In the method proposed by Sampurna et al. [9], the potential drugs for atrioventricular blockage could be studied in detail by the image-based method. However, this ImageJ-based method performed manual counting, which involved multiple steps before obtaining cardiac function. Gaur et al. [20] combined ImageJ with an algorithm written in Microsoft Excel and an online Google spreadsheet. Instead of using Origin Pro software to calculate the heartbeat from the dynamic pixel pattern, the algorithm could be used in smoothening raw heartbeat data, and automatic peak detection to avoid unambiguous peak detection [20].

5. Indirect Measurement from Blood Vessels

The heartbeat in zebrafish embryos could be detected indirectly from its blood cells. Shuk Han Cheng's team at the University of Hong Kong described a non-invasive technique that integrated digital motion analysis and power spectral analysis to determine heart rate and heartbeat regularity in peripheral blood vessels. Pulsatile movement of blood cells was observed in the caudal vasculature of zebrafish embryos. A waveform of dynamic pixels can visualize the posterior cardinal vein (PCV) and blood vessels' oscillatory movement. The heart rate was determined by digital motion analysis and power spectral analysis by extracting the cardiac rhythm's frequency characteristics. This study showed that the program could also detect the changes in the variation of heart rate in zebrafish embryos after exposure to Terfenadine, a known QT-prolonging drug [34]. Heartbeat regularity is an essential parameter for cardiac function and is associated with cardiotoxicity in human beings.

On the other hand, another study proved that the heart rhythm calculation from blood flow velocity could be done using the ImageJ-based method [27]. The dorsal aorta (DA) vessels are directly connected to the heart chamber, making the DA regional blood flow pattern following the ventricle's pumping. Similar to the previous study, the calculation is based on pixel intensity change. The principle of pixel intensity change is based on the cell numbers and differences in the degree of an object affected by speed. During heart pumping, in the DA, the highest peak of blood flow pattern represents the systolic phase, where the dynamic pixel change intensity would be higher, and a higher peak rhythm is formed. On the other hand, at low blood flow velocity, a lower peak rhythm is formed. The study found that the time interval of blood flow patterns to be in agreement with heart rate. Heart rate measurement could also be done indirectly based on the recorded blood flow video. However, heart rate measurement calculated from blood flow patterns may lead to biased results [27]. According to Grimm and colleagues (1996), the variability of heartbeat interval could be determined not only from ECG but also from the blood pressure. Their results showed that waveform data derived from the blood pressure was consistent with the data from ECG [37].

6. Kymograph-Based Method

Kymograph is a two-dimension (2D) plot containing time and space information created from time-lapse images of the region of interest. It can quantify the movement velocity and trajectory of the objects. In measuring velocities based upon kymographs, the moving object's path has to be marked [38]. A kymograph is generated from the fluorescence intensity, presented along the segmented line (x-axis) over time (y-axis). Diagonal lines in kymograph demonstrate moving objects over time, and ventricle lines illustrate stationary objects [39]. In zebrafish, a kymograph was used to quantify heart rhythm. The results of kymograph-based quantification of the cardiac cycle could illustrate bradycardia effect and irregular heart rhythm in *Islet-1(isl1)* mutant zebrafish embryo, as the distance between two dotted lines encompassing a full cardiac cycle is much longer in the mutant than in the sibling [40]. Other research used kymograph to record the frog's myocardial activity [41].

Kymographs have long been used for visualizing intracellular motion. Kymographs can be generated from a time-lapse image sequence using image analysis software, such as MetaMorph (Molecular Devices), NIS-Elements (Nikon), and ImageJ (NIH). By using the ImageJ, the kymographs can be plotted, smoothened, and quantified using the Smoothed Plot Profile and Find Peaks tools provided in the BAR Plugin [42]. The advantage of a kymograph is time-lapse data compressed onto a single image allowing visualization of the motion. For another, the human eye is very good at picking outlines, even in substantial noise. With kymographs' help, it can be much easier to see how many moving particles are present [43]. Freely available kymograph software has been used to visualize live primary cilia dynamics using fluorescence microscopy and in quantitative measurements of intraflagellar transport (IFT) movement within cells [43,44]. Thus far, the implementation was limited in zebrafish and other aquatic animals. Studies on cardiac rhythm detection by using the kymography method can be explored in the future.

7. Laser Confocal Scan Method

A laser-scanning confocal microscope is a sensitive and precise tool for measuring cardiovascular changes in the zebrafish embryo. It is also reported that the measurements are similar to those obtained with Doppler echocardiography [45]. A previous study reported that the heart rate evaluation in transgenic larvae could be obtained from sequential images acquired by a resonant laser scanning confocal microscope. The heart region extracted was based on fluorescence (red/green), and was processed further by morphological operations, based on the threshold values [18]. Another technique, called laser-scanning velocimetry, provided continuous blood cell velocity measurement necessary for estimating cardiac output and other cardiovascular function parameters. Line scans are images constructed with laser-scanning microscopy by repeatedly imaging one pixel-wide line. When the scan line is placed across a vessel, either perpendicular or parallel to blood flow, the resulting line scan image contains information about circulation dynamics. The continuity of velocity information provided by laser-scanning velocimetry makes it possible to measure blood acceleration and deceleration, which are similar parameters that are attainable using Doppler echocardiography [45]. However, this method is only applicable to transgenic embryos with fluorescence-labeled blood cells and requires costly instrumental settings.

8. AI Deep Learning-Based Method

Integrating artificial intelligence (AI) into cardiovascular research shows optimistic promise in generating quantitative diagnostic for clinical implementation. AI integration is not a simple transition since machines replace humans. However, AI could help researchers and clinicians to make better decisions. AI can integrate complex omics data with additional layers of information, including imaging and electronic health data, to provide accurate information and quantitatively analyze large data sets, which would not be feasible manually [46]. Several effective automated heartbeat detection methods have been developed to reduce the workload for larva heartbeat analysis. A previous study utilized a deep learning platform, called Cardiac Functional Imaging Network (CFIN) to design automatic and rapidly segment atrial and ventricular boundaries in live zebrafish embryo hearts and utilize data to calculate other cardiac function parameters. This aspect of CFIN was built in Matlab's underlying architecture of the deep convolutional encoder-decoder SegNet. As a result, CFIN is capable of detecting elevation in cardiac output and sensitivity over fractional shortening. This method was shown to be a powerful new tool to accurately measure heart function in a vertebrate model organism [30]. Custom Matlab-based software, called FishInspector, was created to detect morphological features in zebrafish embryos automatically. The zebrafish heart, as the region of interest (ROI), is identified by comparing the absolute difference in pixel intensity between two consecutive frames. However, this method depends heavily on image quality (camera and microscope settings, resolution, contrast, intensity) [47]. Another automatic method, Zebrafish Heart Rate Automatic Method (Z-HRAM), was developed to detect and track the heartbeats of immobilized, ventrally positioned zebrafish larvae without direct heart observation. This method is well suited for the analysis of low resolution and low-frequency image data. Z-HRAM focused on detecting the body deformation, and computation of the pixel-wise motion images of all images in the video recording to associate zebrafish body deformation frequency with the heartbeat. Heartbeats detected from Z-HRAM were shown to correlate reliably with those determined through corresponding electrocardiogram and manual video inspection. However, Z-HRAM is currently limited to the detection of heart rate and beat-to-beat intervals [31].

In a deep-learning-based method, training was necessary to demonstrate consistency with the overall assessment and compensate for the automated image analysis [47]. Xing et al. [31], conducted training at a variable learning rate beginning at 0.1, which was reduced by a factor of five every two epochs. Using these parameters, they observed an increase in accuracy and decreased in function for both the training and cross-validation datasets, which were consistent with successful training.

9. Electrocardiography Method (ECG)

The optimization of ECG detection in early stage zebrafish larvae has been demonstrated in its utility and detecting the effect of QT-prolonging. Anesthetized zebrafish embryos were transferred to paraffin wax. The glass micropipette was then positioned on the skin surface between the ventricle and atrium with no penetration. As early as 2 dpf (days post-fertilization) of zebrafish could be used for ECG measurements, as the compound action potentials have been generated, and effective cardiac conduction are already present [48]. Electrical Potential Sensing (EPS) technology was established to record in vivo electrocardiogram activity from the heart of the zebrafish embryo at 3 dpf and 5 dpf. This method does not require complex post-processing tools, and importantly, the embryo is maintained alive. The EPS sensor uses a metallic titanium (Ti) based central electrode coated with a titanium dioxide (TiO_2) film/membrane acting as a dielectric [49]. Nonetheless, ECG methods were considered challenging to record heartbeat in zebrafish embryo due to its small size [18]. Moreover, the requirement of using expensive specialized devices and software has kept it inaccessible to many scientists.

10. Overview of Adult Cardiac Rhythm Detection

The cardiac rhythm detection method in adult zebrafish (2–3 months old) is more complicated than techniques applicable to the embryonic stage due to a loss of transparency and dependence on anesthetic drugs. In aquatic toxicity studies, the cardiovascular function has been an indicator of changes in the physical condition of health or stress in response to an environment [50]. Zebrafish is an excellent model for its sensitivity to drug treatment. It can reveal a decreased in heart rate concerning the human *ether-a-go-go* gene (hERG) channel blockade, allowing for drug testing. Moreover, zebrafish also provide an efficient genetic approach to reveal the genetic basis underlying molecular mechanisms of numerous heart diseases [51]. It could be a robust human cardiac electrophysiology model since its heart rate, and action potential morphology are similar, although some differences are apparent [52]. Moreover, adult zebrafish exhibit the amazing regenerative capacity of heart muscle [11], thus making zebrafish a promising model to study cardiovascular disease in humans.

Advanced imaging techniques are required to measure all facets of cardiac function in adult zebrafish. Electrocardiogram (ECG) is a standard diagnostic tool to detect cardiovascular disease in humans. The body surface ECG recording of adult zebrafish was first developed in 2006 by Milan et al. at the Cardiovascular Research Center, Boston, MA, USA [53], followed by several modifications made in the methods of ECG recording in zebrafish. ECG waveforms present a distinct P wave, QRS complex, and T wave. It is reported that the waveform in adult zebrafish is comparable with the waveform presents in humans [54]. High-frequency ultrasound imaging has been proposed as a suitable tool for achieving high-resolution imaging of adult zebrafish tissue structures [55]. The use of echocardiography with a high frequency (50–70 MHz) probe can allow for high resolution, real-time, non-invasive imaging to examine many cardiac structure parameters and function [52]. Magnetic Resonance Imaging (MRI) is also well-established for imaging adult zebrafish as a cardiovascular disease animal model. This method could provide three dimensional (3D) live images to depict the embryonic heart developmental processes in zebrafish and the injury recovery of adult zebrafish skin. However, due to the small size of zebrafish, a high-resolution micro-imaging magnet was required [56,57]. Modern electronic sensor tags were recently established to collect high-resolution data on the movement and physiology of zebrafish. The loggers were surgically inserted into the fish, close to the heart. The application of the loggers is considered difficult or even challenging due to the minuscule scale surgical procedure. Moreover, it may cause stress on the fish. New cordless heart rate bio-loggers were introduced to provide easier tag-deployment and surgery, hence reducing stress for the fish [58,59]. With all the methods mentioned, the advantage of using aquatic creatures like fish is that they can be easily accommodated in a smaller space. Nonetheless, at the same time, the smaller size restricts the researcher from performing several activities, unlike other vertebrates, which allow manipulation with ease [60]. Summary of cardiac rhythm detection method in larvae and adult zebrafish can be found in Figure 1 and the comparison beetwen previously published methods to detect cardiac rhythm in adult zebrafish can be found in Table 2.

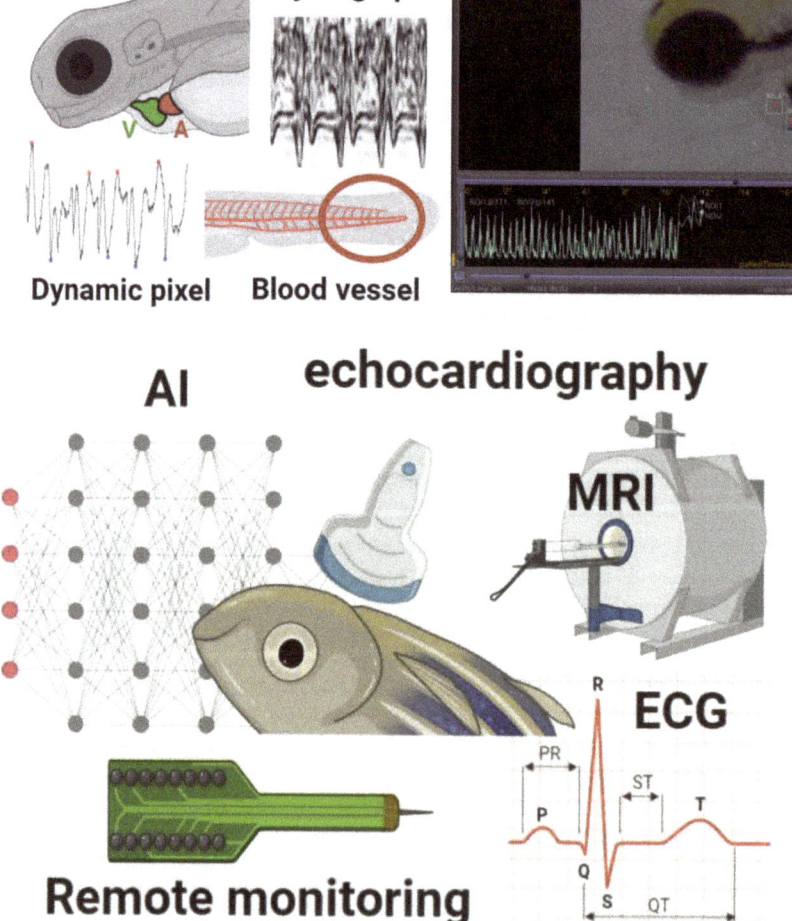

Figure 1. Summary of different methods used to measure cardiac rhythm in either embryo (upper red panel) or adult (bottom green panel) zebrafish. Several methods based on either dynamic pixel change or kymograph are proposed in the embryonic stage of zebrafish. Some commercial third-party software is also available for cardiac rhythm measurement. In adult zebrafish, some instruments like Electrocardiography (ECG), Echocardiography (Echo), and Magnetic Resonance Imaging (MRI) can be used for cardiac rhythm measurement.

Table 2. Comparison of the methods for cardiac rhythm detection in adult zebrafish.

Author and Published Years	Require Special Transgenic Fish Lines?	Require Special Script to Run the Software?	Major Platform to Calculate Heartbeat Regularity	Major Facility to Capture Heartbeat Images	Region of Interests (ROI)	What Kind of Message Can Be Obtained?	Automated Calculation?	References
Electrocardiogram-Based Methods								
Mousavi & Patil (2020)	No	No	ImageJ	Stereoscope (MZ12.5, Leica Microsystems, Wetzlar, Germany) and camera (Dino-Eye Edge series AM7025X)	Whole heart	Heart rate, dominant frequency	No	[61]
Lenning, et al. (2017)	No	Yes	LabView	4-channel MEA membranes for ECG acquisition	Whole heart	Whole heartbeat frequency	Yes	[51]
Vaz da Silva et al. (2017)	Yes	Yes	LabChart program	ECG signals a NeuroLog System	Whole heart	Whole heartbeat frequency	Yes	[62]
Liu et al. (2016)	No	Yes	Clampfit 10.0 software	ECG recording	Whole heart	Heart rate, PR, QRS, and QT intervals	Yes	[54]
Chaudari et al. (2013)	No	Yes	Power lab software	ECG recording	Whole heart	Heart rate, QT, PR and RR intervals	Yes	[63]
Echocardiography-Based Detection Methods								
Chiang, et al. (2020)	No	Yes	Matlab	A 70-MHz ultrasound imaging system and single-element transducer	Heart and dorsal aorta	Blood flow, tissue velocity, and cardiac deformation measurement	Yes	[55]
Yeo, Yoon et al. (2019)	No	Yes	Matlab	Custom-built, 64-channel high-frequency array imaging system and a high-frequency linear array transducer with 256 elements	Heart and dorsal aorta	Blood flow velocity, Heart regeneration	Yes	[64]
Wang, Huttneer et al. (2017)	Yes	Yes	Vevo Lab™ analysis software	Vevo2100® Imaging System and Vevo Imaging Station (VisualSonics) equipped with a high frequency transducer	Whole heart	Cardiovascular function parameters	Yes	[65]
Lee, Genge et al. (2016)	No	Yes	VisualSonics software	Vevo 2100 ultrasound system (VisualSonics1, Toronto, ON, Canada), with a 70 MHz ultrasound transducer	Whole heart	Heart rate, stroke volume (SV), ejection fraction (EF), fractional shorting (FS) and cardiac output (CO)	Yes	[52]

Table 2. *Cont.*

Author and Published Years	Require Special Transgenic Fish Lines?	Require Special Script to Run the Software?	Major Platform to Calculate Heartbeat Regularity	Major Facility to Capture Heartbeat Images	Region of Interests (ROI)	What Kind of Message Can Be Obtained?	Automated Calculation?	References
Magnetic Resonance Imaging (MRI)								
Koth, Maguire, et al. (2017)	Yes	Yes	Matlab	MR scanner	Whole heart	Heart regeneration	Yes	[56]
Kabli, Alia et al. (2006)	No	Yes	Para Vision 3.02pl running on a Silicon Graphics O2 workstation with the Irix 6.5.3 operating system and using Linux XWinNMR 3.2	Magnetic Resonance Microscopy (MRM) consist of microimaging probe, MR magnet	Whole body	Developmental process in zebrafish	Yes	[57]
Remote Monitoring Methods								
Norling (2017)	No	Yes	Software AcceleRater (python-based web application)	DST micro-HRT logger	Whole heart	Heart rate, Behavior performance	Yes	[58]
Brijs, Sandblom et al. (2019)	No	Yes	LabChart Pro software	Custom-built Logger	Heart and coeliacomesenteric artery	Blood flow, Heart rate	Yes	[59]

11. ECG-Based Detection Methods

Electrocardiogram (ECG), including up to five embryones/well, has become the most extensively used non-invasive diagnostic tool for evaluating cardiac diseases. Measurement of ECG intervals is considered one of the most important and gold standard techniques because ECG interval provides an indirect assessment of the heart's state and can be indicative of certain cardiac conditions. So far, ECG has been an excellent way to record the heartbeat in adult zebrafish with less harm to the fish. The results were also proved to be very accurate without a requirement for additional reading and formula [66]. In ECG, three components are crucial for detection: T wave, P wave, and the QRS complex. The P wave represents the depolarization of the atrium; QRS complex represents depolarization of the ventricle, and the T wave, represents the repolarization of the ventricle [67]. In addition, the QT interval is the most important time interval in the ECG waveform, defined as the time from the upstroke of the QRS complex to the end of the T wave. This interval represents the duration of the ventricle's electrical activity (depolarization and repolarization) in a given heartbeat. The reported QT intervals of adult zebrafish in previous studies ranged from 250 ms to 600 ms with multiform ECG signals [54]. The overall ECG waveform can be seen in Figure 1. In establishing the authenticity of ECG signals in fish, several different recordings were taken. A study by Haverkamp et al. [68] showed that the average heart rate of the zebrafish is around 148 beats per minute; the QRS interval recorded was 44 ± 3 ms. The average PR interval was about 62 ms, and the RR interval was around 469 ms. Lastly, the QT interval recorded was 269 ± 60 ms. The results were consistent with the past ECG systems and paved the way for more complex types of ECG experiments.

Leor-Librach et al. [69] developed a computerized system for the controlled increase of heart rate by Isoproterenol based on a modified proportional-integral controller. Previous references and protocols were used to carry out some important steps for developing a pharmacodynamic model for model-based, adaptive control systems, and as a part of larger cardiovascular models [69]. In optimizing the adult zebrafish ECG method for assessing drug-induced QTc prolongation, specific procedures using the histamine receptor antagonist, Terfenadine as a test drug, were carried out for ECG recording in the adult zebrafish. The fish were anesthetized and mounted in a wet sponge, so thatthe upper side could be easily analyzed. The sponge had been cut into a triangle to preventing the water from infiltrating the gill. The scales which cover the heart were removed; thus the electrode could penetrate the skin vividly [63]. The dermis peeling on the chest significantly enhanced signal recording from the muscle layer on the chest. In addition, opening the pericardial sac further enhanced the ECG signal's surface without changes to the electrophysiology [54]. The experiment's region of interest was below the fishes' fins, and it was constantly monitored through a microscope. The electrode responsible for recording the ECG signal was carefully inserted without damaging any tissue or muscle. The positive needle electrode was inserted between the pectoral fins. The negative electrode was placed in two-third of the body length down from the head and positioned near the anal region or reproductive cavity. Another grounding electrode, used as a reference electrode, was placed at the sponge's left corner. The penetration depth of the needle electrodes was about 1–1.5 mm [63]. The pectoral electrode was constantly moved so that a stronger P wave, T wave, and QRS complex were clearly detected and recorded accurately. The timing of the experiment depended on the objectives and the response time for the ECG recording.

There are several limitations in the ECG acquisition systems as only a short period can be recorded, and it requires the use of an anesthetized animal [70,71]. Notably, the anesthetics could only sedate the fish for about 30 m, after which, it is needed to be transferred to a recovery tank [69]. These two factors could lead to the inconsistency of results. The appropriate type of anesthetic drugs and a precise dose should be carefully chosen to avoid unreliable results. The ECG is only suitable for manual measurement of fish, one at a time, which is another limitation when screening multiple fish. Moreover, long-term ECG monitoring with repeated experiments will stress zebrafish, and weak ECG signals generated [51].

T-wave is the most significant ECG wave that shows the cardiac cycle's repolarization from beat to beat. ECG acquisition method improved with the development of microelectrode array (MEA) membranes that can provide an appropriate signal-to-noise ratio (SNR) with complete P wave features, QRS complex, and T-wave. This method has recorded ECG signals that exhibit a clear difference between injured heart muscle ECG and normal heart ECG reading [72]. The additional limitation for ECG recordings in adult zebrafish is in the application of drug discovery where the dosage of the drug could not be determined precisely, making the data difficult to interpret. Differences in acclimatization and flow rate of oral perfusion may differ significantly between various laboratories, adding the result's high variances [63].

The lack of well-defined diagnostic parameters for specific-disease patterns is one of the big challenges in doing ECG recording. This makes the traditional methods of algorithmic identification even harder to do. Despite this, a trained eye can identify abnormal features, even when an algorithm fails. Therefore, the new current methods which make use of machine learning were proposed for ECG waveforms. In recent studies, computational analysis on surface ECG recording and Deep Neural Network (DNN) achieved much more accuracy in detecting the premature ventricular contractions than Artificial Neural Network (ANN). It has been established that ANN shows accurate results in small datasets, and both of the ECG analysis tools are based on Image processing techniques. Zebrafish ECG images can be transformed in Matlab software to the digitized values as in Human ECG. Most of the experiments performed on awake zebrafish compared to anesthetized fish and artifacts dominated the raw signals. Moreover, the noise was removed by using Wavelet transform [51].

11.1. Noise Interfaces for ECG

The ECG recording methods used in adult zebrafish showed similar noise interference as in human ECG recording. However, the high noise level inherent in the signal is an essential challenge to identify ECG recording in adult zebrafish. The noise sourced could be influenced by the power line artifact, electrode contact noise, and muscle movement [73]. A protocol has been proposed for noise-free signals propagation and obtaining raw ECG signals without any data preprocessing as a wavelet transform. Thus, making the characteristic peaks of the P wave, QRS Complex, and T-wave easily identifiable [54].

The significance of the conventional method used in practice in ECG recording of adult zebrafish has been incorporated with of ECG analysis efficiency using an electrophysiology software package. ECG recording in zebrafish has a high-frequency ECG signal, which varies in a range of 50 Hz power line interference. The components are having low frequency exhibit muscle and movement artifacts. It has been demonstrated that pericardial sac with the dermis and silvery affect the ECG recording of adult zebrafish as zebrafish dermis is densely composed with a pack of collagen fibers [74].

EZ-Instrument Technology Co, Taiwan, has developed a simple ECG kit for teaching and research to make the extent of recording in zebrafish easy and simple. The zebrafish ECG kit comprises an integrated signal receiver and amplifier with the software package used for data processing. The specialized electrodes were also designed for anesthetized adult zebrafish. The design of three needlepoint electrode probes is comprised of the pectoral, abdominal, and grounding electrodes [56]. In reducing the noise in an aqueous environment, insulating paint was used on the electrodes' surface with a harbored stainless-steel needle. The area of signal detection was defined to 1 to 1.5 mm on the head of the needle. The tail of the needle was welded with the connecting wire having a 3-pole auxiliary connector cluster. Zebrafish ECG recording by this method exhibited two micromanipulators that hold the pectoral and abdominal needles and a computer system with the software package for the analysis [75].

It must be noted that the background noise was more pronounced in adults than the optically transparent embryos. Therefore, appropriate normalization and validation of data may be required for comparative purposes. Acclimatization for 16 h in a recirculation system then 2 h of acclimatization in a semi-static tank used to immobilize the fish before recording ECG was found to be the best acclimatization time to produce consistent ECG signal. Regular, stable, reproducible, and noise-free ECG with nearly similar R–R intervals were considered consistent ECG [63]. Grounded Faraday cage was commonly used in some methods to minimize the background noise [48,51,63,76]. On the other hand, in a previous study, background noise was effectively reduced by applying the optimum signal threshold and Savitzky-Golay smoothing. The Savitzky–Golay algorithm also allows unbiased smoothing and real-time data calculation without a need for noise statistics [61].

11.2. Comparison of Human ECG with Zebrafish ECG and Application for Toxicity Assessment

Similar to humans' experience, the different placement of the electrode in adult zebrafish ECGs is thought to account for the variations in T wave morphology and amplitude between different fish. Liu et al. [54] recorded a zebrafish ECG in the presence of hyperkalemia and found the similarity with human ECG during hyperkalemia. They also investigated the change in ventricular repolarization during heart regeneration in an amputation and cryoinjury model and a zebrafish mutant as a human long QT syndrome model. Moreover, in the context of the cardiac action potential in zebrafish, ECG shows similarity with the human cardiac action potential [76]. The anatomy of human ECG and zebrafish is shown in Figure 2.

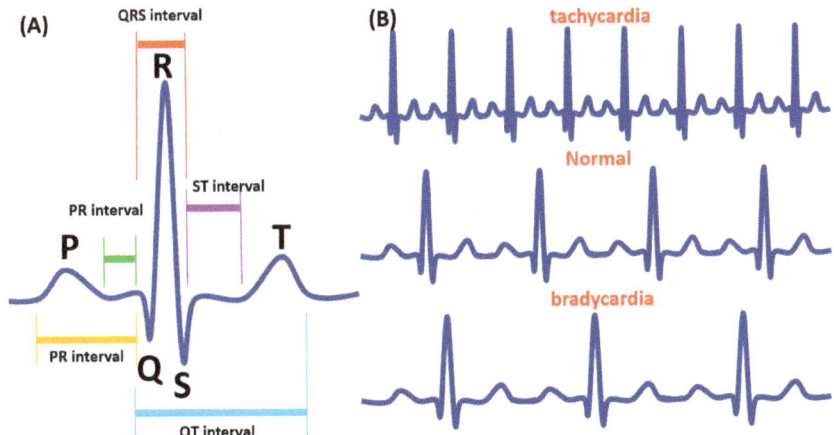

Figure 2. The Electrocardiography (ECG) waveform in adult zebrafish. (**A**) The waveform analysis of ECG. (**B**) Tachycardia (upper panel), normal (middle panel), and bradycardia (lower panel) heart pattern was shown according to a previous publication [73].

In adult zebrafish, the technique of needle electrodes is used with the anesthetic model incorporated [76,77]. Anesthetic drugs are commonly used in animal model assay before the experiment is conducted. However, anesthetic drugs were reported to affect the adult zebrafish's circulatory system and cardiac physiology. A previous study has reported that MS-222 could induce bradycardia. However, isoproterenol, other anesthetic drugs, could increase the heart rate of the fish. The injection of MS-222 caused a heart rate reduction from 160 to 130 beats per minute in one minute. Afterward, injection with isoproterenol has increased the heart rate from 130 to 155 beats per minute. Therefore, the combinational effect of those two anesthetic drugs was studied, and less heart rate alteration was observed. Afterward, in 10 minutes, the heart rate dropped to 64 beats per minute after exposure with MS-222. On the other hand, the heart rate only dropped from 148 to 131 bpm after exposure to MS-222 and Isoflurane combination. In addition, most of the zebrafish in the MS-222 treated group did not recover after sedation. This result suggested that a combination of anesthetic drugs is safer for sedating the zebrafish [68].

Aftereffect of different anesthetic drugs could be observed using the ECG system. A new approach by using other drugs was then performed to see the alteration on cardiovascular performances. Isoproterenol, the agonist of the beta-adrenergic, an amine analog of adrenaline [78], has been widely used for pharmaceutical purposes and has been prescribed to people who have bradycardia [48], as it is known to increase the heart rate of patients. In fish, it is reported that the result was dose-dependent. A dose of 5 µM of the drug caused an increment of heart rate by 1.25-fold. However, in low concentration, 0.5 µM, the recorded heart rate could only increase by 1.04-fold [79].

On the other hand, Mousavi and the colleagues used a recording chamber with a high-resolution camera mounted on the underside coupled with automated recording, heart detection, movement correction, and advanced noise reduction algorithms could allow monitoring the heart rate of swimming fish in real-time without the need for anesthesia [61]. Lauridsen et al.'s findings also supported this study, demonstrating the possibility of measuring heart rate without masking its frequencies even with rapid fish movements [80].

12. Light-Cardiogram Methods

Although the body-surface ECG recording method has been proposed in adult zebrafish, it remained inaccessible to other scientists due to the expensive specialized devices and software, low signal-to-noise ratio. In addition, electrode placement's subjectivity often requires specialist expertise and not readily transferable to other laboratories for routine assessment [81]. Mousavi and Patil established a simple, non-invasive, and inexpensive light-cardiogram technique to assess heart rate and frequency in adult zebrafish. A Bright-field microscope equipped with a high-resolution camera and ImageJ software was used for recording and processing. Collectively, the technique can measure heartbeats and record relative cardiac outputs and compare differences between physiological states (e.g., sexes). Isosceles triangle, as the region of interests (ROI), was placed between opercula and the perpendicular ventral midline. The dynamic pixel change method from ImageJ software was used for heartbeat measurement. The cardiograms generated reverse light signal oscillations. Contraction decreased average brightness within the corresponding ROI; conversely, relaxation increased average brightness. The heartbeat detected by this method was 120 bpm (male 122.58 ± 2.15 and female 121.37 ± 2.63 beats/min), as it is comparable with ECG recording [61]. The approach could be amenable to automation and applicable to other fish species.

13. Echocardiography-Based Detection Methods

Echocardiography, which makes use of ultrasound imaging method, has recently been explored to capture the heart image of adult zebrafish. The ultrasound energy is applied to the body through a transducer with piezo-electric transmit and receive ultrasound crystals [82]. A conventional ultrasound imaging device at 8.5 MHz was used to image adult zebrafish hearts [55]. Single-element transducers, a 30-MHz high-frequency ultrasound array system with duplex imaging, were used to measure adult zebrafish hearts and blood flow velocities. Recently, a dual-pulsed wave Doppler imaging method that acquired both spectral and tissue Doppler waveforms simultaneously was developed to enable real-time measurement of the functional change during heart regeneration and adult cardiac structure zebrafish [64]. Most clinical ultrasound scanners can acquire B-mode (brightness) images, M-mode (motion) images, and Doppler (velocity) images. In B-mode imaging, a 2D sector scan is used to create an image where pixel brightness in the image is proportional to the received echo signal's strength. In M-mode imaging, a 2D image is formed where one image axis is the transducer's distance, and the other axis is time. As with B-mode, pixel intensities in the M-mode image are proportional to the received echo signal's strength. M-mode images can be used to track myocardial wall and valve motion. Doppler imaging uses the frequency shift in the received signal to estimate the velocity of ultrasound scatters. Doppler imaging can measure wall and valve motion and assess blood flow through the arteries and heart [82]. In a previous study, two-chamber B-mode images were used to obtain cardiac functional parameters measurement in adult zebrafish, such as stroke volume (SV), ejection fraction (EF), fractional shortening (FS), and cardiac output (CO). Ordinarily, in clinical echocardiography, an image captured from the parasternal short-axis in M-mode would be the most accurate, thus measurement of fractional shortening is the best choice. However, the small size of the zebrafish's heart (~1.5 mm) makes the M-mode image not easily obtainable [52]. However, other research showed that M-mode imaging was used to analyze the blood flow and tissue motion velocity within the ventricle [55]. High-frequency echocardiography (HFE) has recently allowed the study of cardiac rates in adult zebrafish in 6–9 months old with a body length of ≥20 mm. Nevertheless, the image quality was sex-dependent. The adult female zebrafish often was compromised compared to males due to gravidity in females [65].

14. Magnetic Resonance Imaging (MRI)

Echocardiography is an inexpensive and widely available technique, but it usually provides only one- or two-dimensional information and is limited to morphological and functional investigations. CT (Computed Tomography) can provide excellent spatial resolution, but relies on ionizing radiation and the application of dedicated stains to achieve soft-tissue contrast. On the other hand, MRI is a well-established clinical diagnostic imaging as it provides multi-parametric information on the heart radiation-free and non-invasively. MRI also is frequently used for in vivo imaging in non-aquatic animal models of cardiovascular disease, including small (e.g., rodents) and large (e.g., sheep, pigs) mammals. Previously, in vivo MRI has been applied to image early developmental stages of frog embryos [56]. The small size of adult zebrafish and optically non-transparent bodies has been challenging to imagine at sufficient resolution. MRM (Magnetic Resonance Microscopy) is established with the same principle as MRI but produces images with a higher resolution because it uses stronger magnetic field gradients (200–1000 mT/m) and specialized radio frequency (RF) coils. Combining high-resolution MRM with 3D image reconstruction makes possible image acquisition of a live adult fish non-invasively, which is impossible using other imaging techniques [57].

Another study by Koth et al. [56] combined cutting-edge technical developments in MRI, novel data processing approaches, and 3D-printing for resolving minimal changes in vivo during zebrafish heart regeneration. To validate the method, they used investigated uninjured, sham-injured, cryo-injured, and resection-injured Tg(*hsp70l:dnfgfr1-EGFP*) transgenic fish which can be conditionally activated dominant-negative *fgfr1* signaling after heat shock treatment. They were able to scan live adult zebrafish under anesthesia and physiological conditions for several hours and with a 100% recovery rate. Thus, they were able to image the same fish repeatedly during the repair process.

The limitation of this method is the small size of zebrafish, in which additional precautions and high-resolution micro-imaging magnet are required to get a good resolution. It has limited space for a flow-through chamber for imaging. The small flow-through chamber cannot support the high water flow, which is needed if noise from surrounding water is to be avoided. Furthermore, zebrafish cannot tolerate a high flow of water. The experimental time should be kept as short as possible since the zebrafish has a relatively low tolerance to anesthetic [57].

15. Remote Monitoring Methods

Cardiovascular performances in big fish could also be performed by remote monitoring [58,59]. Modern electronic sensor tags (Bio-loggers) can collect high-resolution data on movement and physiological fish. Electronic sensor tags measure depth, temperature, fluorescence, heart rate, swimming speed, stroke frequency, heat flux, muscle oxygen, acceleration, and many other parameters. Some of these parameters can be used to quantify feeding events and predator-prey interactions. Bio-loggers are often used to measure cardiac performance in big fish. The loggers were surgically inserted into the fish, where the heart's location provided substantially higher data quality than when the logger was positioned in the fish belly [58]. However, the loggers' application is considered difficult due to the surgical operation; the cord-based bio-electrodes are invasive and may increase stress to the fish [83]. Recently, new cordless heart rate bio-loggers, which are easier to the implant, were introduced on the market to provide easier tag-deployment and surgery while inducing less stress for the fish [58].

Bio-logging and bio-telemetric devices were commonly used to study stress physiology. The alteration of heart rate and other cardiovascular variables, mostly affected by behavioral responses and environmental perturbations, has been widely used to determine and quantify acute stress responses of fish. Another early physiological indicator of stress; and potential method for assessing farmed fish's welfare is the changes in gastrointestinal blood flow (GBF). GBF is known to decrease dramatically in fish in response to acute stress, as blood flow is prioritized for oxygen demanding organs and muscle tissues. A previous study has positioned bio-loggers within the abdominal cavity. GBF was measured from the coeliac mesenteric artery, the first caudal branch of the dorsal aorta that divides progressively to supply the stomach, intestine, liver, and gonads [59]. The major disadvantage of bio-logger is the requirement of invasive surgery, as precise placement of tags is required to have high featured data. Generally, when studying fish in the wild, there is a need to recapture the fish to collect the data [84]. Nevertheless, this method is still applicableto big fish, and the application on zebrafish remains unexplored.

16. Conclusions

This is the first review of recent and advanced cardiac rhythm detection methods in adult and embryonic stages of zebrafish (methods are summarized in Figure 1. All the proposed methods in detecting heart rate in zebrafish have some advantages and limitations. The heartbeat detection in the zebrafish embryo was mostly performed by a dynamic pixel change method. This method could be performed by open source and user-friendly software, Image-J, or automatically common software Matlab. A laser-scanning confocal microscope is another approach that has been proved to be a sensitive and precision tool for measuring cardiovascular changes in the zebrafish embryo. However, this method is only applicable for transgenic embryos, and it requires costly equipment. While electrocardiography (ECG) is not easy to be conducted in zebrafish embryos, it has been widely used as a gold standard method for the heartbeat and cardiac rhythm detection in adult zebrafish. It is reported that the waveform in adult zebrafish is comparable with the waveform presents in humans. High-frequency ultrasound imaging has also been proposed as a suitable tool for acquiring high-resolution imaging of adult zebrafish tissue structures. Modern electronic sensor tags were established to collect high-resolution data on movement and physiological fish. The loggers were surgically inserted into the fish, close to the heart. However, it is considered difficult due to the surgical procedure and might cause stress on the fish. In conclusion, the cardiac rhythm can be measured at either embryonic or adult zebrafish by utilizing the methods mentioned above. However, the embryonic stage can be better to study cardiovascular function due to its body transparency, independent of anesthetic drugs, facilitate high-throughput heart assay, can be used to detect heart developmental process, and the ability to survive for several days without circulation. The methodology to perform heartbeat and other cardiovascular function parameters can be chosen based on each laboratory capacity. Overall, zebrafish have proven a promising research model for human cardiovascular diseases, pharmaceutical, and toxicological research.

Funding: This study was funded by grants sponsored by the Ministry of Science Technology (MOST 105-2313-B-033-001-MY3 and MOST107-2622-B-033-001-CC2) to C.-D.H., and (MOST106-2633-B153-001 and MOST107-2633-B153-001) J.-C.H.

Acknowledgments: We appreciate Jimmy Tseng from Zgenebio company and Daniel Lu from RasVector Technology on providing RvVisualPulse software for cardiac rhythm testing in zebrafish. We appreciate Marri Jmelou Roldan from the University of Santo Tomas for providing English editing to enhance the quality of the paper.

Conflicts of Interest: The authors declare no conflict of interest.

References

1. Redfern, W.; Carlsson, L.; Davis, A.; Lynch, W.; MacKenzie, I.; Palethorpe, S.; Siegl, P.; Strang, I.; Sullivan, A.; Wallis, R. Relationships between preclinical cardiac electrophysiology, clinical QT interval prolongation and torsade de pointes for a broad range of drugs: Evidence for a provisional safety margin in drug development. *Cardiovasc. Res.* **2003**, *58*, 32–45. [CrossRef]
2. Caballero, M.V.; Candiracci, M. Zebrafish as screening model for detecting toxicity and drugs efficacy. *J. Unexplored Med. Data* **2018**, *3*. [CrossRef]
3. Giardoglou, P.; Beis, D. On zebrafish disease models and matters of the heart. *Biomedicines* **2019**, *7*, 15. [CrossRef] [PubMed]
4. MacRae, C.A.; Peterson, R.T. Zebrafish as tools for drug discovery. *Nat. Rev. Drug Discov.* **2015**, *14*, 721–731. [CrossRef]
5. Cassar, S.; Adatto, I.; Freeman, J.L.; Gamse, J.T.; Iturria, I.; Lawrence, C.; Muriana, A.; Peterson, R.T.; Van Cruchten, S.; Zon, L.I. Use of zebrafish in drug discovery toxicology. *Chem. Res. Toxicol.* **2019**, *33*, 95–118. [CrossRef]
6. Incardona, J.P.; Collier, T.K.; Scholz, N.L. Defects in cardiac function precede morphological abnormalities in fish embryos exposed to polycyclic aromatic hydrocarbons. *Toxicol. Appl. Pharmacol.* **2004**, *196*, 191–205. [CrossRef]
7. Chen, J.-N.; Haffter, P.; Odenthal, J.; Vogelsang, E.; Brand, M.; Van Eeden, F.; Furutani-Seiki, M.; Granato, M.; Hammerschmidt, M.; Heisenberg, C.-P. Mutations affecting the cardiovascular system and other internal organs in zebrafish. *Development* **1996**, *123*, 293–302.
8. Stainier, D.Y. Zebrafish genetics and vertebrate heart formation. *Nat. Rev. Genet.* **2001**, *2*, 39–48. [CrossRef]
9. Sarasamma, S.; Audira, G.; Juniardi, S.; Sampurna, B.; Liang, S.-T.; Hao, E.; Lai, Y.-H.; Hsiao, C.-D. Zinc Chloride Exposure Inhibits Brain Acetylcholine Levels, Produces Neurotoxic Signatures, and Diminishes Memory and Motor Activities in Adult Zebrafish. *Int. J. Mol. Sci.* **2018**, *19*, 3195. [CrossRef]
10. Sarmah, S.; Marrs, J.A. Zebrafish as a vertebrate model system to evaluate effects of environmental toxicants on cardiac development and function. *Int. J. Mol. Sci.* **2016**, *17*, 2123. [CrossRef]
11. Poss, K.D.; Wilson, L.G.; Keating, M.T. Heart regeneration in zebrafish. *Science* **2002**, *298*, 2188–2190. [CrossRef] [PubMed]
12. Gut, P.; Reischauer, S.; Stainier, D.Y.; Arnaout, R. Little fish, big data: Zebrafish as a model for cardiovascular and metabolic disease. *Physiol. Rev.* **2017**, *97*, 889–938. [CrossRef] [PubMed]
13. Burggren, W.W.; Gore, M. Cardiac and metabolic physiology of early larval zebrafish (*Danio rerio*) reflects parental swimming stamina. *Front. Physiol.* **2012**, *3*, 35.
14. Fishman, M.C.; Stainier, D.Y.; Breitbart, R.E.; Westerfield, M. Zebrafish: Genetic and Embryological Methods in a Transparent Vertebrate Embryo. In *Methods in Cell Biology*; Elsevier: Amsterdam, The Netherlands, 1997; Volume 52, pp. 67–82.
15. Burns, C.G.; Milan, D.J.; Grande, E.J.; Rottbauer, W.; MacRae, C.A.; Fishman, M.C. High-throughput assay for small molecules that modulate zebrafish embryonic heart rate. *Nat. Chem. Biol.* **2005**, *1*, 263–264. [CrossRef]
16. Staudt, D.; Stainier, D. Uncovering the molecular and cellular mechanisms of heart development using the zebrafish. *Annu. Rev. Genet.* **2012**, *46*, 397–418. [CrossRef] [PubMed]
17. Brown, D.R.; Samsa, L.A.; Qian, L.; Liu, J. Advances in the study of heart development and disease using zebrafish. *J. Cardiovasc. Dev. Dis.* **2016**, *3*, 13. [CrossRef]
18. De Luca, E.; Zaccaria, G.M.; Hadhoud, M.; Rizzo, G.; Ponzini, R.; Morbiducci, U.; Santoro, M.M. ZebraBeat: A flexible platform for the analysis of the cardiac rate in zebrafish embryos. *Sci. Rep.* **2014**, *4*, 4898. [CrossRef]
19. Kang, C.-P.; Tu, H.-C.; Fu, T.-F.; Wu, J.-M.; Chu, P.-H.; Chang, D.T.-H. An automatic method to calculate heart rate from zebrafish larval cardiac videos. *BMC Bioinform.* **2018**, *19*, 169. [CrossRef]
20. Gaur, H.; Pullaguri, N.; Nema, S.; Purushothaman, S.; Bhargava, Y.; Bhargava, A. ZebraPace: An open-source method for cardiac-rhythm estimation in untethered zebrafish larvae. *Zebrafish* **2018**, *15*, 254–262. [CrossRef]
21. Fink, M.; Callol-Massot, C.; Chu, A.; Ruiz-Lozano, P.; Belmonte, J.C.I.; Giles, W.; Bodmer, R.; Ocorr, K. A new method for detection and quantification of heartbeat parameters in Drosophila, zebrafish, and embryonic mouse hearts. *Biotechniques* **2009**, *46*, 101–113. [CrossRef]
22. Ocorr, K.; Fink, M.; Cammarato, A.; Bernstein, S.I.; Bodmer, R. Semi-automated optical heartbeat analysis of small hearts. *JOVE J. Vis. Exp.* **2009**, *31*, e1435. [CrossRef] [PubMed]

23. Ohn, J.; Liebling, M. In Vivo, High-Throughput Imaging for Functional Characterization of the Embryonic Zebrafish Heart. In Proceedings of the 2011 IEEE International Symposium on Biomedical Imaging: From Nano to Macro, Chicago, IL, USA, 30 March–2 April 2011; pp. 1549–1552.
24. Gierten, J.; Pylatiuk, C.; Hammouda, O.T.; Schock, C.; Stegmaier, J.; Wittbrodt, J.; Gehrig, J.; Loosli, F. Automated high-throughput heart rate measurement in medaka and zebrafish embryos under physiological conditions. *BioRxiv* **2019**, 548594. [CrossRef]
25. Krishna, S.; Chatti, K.; Galigekere, R.R. Automatic and robust estimation of heart rate in zebrafish larvae. *IEEE Trans. Autom. Sci. Eng.* **2017**, *15*, 1041–1052. [CrossRef]
26. Pylatiuk, C.; Sanchez, D.; Mikut, R.; Alshut, R.; Reischl, M.; Hirth, S.; Rottbauer, W.; Just, S. Automatic zebrafish heartbeat detection and analysis for zebrafish embryos. *Zebrafish* **2014**, *11*, 379–383. [CrossRef] [PubMed]
27. Santoso, F.; Sampurna, B.P.; Lai, Y.-H.; Liang, S.-T.; Hao, E.; Chen, J.-R.; Hsiao, C.-D. Development of a Simple ImageJ-Based Method for Dynamic Blood Flow Tracking in Zebrafish Embryos and Its Application in Drug Toxicity Evaluation. *Inventions* **2019**, *4*, 65. [CrossRef]
28. Sampurna, B.; Audira, G.; Juniardi, S.; Lai, Y.-H.; Hsiao, C.-D. A Simple ImageJ-Based Method to Measure Cardiac Rhythm in Zebrafish Embryos. *Inventions* **2018**, *3*, 21. [CrossRef]
29. van Opbergen, C.J.; Koopman, C.D.; Kok, B.J.; Knöpfel, T.; Renninger, S.L.; Orger, M.B.; Vos, M.A.; van Veen, T.A.; Bakkers, J.; de Boer, T.P. Optogenetic sensors in the zebrafish heart: A novel in vivo electrophysiological tool to study cardiac arrhythmogenesis. *Theranostics* **2018**, *8*, 4750. [CrossRef]
30. Akerberg, A.A.; Burns, C.E.; Burns, C.G.; Nguyen, C. Deep learning enables automated volumetric assessments of cardiac function in zebrafish. *Dis. Models Mech.* **2019**, *12*. [CrossRef]
31. Xing, Q.; Huynh, V.; Parolari, T.G.; Maurer-Morelli, C.V.; Peixoto, N.; Wei, Q. Zebrafish larvae heartbeat detection from body deformation in low resolution and low frequency video. *Med Biol. Eng. Comput.* **2018**, *56*, 2353–2365. [CrossRef]
32. Martin, W.K.; Tennant, A.H.; Conolly, R.B.; Prince, K.; Stevens, J.S.; DeMarini, D.M.; Martin, B.L.; Thompson, L.C.; Gilmour, M.I.; Cascio, W.E. High-Throughput Video Processing of Heart Rate Responses in Multiple Wild-type Embryonic Zebrafish per Imaging Field. *Sci. Rep.* **2019**, *9*, 1–14. [CrossRef]
33. Yozzo, K.L.; Isales, G.M.; Raftery, T.D.; Volz, D.C. High-content screening assay for identification of chemicals impacting cardiovascular function in zebrafish embryos. *Environ. Sci. Technol.* **2013**, *47*, 11302–11310. [CrossRef] [PubMed]
34. Chan, P.K.; Lin, C.C.; Cheng, S.H. Noninvasive technique for measurement of heartbeat regularity in zebrafish (*Danio rerio*) embryos. *BMC Biotechnol.* **2009**, *9*, 11. [CrossRef]
35. Lin, S.-J. *Role of Endoplasmic Reticulum Calcium Pump in Alternation of Heart Failure Membrane Potential Heartbeat in Zebrafish*; Department of Medicine, National Taiwan University Taiwan: Taipei, Taiwan, 2016.
36. Rueden, C.T.; Schindelin, J.; Hiner, M.C.; DeZonia, B.E.; Walter, A.E.; Arena, E.T.; Eliceiri, K.W. ImageJ2: ImageJ for the next generation of scientific image data. *BMC Bioinform.* **2017**, *18*, 529. [CrossRef] [PubMed]
37. Grimm, W.; Steder, U.; Menz, V.; Hoffmann, J.; Maisch, B. QT dispersion and arrhythmic events in idiopathic dilated cardiomyopathy. *Am. J. Cardiol.* **1996**, *78*, 458–461. [CrossRef]
38. Nitzsche, B.; Bormuth, V.; Bräuer, C.; Howard, J.; Ionov, L.; Kerssemakers, J.; Korten, T.; Leduc, C.; Ruhnow, F.; Diez, S. Studying Kinesin Motors by Optical 3D-Nanometry in Gliding Motility Assays. In *Methods in Cell Biology*; Elsevier: Amsterdam, The Netherlands, 2010; Volume 95, pp. 247–271.
39. Marra, M.H.; Tobias, Z.J.; Cohen, H.R.; Glover, G.; Weissman, T.A. In vivo time-lapse imaging in the zebrafish lateral line: A flexible, open-ended research project for an undergraduate neurobiology laboratory course. *J. Undergrad. Neurosci. Educ.* **2015**, *13*, A215. [PubMed]
40. Tessadori, F.; van Weerd, J.H.; Burkhard, S.B.; Verkerk, A.O.; de Pater, E.; Boukens, B.J.; Vink, A.; Christoffels, V.M.; Bakkers, J. Identification and functional characterization of cardiac pacemaker cells in zebrafish. *PLoS ONE* **2012**, *7*, e47644. [CrossRef] [PubMed]
41. Waziri, B.; Shahzad, A. Direct effects of glucose administration on heart rate, myocardial contraction, and duration of cardiac cycle in frog's heart. *J. Pract. Cardiovasc. Sci.* **2018**, *4*, 29. [CrossRef]
42. Ferreira, T.; Miura, K.; Chef, B.; Eglinger, J. Scripts: BAR 1.1.6. Available online: https://zenodo.org/record/28838#.X1CaPnkzYuU (accessed on 3 August 2020).

43. Ishikawa, H.; Marshall, W.F. Efficient Live Fluorescence Imaging of Intraflagellar Transport in Mammalian Primary Cilia. In *Methods in Cell Biology*; Elsevier: Amsterdam, The Netherlands, 2015; Volume 127, pp. 189–201.
44. Ott, C.; Lippincott-Schwartz, J. Visualization of live primary cilia dynamics using fluorescence microscopy. *Curr. Protoc. Cell Biol.* **2012**, *57*, 4–26. [CrossRef]
45. Malone, M.H.; Sciaky, N.; Stalheim, L.; Hahn, K.M.; Linney, E.; Johnson, G.L. Laser-scanning velocimetry: A confocal microscopy method for quantitative measurement of cardiovascular performance in zebrafish embryos and larvae. *BMC Biotechnol.* **2007**, *7*, 40. [CrossRef]
46. Rogers, M.A.; Aikawa, E. Cardiovascular calcification: Artificial intelligence and big data accelerate mechanistic discovery. *Nat. Rev. Cardiol.* **2019**, *16*, 261–274. [CrossRef]
47. Teixidó, E.; Kießling, T.R.; Krupp, E.; Quevedo, C.; Muriana, A.; Scholz, S. Automated morphological feature assessment for zebrafish embryo developmental toxicity screens. *Toxicol. Sci.* **2019**, *167*, 438–449. [CrossRef] [PubMed]
48. Dhillon, S.S.; Dóró, É.; Magyary, I.; Egginton, S.; Sík, A.; Müller, F. Optimisation of embryonic and larval ECG measurement in zebrafish for quantifying the effect of QT prolonging drugs. *PLoS ONE* **2013**, *8*, e60552. [CrossRef] [PubMed]
49. Rendon-Morales, E.; Prance, R.; Prance, H.; Aviles-Espinosa, R. Non-invasive electrocardiogram detection of in vivo zebrafish embryos using electric potential sensors. *Appl. Phys. Lett.* **2015**, *107*, 193701. [CrossRef]
50. Cooke, S.; Chandroo, K.; Beddow, T.; Moccia, R.; McKinley, R. Swimming activity and energetic expenditure of captive rainbow trout *Oncorhynchus mykiss* (Walbaum) estimated by electromyogram telemetry. *Aquac. Res.* **2000**, *31*, 495–505. [CrossRef]
51. Lenning, M.; Fortunato, J.; Le, T.; Clark, I.; Sherpa, A.; Yi, S.; Hofsteen, P.; Thamilarasu, G.; Yang, J.; Xu, X. Real-time monitoring and analysis of zebrafish electrocardiogram with anomaly detection. *Sensors* **2018**, *18*, 61. [CrossRef] [PubMed]
52. Lee, L.; Genge, C.E.; Cua, M.; Sheng, X.; Rayani, K.; Beg, M.F.; Sarunic, M.V.; Tibbits, G.F. Functional assessment of cardiac responses of adult zebrafish (*Danio rerio*) to acute and chronic temperature change using high-resolution echocardiography. *PLoS ONE* **2016**, *11*, e0145163. [CrossRef]
53. Milan, D.J.; Jones, I.L.; Ellinor, P.T.; MacRae, C.A. In vivo recording of adult zebrafish electrocardiogram and assessment of drug-induced QT prolongation. *Am. J. Physiol. Heart Circ. Physiol.* **2006**, *291*, H269–H273. [CrossRef]
54. Liu, C.C.; Li, L.; Lam, Y.W.; Siu, C.W.; Cheng, S.H. Improvement of surface ECG recording in adult zebrafish reveals that the value of this model exceeds our expectation. *Sci. Rep.* **2016**, *6*, 1–13. [CrossRef]
55. Ho-Chiang, C.; Huang, H.; Huang, C.-C. High-frequency ultrasound deformation imaging for adult zebrafish during heart regeneration. *Quant. Imaging Med. Surg.* **2020**, *10*, 66. [CrossRef]
56. Koth, J.; Maguire, M.L.; McClymont, D.; Diffley, L.; Thornton, V.L.; Beech, J.; Patient, R.K.; Riley, P.R.; Schneider, J.E. High-resolution magnetic resonance imaging of the regenerating adult zebrafish heart. *Sci. Rep.* **2017**, *7*, 1–12. [CrossRef]
57. Kabli, S.; Alia, A.; Spaink, H.P.; Verbeek, F.J.; De Groot, H.J. Magnetic resonance microscopy of the adult zebrafish. *Zebrafish* **2006**, *3*, 431–439. [CrossRef] [PubMed]
58. Norling, T.A. Remotely Monitor Heart-Rate and Feeding Behaviour of Fish by Using Electronic Sensor-Tags. Available online: https://stud.epsilon.slu.se/10662/1/arvennorling_t_170831.pdf (accessed on 3 August 2020).
59. Brijs, J.; Sandblom, E.; Axelsson, M.; Sundell, K.; Sundh, H.; Kiessling, A.; Berg, C.; Gräns, A. Remote physiological monitoring provides unique insights on the cardiovascular performance and stress responses of freely swimming rainbow trout in aquaculture. *Sci. Rep.* **2019**, *9*, 1–12. [CrossRef] [PubMed]
60. Ho, D.; Zhao, X.; Gao, S.; Hong, C.; Vatner, D.E.; Vatner, S.F. Heart rate and electrocardiography monitoring in mice. *Curr. Protoc. Mouse Biol.* **2011**, *1*, 123–139.
61. Mousavi, S.E.; Patil, J.G. Light-cardiogram, a simple technique for heart rate determination in adult zebrafish, *Danio rerio*. *Comp. Biochem. Physiol. Part A Mol. Integr. Physiol.* **2020**, *246*, 110705. [CrossRef] [PubMed]
62. da Silva, V.V.; Napoleão, P.; Geraldes, V.; Rocha, I. Non-invasive ECG recording for zebrafish. In Proceedings of the 2017 IEEE 5th Portuguese Meeting on Bioengineering (ENBENG), Coimbra, Portugal, 16–18 February 2017; pp. 1–4.

63. Chaudhari, G.H.; Chennubhotla, K.S.; Chatti, K.; Kulkarni, P. Optimization of the adult zebrafish ECG method for assessment of drug-induced QTc prolongation. *J. Pharmacol. Toxicol. Methods* **2013**, *67*, 115–120. [CrossRef]
64. Yeo, S.; Yoon, C.; Lien, C.-L.; Song, T.-K.; Shung, K.K. Monitoring of Adult Zebrafish Heart Regeneration Using High-Frequency Ultrasound Spectral Doppler and Nakagami Imaging. *Sensors* **2019**, *19*, 4094. [CrossRef]
65. Wang, L.W.; Huttner, I.G.; Santiago, C.F.; Kesteven, S.H.; Yu, Z.-Y.; Feneley, M.P.; Fatkin, D. Standardized echocardiographic assessment of cardiac function in normal adult zebrafish and heart disease models. *Dis. Models Mech.* **2017**, *10*, 63–76. [CrossRef]
66. Leong, I.U.S.; Skinner, J.; Shelling, A.; Love, D. Zebrafish as a model for long QT syndrome: The evidence and the means of manipulating zebrafish gene expression. *Acta Physiol.* **2010**, *199*, 257–276. [CrossRef]
67. Aehlert, B.J. *ECGs Made Easy-E-Book*; Elsevier Health Sciences: Amsterdam, The Netherlands, 2015.
68. Haverkamp, W.; Breithardt, G.; Camm, A.J.; Janse, M.J.; Rosen, M.R.; Antzelevitch, C.; Escande, D.; Franz, M.; Malik, M.; Moss, A. The potential for QT prolongation and pro-arrhythmia by non-anti-arrhythmic drugs: Clinical and regulatory implications: Report on a Policy Conference of the European Society of Cardiology. *Cardiovasc. Res.* **2000**, *47*, 219–233. [CrossRef]
69. Leor-Librach, R.J.; Bobrovsky, B.-Z.; Eliash, S.; Kaplinsky, E. Computer-controlled heart rate increase by isoproterenol infusion: Mathematical modeling of the system. *Am. J. Physiol. Heart Circ. Physiol.* **1999**, *277*, H1478–H1483. [CrossRef]
70. Langheinrich, U.; Vacun, G.; Wagner, T. Zebrafish embryos express an orthologue of HERG and are sensitive toward a range of QT-prolonging drugs inducing severe arrhythmia. *Toxicol. Appl. Pharmacol.* **2003**, *193*, 370–382. [CrossRef] [PubMed]
71. Bournele, D.; Beis, D. Zebrafish models of cardiovascular disease. *Heart Fail. Rev.* **2016**, *21*, 803–813. [CrossRef] [PubMed]
72. Milan, D.J.; MacRae, C.A. Animal models for arrhythmias. *Cardiovasc. Res.* **2005**, *67*, 426–437. [CrossRef] [PubMed]
73. Biomedical, D. Introductory Guide to Identifiying ECG Irregularities. Available online: https://www.dcbiomed.com/proimages/materials/Brochures_and_related_Articles/Introductory_guide_to_ECG_E2_0-950820.pdf (accessed on 3 August 2020).
74. Yu, F.; Huang, J.; Adlerz, K.; Jadvar, H.; Hamdan, M.H.; Chi, N.; Chen, J.-N.; Hsiai, T.K.J.B.m. Evolving cardiac conduction phenotypes in developing zebrafish larvae: Implications to drug sensitivity. *Zebrafish* **2010**, *7*, 325–331. [CrossRef] [PubMed]
75. Baer, H.U.; Hendrawan, S.; The, S.; Lelosutan, S.A.; Salim, G.; Lindl, T.; Mathes, S.; Graf-Hausner, U.; Weber, U.; Watson, R.; et al. The Intracorporeal Autologous Hepatocyte Matrix Implant for the Treatment of Chronic Liver Disease: A Modified Clinical Phase I Study. *World J. Surg. Surg. Res.* **2018**, *1*, 1067.
76. Forouhar, A.; Hove, J.; Calvert, C.; Flores, J.; Jadvar, H.; Gharib, M. Electrocardiographic Characterization of Embryonic Zebrafish. In Proceedings of the 26th Annual International Conference of the IEEE Engineering in Medicine and Biology Society, San Francisco, CA, USA, 1–4 September 2004; pp. 3615–3617.
77. Van der Linde, H.; Van Deuren, B.; Teisman, A.; Towart, R.; Gallacher, D. The effect of changes in core body temperature on the QT interval in beagle dogs: A previously ignored phenomenon, with a method for correction. *Br. J. Pharmacol.* **2008**, *154*, 1474–1481. [CrossRef]
78. Parker, T.; Libourel, P.-A.; Hetheridge, M.J.; Cumming, R.I.; Sutcliffe, T.P.; Goonesinghe, A.C.; Ball, J.S.; Owen, S.F.; Chomis, Y.; Winter, M.J. A multi-endpoint in vivo larval zebrafish (*Danio rerio*) model for the assessment of integrated cardiovascular function. *J. Pharmacol. Toxicol. Methods* **2014**, *69*, 30–38. [CrossRef]
79. Vornanen, M.; Hassinen, M.J.C. Zebrafish heart as a model for human cardiac electrophysiology. *Channels* **2016**, *10*, 101–110. [CrossRef]
80. Lauridsen, H.; Gonzales, S.; Hedwig, D.; Perrin, K.L.; Williams, C.J.; Wrege, P.H.; Bertelsen, M.F.; Pedersen, M.; Butcher, J.T. Extracting physiological information in experimental biology via Eulerian video magnification. *BMC Biol.* **2019**, *17*, 103. [CrossRef]
81. Zhao, Y.; Yun, M.; Nguyen, S.A.; Tran, M.; Nguyen, T.P. In Vivo Surface Electrocardiography for Adult Zebrafish. *JOVE J. Vis. Exp.* **2019**, *150*, e60011. [CrossRef]
82. Bovik, A.C. *Handbook of Image and Video Processing*; Academic Press: Burlington, VT, USA, 2010.

83. Relić, R.R.; Hristov, S.V.; Vučinić, M.M.; Poleksić, V.D.; Marković, Z.Z. Principles of fish welfare assessment in farm rearing conditions. *J. Agric. Sci.* **2010**, *55*, 273–282.
84. Baras, E.; Lagardère, J.-P. Fish telemetry in aquaculture: Review and perspectives. *Aquac. Int.* **1995**, *3*, 77–102. [CrossRef]

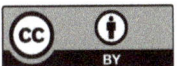

© 2020 by the authors. Licensee MDPI, Basel, Switzerland. This article is an open access article distributed under the terms and conditions of the Creative Commons Attribution (CC BY) license (http://creativecommons.org/licenses/by/4.0/).

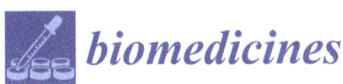

Review

Zebra-Fishing for Regenerative Awakening in Mammals

Laura Massoz †, Marie Alice Dupont † and Isabelle Manfroid *

Zebrafish Development and Disease Models Laboratory, GIGA-Stem Cells, University of Liège, B-4000 Liège, Belgium; laura.massoz@doct.uliege.be (L.M.); marie.dupont@uliege.be (M.A.D.)
* Correspondence: isabelle.manfroid@uliege.be; Tel.: +32-4-366-3374
† These authors contributed equally to this work.

Abstract: Regeneration is defined as the ability to regrow an organ or a tissue destroyed by degeneration or injury. Many human degenerative diseases and pathologies, currently incurable, could be cured if functional tissues or cells could be restored. Unfortunately, humans and more generally mammals have limited regenerative capabilities, capacities that are even further declining with age, contrary to simpler organisms. Initially thought to be lost during evolution, several studies have revealed that regenerative mechanisms are still present in mammals but are latent and thus they could be stimulated. To do so there is a pressing need to identify the fundamental mechanisms of regeneration in species able to efficiently regenerate. Thanks to its ability to regenerate most of its organs and tissues, the zebrafish has become a powerful model organism in regenerative biology and has recently engendered a number of studies attesting the validity of awakening the regenerative potential in mammals. In this review we highlight studies, particularly in the liver, pancreas, retina, heart, brain and spinal cord, which have identified conserved regenerative molecular events that proved to be beneficial to restore murine and even human cells and which helped clarify the real clinical translation potential of zebrafish research to mammals.

Keywords: zebrafish; regeneration; mammal; liver; pancreas; heart; retina; brain; spinal cord

1. Introduction

Humankind has been fascinated with regeneration abilities since the times of the Ancient Greece. In Greek mythology, one of the labors of Hercules was to kill the Hydra, which is able to regrow two heads when one is ablated. In another myth, Prometheus' liver is renewed every night. However, it was only in the late seventeenth century that scholars paid formal attention to regeneration. Abraham Trembley became a pioneer in this field with his work on fresh water polyps. He described that after cutting a polyp in pieces, each of them was able to regrow an entire organism. He named the polyp "hydra" for its regenerative capacities. After that, regenerative biology had a major influence in the history of biological sciences as it contributed to legitimize biology as an experimental discipline rather than a descriptive science [1].

In recent decades, new technologies such as imaging, genetic engineering and stem cells have enabled the development of regenerative biology, which laid the foundation of a new branch of medicine, i.e., regenerative medicine. Many human diseases and pathologies such as diabetes, Alzheimer's disease, blindness, heart failure or spine injuries, today incurable, could be cured if functional tissues or cells could be restored by regeneration. However, humans, and more generally mammals, possess limited regenerative capabilities, capacities that even further decline with age. In contrast, invertebrates and phylogenetically primitive vertebrates are able to regenerate full tissues after injury. Even though species with strong regenerative capacities are non-uniformly widespread across the phylogenetic tree, simpler organisms generally perform better in this respect [2]. For this reason, it has been assumed that regenerative potential has been lost during evolution. However, in the last years, several studies have revealed that regenerative mechanisms are still present in mammals but are latent or dormant, and thus it would be possible to stimulate them. This is why elucidating the regenerative mechanisms in competent species is important to permanently cure patients.

Classical models of regeneration are found in invertebrate and vertebrate phylum such as the *hydra*, *planarian*, *drosophila*, *zebrafish*, *axolotl* and *newt*. First exploited to study embryonic development, the zebrafish became in the last 40 years a powerful model organism for deciphering regenerative mechanisms [3]. In 2013, the keyword "regeneration" was the 20th most frequently used in publications using zebrafish [4]. Its success is also due to its fast and external development, the abundant number of eggs and its transparency in the first development stages, making easier the observation of organs and live imaging. Recent technologies, such as CRISPR/Cas9 and TALENs to generate mutant or transgenic lines [5] and high throughput drug screenings [6], have facilitated the study of regeneration in zebrafish. Moreover, its genome is well characterized: 71.4% of the human genes possess at least one or two orthologs in zebrafish and 82% of disease-linked genes listed in the Online Mendelian Inheritance in Man (OMIM) database can be related to at least one zebrafish orthologue [7]. As it has been shown that most of the studied mechanisms in zebrafish implicate the same factors as in mammals, the genetic cascades implicated in a given regenerative process in zebrafish are most likely to be conserved in mammals, rendering possible their manipulation to stimulate regeneration in mammals.

Here we focused on several organs (the heart, liver, pancreas and central nervous system) where research performed in zebrafish clearly helped promote regeneration in murine and human models. These zebrafish studies were selected based on direct evidence of experimental validation in mammalian models (in the same study or in citing references). The overview of these studies also contributes to understanding why the response to tissue damage differs between organs and species and how mechanisms detrimental to regeneration could be overcome.

2. Awakening the Regenerative Capacity in Different Organs

2.1. The Heart

Unsurprisingly, healthy cardiac function is essential for survival and heart failure remains one of the leading cause of death worldwide [8]. In mammals, even if cardiomyocyte self-renewal does occur, the annual turnover is low, decreasing from 1% to 0.3% between 20 and 75 years old [9], and it is not sufficient to repair injured hearts. Instead, after a myocardial infarction, the damaged myocardium is replaced by fibrotic scar tissue, which tampers cardiac function, ultimately leading to fatal heart failure [10]. By contrast, following a 20% ventricular ablation by resection or cryoinjury, the zebrafish fully regenerates a functional myocardium within a few months without scarring, even at the adult stage (Table 1) [10–15]. Although this regenerative capacity is also observed in neonatal mice, in contrast to zebrafish, it is lost after the first week of postnatal life [16].

Using cardiomyocyte lineage tracing systems in adult fish and neonatal mice, regenerated cardiomyocytes were shown to derive from dedifferentiation of pre-existing mature cardiomyocytes followed by proliferation and redifferentiation, rather than from progenitor or stem cells [16,17]. The ploidy of cardiomyocytes is one of the major differences between adult zebrafish and mice. Adult zebrafish cardiomyocytes are mainly diploid and mononucleated with a high proliferative potential during regeneration [18], whereas the non-regenerative myocardium of adult rodents and humans is largely composed of polyploid mono- or binucleated cardiomyocytes [19–21]. Polyploidy has been proposed to account for the decreased regenerative potential of these species [22].

The RhoGEF Ect2 is required for cytokinesis initiation [23] and its expression in murine cardiomyocytes decreases during the first week of postnatal life [18] correlating with the binucleation event and the loss of regenerative ability [16,24]. However, its expression remains high in zebrafish [18]. Using a transgenic line inhibiting *ect2*, Gonzalez-Rosa et al. managed to induce cardiomyocyte polyploidization in zebrafish. After heart injury, they observed that an excess of 50% of polyploid cardiomyocytes dampens the proliferation of remaining cells, and thus the regeneration of the organ, while it induces a persistent scarring. This highlighted an inverse correlation between the percentage of polyploid cells and the regeneration ability of the heart [18]. The mobilization of diploid instead of polyploid cardiomyocytes in mammals, by maintaining the expression of *ect2*, would offer a therapeutic alternative to stimulate the proliferation of cardiac cells and heart regeneration.

Table 1. Overview of injury models presented in the review.

Organ	Model Organism	Injury Model	Type of Injury	Mechanism of Regeneration	Characteristics	References
Heart	Zebrafish	Ventricular resection	Surgical	Proliferation from pre-existing myocytes	-	[11]
		Cryoinjury	Surgical	Proliferation from pre-existing myocytes	Clinically relevant to mammalian infarcts with massive cell death	[13]
	Mouse	Ventricular resection	Surgical	Proliferation from pre-existing myocytes	Fully regenerates a functional myocardium in 1–2 months without scarring	[11,12]
		Myocardial infarction	Surgical	Proliferation from pre-existing myocytes	Left anterior descending coronary artery occluded with a nylon suture	[25]
Liver		Partial hepatectomy	Surgical	Hepatocyte-driven	Clinically relevant	[26]
		APAP overdose	Chemical	BEC-driven regeneration	Paracetamol overdose	[26]
	Zebrafish	Nitroreductase (NTR)-mediated ablation	Genetic/Chemical	Hepatocyte-driven BEC-driven regeneration	Tg(fabp10a:CFP-NTR)	[27–29]
		CDE diet	Chemical	BEC-driven regeneration	Ethionine, a toxic analog of methionine, in association with choline deficiency, leads to hepatocyte death and liver inflammation	[30]
		Ctnnb1 hepatocyte KO	Genetic	BEC-driven regeneration	Represses hepatocyte proliferation—in an injury model	[29]
	Mouse	Mdm2 deletion (hepatocyte-specific)	Genetic	BEC-driven regeneration	AhCreMdm2flox/floxInducible, represses hepatocyte proliferation	[30]
	Zebrafish	NTR-mediated ablation	Genetic/Chemical	Beta cell proliferation/alpha cell transdifferentiation; Neogenesis from ductal progenitors	Tg(ins:CFP-NTR) In cells expressing NTR, reduces non-toxic pro-drug into cytotoxic products causing targeted cell apoptosis	[31–34]
Beta cell/Pancreas		Pancreatic Duct Ligation (PDL)	Surgical	Neogenesis from ductal progenitors	Induces acinar cell death and acute inflammation without destruction of beta cells	[35–37]
		Streptozotocin (STZ)	Chemical	Beta cell proliferation; Neogenesis from ductal progenitors	Toxic glucose analogue that enters into beta cells via the GLUT2 transporter causing their death	[31,38]
	Mouse	Diphtheria Toxin Analogue (DTA)	Genetic/Chemical	Alpha cell transdifferentiation (adult only) Delta cell transdifferentiation (neonatal only)	Tg(RIP:DTR) The toxin enters in cells expressing the DTR and inhibits protein synthesis, leading to cell apoptosis. Here targeted in beta cells with the Rat Insulin Promoter (RIP).	[39,40]
Spinal Cord	Zebrafish	Spinal cord transection	Surgical	Glial bridge	Complete cutting of the vertebral column	[41]
	Mouse	Laminectomy and spinal cord hemisection	Surgical	-	Hemisection leading to complete paralysis of the ipsilateral limb	[42]
Brain	Zebrafish	Stab-lesion assay	Surgical	Regeneration from radial cells	Injury in the telencephalon parenchyma	[43]
		Bβ42 mediated injury	Surgical/Chemical	Regeneration from radial cells	Alzheimer's-disease-like	[44]
	Mouse	AD-like model	Genetic	No regeneration	APP/PS1dE9 transgenic	[45]
Retina	Zebrafish	Needle poke	Surgical	From Muller cells	-	[46]
		Optic nerve lesion	Surgical	From Muller cells	-	[47]
		NMDA	Chemical	From Muller cells	-	[46,48]
	Mouse	Excessive light	Surgical	From Muller cells	-	[46]
		AD-like model	Genetic	No regeneration	APP/PS1dE9 transgenic	[45]

In order to identify other mechanisms underlying heart regeneration in adult zebrafish and potentially conserved but dormant mechanisms in mammals, Aguirre and colleagues focused on the microRNAs (miRNAs) differentially regulated after amputation of the ventricular apex in adult zebrafish [25]. They identified miR99/100 and let-7a/c that are downregulated during regeneration. These miRs are known to be implicated in proliferation, chromatin remodeling and morphogenesis, including cardiomyogenesis. Downregulation of miR99/100 during the cardiac regenerative process in zebrafish allows a significant de-repression of their targets *fntb* and *smarca5* in cardiomyocytes, associated with increased cell cycle entry. By contrast, in adult mouse and in human heart tissue, the expression of miR-99/100 stays high after injury, inhibiting the expression of *Fntb* and *Smarca5*. Silencing of miR99/100 or let-7a/c in isolated primary murine adult cardiomyocytes or in murine organotypic slices induced cardiomyocyte dedifferentiation and the acquisition of a proliferative phenotype similar to what was observed in zebrafish. Similar results were obtained in vivo by intracardiac injection of anti-miR-99/100 and anti-Let-7a/c in a murine model of myocardial infarction. More importantly, this led to an improvement of functional heart parameters after 15 days and to the reduction of fibrotic scarring and of the infarct size compared to scrambled controls. Of note, the dedifferentiation observed after miR99/100 downregulation in mammalian cardiomyocytes is limited to the mononucleated cells. Either the polyploid cardiomyocytes are able to convert to a mononucleated state or the mononucleated cardiomyocyte population is more responsive to the regenerative pathway [25]. It would be interesting to answer this question in order to find the best strategy to induce cardiomyocyte proliferation in mammals. In conclusion, the limited cardiac regeneration in mice is at least due to the failure to modulate the miR99/100 and let-7a/c/FNTB and SMARCA5 axis and anti-miR delivery can reactivate this dormant pathway in mammals [25,49].

In the same way, comparison of gene and miRNA profiling of injured zebrafish and mouse adult hearts identified miR-26a [50]. miR-26a represses expression of *ezh2*, a key component of the polycomb repressive complex involved in the methylation of histone H3K27 that is implicated in cardiomyocyte proliferation and in the maintenance of cardiac identity in mice. After ventricular resection in zebrafish, *ezh2* expression is induced due to the downregulation of miR-26a whereas, in the murine heart, miR-26a expression remains high after injury and maintains inhibition of *Ezh2*. Knock-down of miR26a in neonatal mice via injection of anti-miR-26a oligonucleotides increased expression of *Ezh2* and augmented the number of proliferating cardiomyocytes [50].

Together, miR-99/100 and miR-26a are downregulated during the regenerative process in zebrafish whereas their expression is high in adult mice [25,50]. As their expression can be inhibited by antagomir therapy in the mammals, miRNAs could constitute clinical targets to stimulate cardiac regeneration [25,49,50].

Other transcriptomic analyses from adult zebrafish have shown that leptin B (*lepB*), a paralog of mammalian leptin, is induced in the regenerating tail fin and heart [51]. By epigenetic profiling, Kang et al. have identified a short sequence upstream the *lepB* promoter, called *lepb-linked enhancer* (LEN), which acquires H3K27ac marks and open chromatin marks during regeneration [51]. Moreover, the authors showed that LEN can direct regeneration-activated gene expression not only from *lepB* but also from different promoters such as *cmlc2* (cardiomyocytes) or α-*cry* (lens). They exploited this LEN sequence to overexpress *neuregulin 1* (*nrg1*), known to be implicated in cardiomyocyte proliferation and regeneration [52], in adult zebrafish via transgenesis using a promoter combining LEN and the *lepB* minimal promoter. After ventricular resection, these fish strongly activated *nrg1* expression at the injured area and exacerbated cardiomyocyte proliferation. In contrast, control fish did not induce expression of *nrg1* under the *lepB* minimal promoter only without the LEN sequence, showing that LEN can modulate heart regeneration. Even if the LEN sequence is poorly conserved in mammals, LEN-hsp68::lacZ transgenic mice where the zebrafish LEN was fused to the murine *hsp68* promoter revealed injury-dependent LEN activity in wounds after heart resection or even digit amputation in neonates [51]. This result shows that mammalian gene regulatory networks have the potential to activate zebrafish LEN enhancer and to enable injury-induced expression in mice [53], suggesting that similar constructs could be designed to stimulate timely regeneration of different organs in mammals. It remains to determine whether overexpression of *Nrg1*, or of other positive regulators, under the LEN promoter could give similar results.

2.2. The Liver

Despite their poor regenerative capabilities, mammals are able to efficiently regrow their liver. After partial hepatectomy or mild injury, liver regeneration is mainly achieved by proliferation of pre-existing hepatocytes. However, this process is impaired after acute injury or in hepatic chronic diseases such as liver cirrhosis, viral hepatitis and liver cancer. These diseases are characterized by inflammation, fibrosis and exhaustion of the proliferative potential and finally the death of the hepatocytes. In these situations, activation and expansion of biliary ductular cells, the so-called "ductular response", takes place. Oval cells have been observed in mammals next to these ducts [54] and it has been hypothesized that they could represent liver progenitors deriving from ducts able to restore hepatocytes. Many rodent models of chronic liver injury have been developed to study this process (Table 1). One category of models involves hepatotoxins such as ethionine, CCl4 or N-acetyl-p-aminophenol (APAP), (also called paracetamol or acetaminophen), which are repeatedly injected or delivered in association with specific pro-inflammatory diets, causing chronic death of hepatocytes. The second category of models consists of mutant models (*Mdm2, Ctnnb1, Itgb1, p21/Cdkn1a*) with impaired hepatocyte proliferation. Models to study liver regeneration from the ducts usually combine chronic hepatocyte injury and repression of replication. Previously the subject of controversy, mainly owing to the diversity of the models, there is now strong evidence that biliary epithelial cells (BECs), also known as cholangiocytes, are able to dedifferentiate into liver progenitor cells (LPCs), or oval cells, when hepatocyte-driven regeneration is compromised [30]. These LPCs are bipotent progenitors able to redifferentiate into BECs or hepatocytes. It is of utmost clinical importance to identify the molecular regulation of this process, still not yet fully understood, to improve liver regrowth in chronic hepatic disease patients. This particular topic has been recently reviewed [55,56].

The zebrafish can efficiently replenish its liver with new hepatocytes through both hepatocyte-driven (i.e., replication) or BEC-driven regeneration, providing a valuable model to decipher the mechanisms of both types of liver regeneration. A chemical screening performed in the zebrafish *Tg(fabp10a:CFP-NTR)* line, based on nitroreductase (NTR)-mediated near-total ablation of hepatocytes, pinpointed that the bromodomain and extra-terminal proteins (BET) are required for BEC-driven regeneration [28]. BETs recognize lysine acetylation in histones and other transcription factors, thereby positively or negatively regulating transcription. They mediate different steps of BEC-driven regeneration in zebrafish, BEC dedifferentiation into LPC, proliferation of LPC and redifferentiation into new hepatocytes and their maturation [28]. In addition, BET proteins also promote hepatocyte-driven liver regeneration in a zebrafish liver injury model of paracetamol (APAP) overdose (Table 1) [26]. Importantly, the requirement for BET proteins in both types of liver regeneration is conserved in mice. In the choline-deficient ethionine-supplemented CDE-diet mouse model of chronic liver injury that induces BEC-driven regeneration, BET proteins are required for activation of LPC [28]. In mice after partial hepatectomy, BET proteins are required for hepatocyte proliferation [26]. These data are of high clinical relevance as the same BET inhibitor, JQ1, has been used in a clinical trial for cancer therapy, including liver cancer. The authors stressed that, even though such drugs could be beneficial in this specific context, they would also inhibit liver regeneration, thereby limiting their therapeutic use [26]. Given the importance of BET proteins as epigenetic regulators, a second chemical screen with a library of compounds targeting epigenetic factors has been conducted with the same zebrafish NTR-mediated liver ablation model [29]. This screening identified the histone deacetylase HDAC1 as a potential regulator of BEC-driven regeneration. HDAC1 was already known to be involved in liver regeneration in mouse models of hepatocyte-driven regeneration [57]. Ko et al. 2019 showed that *hdac1* regulates LPC differentiation into hepatocytes and BECs during BEC-driven regeneration in zebrafish [29]. More exactly, the loss of *hdac1* impairs LPC differentiation into hepatocytes by increasing the expression of *sox9b*, and into BECS via the increased expression of *cdk8*, a negative regulator of Notch signaling. Administration of the HDAC1 inhibitor MS-275 to a mouse model of chronic liver injury combining hepatocyte-specific loss of *ctnnb1* (β-catenin) and a choline-deficient, methionine-supplemented diet impairs differentiation of LPCs into hepatocytes [29]. Interestingly, *HDAC1* is expressed in liver tissues from patients with cirrhosis, suggesting a conserved role of *Hdac1* from zebrafish to human in LPC differentiation [29].

Another approach to decipher regenerative molecular mechanisms is the identification of candidates by RNA sequencing. Using this approach and the zebrafish NTR-mediated ablation model, the Bone Morphogenetic Protein (BMP) pathway was found to be modulated during liver regeneration [27] and BMP inhibition impaired BEC-driven regeneration. Based on these findings, BMP2 treatment was shown to increase the differentiation of a murine liver progenitor cell line into hepatocytes in vitro. To conclude, screenings conducted in zebrafish enabled us to identify mechanisms of both hepatocyte- and BEC-driven liver regeneration, which seems conserved in mammals.

2.3. The Pancreas

Diabetes is a leading health issue worldwide with an incidence of 1 out of 11 people, and causes 1.5 million of deaths per year according to the WHO. The disease is characterized by a dysfunction of blood glucose regulation and various consequent life threatening health conditions. In type 1 diabetes (T1D) or in late stages of type 2 diabetes (T2D), the insulin-producing beta cell mass is dramatically decreased, resulting in a lack of insulin. Besides therapeutic strategies to preserve the beta cell mass and its function and to improve insulin treatments, beta cell regeneration constitutes a promising alternative to replenish the pancreas with functional beta cells. This process is extensively studied in mice, using a model of pancreas injuries. In rodents, the main models of beta cell regeneration consist of injections of a toxic glucose analogue streptozotocin (STZ), expression of the diphtheria toxin A (DTA) suicide transgene, and the pancreatic duct ligation (PDL) model which is characterized by high levels of inflammation in the pancreas but no destruction of beta cells per se (Table 1). Using these models, mice revealed a certain plasticity of mammalian pancreatic cells despite the poor regenerative capacity of mammals. Besides replication of remaining beta cells [58], neogenesis can proceed from alpha cells [40], delta cells [39] or acinar cells [59]. Duct-associated pancreatic progenitors have also been proposed [37,38] even though this source is under controversy [35,36]. These studies underline the importance of the injury model and of age in regeneration efficiency and cellular origin of new beta cells.

To get new insights into beta cell regeneration and to overcome the limited regeneration ability of rodent models, researchers have exploited the zebrafish model. One of the strategies was to identify pharmacological compounds able to enhance beta cell proliferation. Several groups performed medium or high-throughput drug screenings using zebrafish larvae and the inducible NTR-mediated ablation model [31,32,60]. Two independent studies discovered that drugs stimulating the production of cAMP promote beta cell regeneration by proliferation. One class of compounds activates the adenosine/cAMP pathway and promotes beta cell proliferation after beta cell ablation [31], of which the more potent is the *50-N-ethylcarboxamidoadenosine* (NECA), an adenosine agonist activating GPCR signaling. The other study identified the TBK1 and IKKε inhibitor *(E)-3-(3-phenylbenzo[c]isoxazol-5-yl) acrylic acid* (PIAA), which appeared to activate the cAMP-PKA-mTOR pathway leading to increased beta cell proliferation after ablation [32]. Importantly, both drugs, NECA and PIAA, also increased beta cell proliferation in mammalian ex vivo models, NECA being validated in mouse islets and PIAA in both rat and human islets. NECA and PIAA were also able to enhance beta cell regeneration in vivo in STZ-treated mice. Moreover, these drugs led to functional improvement by lowering glycemia in mice [31,32]. By coupling the advantage of assessing the effect of various compounds on a given phenotype (here beta cell regeneration) with toxicological assays, the zebrafish allows not only the pinpointing of the adenosine pathway but also the identification of, among the numerous cAMP modulators, the non-toxic compounds most promising for further clinical studies. Validations in human models are particularly critical in the context of beta cell replication as adult human beta cells are extremely resistant to cell cycle re-entry compared to mice [61]. In addition, beta cell replication is inversely correlated with functional maturation, thus such a strategy should be used with caution.

Besides beta cell proliferation, other pancreatic cells can give rise to new beta cells. The glucagon-producing alpha cells are able to transdifferentiate into beta cells in various mouse models [40], though the regeneration is very slow and low, as well as in the zebrafish NTR model [34]. After a transcriptomic profiling by microarray of zebrafish islets isolated during regeneration following NTR-mediated ablation, secreted proteins were selected as candidate enhancers of beta cell regeneration [33]. One of them, the insulin-like growth factor (Igf) binding-protein 1 (*igfbp1*), was shown to increase transdifferentiation of alpha cells into beta cells when overexpressed by transgenesis, leading to potentiation of beta cell regeneration and accelerated restoration of normoglycemia. Furthermore, IGFBP1 could also promote alpha cell transdifferentiation in mouse and human islets ex vivo. Since *igfbp1* is known to be repressed by insulin, the study also showed that patients with insulin resistance have a lower level of IGFBP1 in their blood while those with a high level of IGFBP1 have a lower risk to develop T2D [33]. In T1D or in late stages of T2D, when the beta cell mass is reduced, the level of IGFBP1 is elevated due to the lack of insulin [62]. These observations demonstrate that IGFBP1 could be a potential biomarker for insulin resistance/diabetes in addition to be a good candidate for beta cell regeneration in (pre)clinical studies.

Another axis of regeneration is to harness pancreatic progenitors. As endocrine cells arise from the pancreatic ductal tree during the development, it has been hypothesized that progenitors could still be associated to the pancreatic ducts in adults. Although beta cell neogenesis from ducts in the adult is under controversy in mammals [35–38,63], it is well established in the zebrafish [64–66]. A drug screening performed without regeneration but in conditions boosting beta cell formation from the ducts in zebrafish larvae, pinpointed two inhibitors of CDK5, roscovitine and DRF, as enhancers of beta cell differentiation from ductal-associated progenitors [67]. Inhibition of *cdk5* has then been shown to stimulate regeneration after beta cell ablation. This finding has been validated in mouse embryonic pancreatic explants, in human iPSCs and in vivo in the PDL mouse model, though glycemia and glucose tolerance were not improved. To summarize, with one unique zebrafish model (the NTR-mediated ablation) it was possible to explore beta cell regeneration from different cellular origins and to identify pharmacological compounds and signaling pathways able to promote beta cell regeneration in mammals.

2.4. The Central Nervous System (CNS)

The central nervous system (CNS) is composed of two main cell types: neurons and glial cells. Neuronal cells are the basic functional units of the CNS capable of sensing and transmitting information via electrochemical pulses. The main roles of glial cells are to maintain homeostasis and to support and protect neurons. The earliest glial cells formed during embryonic development are the radial cells. These cells act as neuronal progenitors and thus give rise to neurons and intermediate progenitors. However, their neurogenic capacity decreases while they differentiate into star-shaped astrocytes. In the adult mammalian brain, the neurogenic capacity of the glia is restricted to few specific regions, called neurogenic niches, where the astroglia can still give rise to a few new neurons. Some of the astroglial cells in these neurogenic niches are considered as neural stem cells. Although it is possible to observe star-shaped cells in zebrafish, there are no clearly defined astroglial cells in this species, and glial cells in zebrafish retain their radial identity through life. Thus these radial/astroglial cells have important neurogenic capacities. These cells can give rise to new neurons not only in the neurogenic niches but more broadly in the CNS [68], and they constitute the basis of regeneration in the CNS, i.e., the spinal cord, the brain and the retina.

2.4.1. The Spinal Cord

Spinal cord injury in mammals is followed by formation of a dense and heterogenous network composed of hypertrophic stellate astrocyte gliosis, fibroblasts and inflammatory immune cells, called the glial scar. This scar establishes a mechanical and impenetrable barrier impeding the regeneration of severed axons and repair of neuronal circuits [69–71]. In zebrafish, complete transection of the spinal cord (Table 1) results in tissue discontinuity and loss of glial and axonal connections. Then, glial cells proliferate and migrate to the injured area and acquire a bipolar and elongated morphology, forming a glial bridge. This allows, by 5 weeks, the regeneration of axons from viable neurons across the lesion site and their reconnection to the central canal, and fish recover their normal swimming behavior [72]. Notably, unlike mammals, this regeneration process is not accompanied by formation of a scar [72–74]. The formation of this bridge results from differential regulations compared to mammals allowing the presence of a permissive pro-regenerative microenvironment in zebrafish. One of these key regulations is a dynamic transient inflammatory response in zebrafish. Indeed, 2–3 days after spinal cord injury, the initially proinflammatory environment switches to an anti-inflammatory one with notably the presence of M2 macrophages, whereas, in mammals, pro-inflammatory macrophages persist at the wound site for a long time after injury [74].

A key regulator of the formation of the glial bridge is Fibroblast Growth Factor (FGF) signaling. Indeed, in zebrafish, the expression of several FGF ligands (*Fgf2, 3, 8*) and their downstream targets (*spry4, pea3* and *erm*) are increased at the injured site [72,75]. Using several models of gain or loss of function, Goldshmit and colleagues have examined the role of FGF during spinal cord regeneration in a series of studies from zebrafish to in vitro and in vivo mammalian models [42,72,76]. They first established in zebrafish that the FGF signaling is necessary for the formation of the glial bridge and for axonal regeneration. Next, they showed that in vitro treatment of primate primary astrocytes with recombinant human Fgf2 (hFgf2) recapitulated some of the characteristics of zebrafish glia cells during spinal cord regeneration such as acquisition of a bipolar elongated shape [72]. In mice, hFgf2 injection after spinal cord hemisection promotes formation of a glial bridge rather than a scar, allowing the growth of neurites and axonal regeneration through the lesion site. Mice injected with hFgf2 also displayed reduced inflammation, less macrophage and microglia activation and reduced leukocyte infiltration [42]. Moreover, these mice showed an improved functional recovery compared to control animals. These results are consistent with previous studies showing that acidic FGF and FGF2 are implicated in locomotor recovery in rodents [77,78]. Interestingly, similar observations were made with endogenous increase of FGF signaling in $spry4^{-/-}$ mutant mice, *spry4* being a feedback inhibitor of this pathway [76].

One promising cellular therapy following a spinal cord injury is the transplantation of stem cells directly into the injured site. Dental pulp cells (DPC) are composed of many types of stem cells and their transplantation induced an enhanced improvement of the functional recovery in a rodent spinal cord injury model compared to bone marrow-derived stromal cells transplantation [79]. These results are even more promising when human DPC are pretreated with FGF2 for several consecutive serial passages and then directly transplanted into the injury site with, notably, an improvement of axonal regeneration and of the locomotor recovery of the hind limbs by improving the survival rate of DPC at the lesion site [80].

Altogether, these results demonstrate a conserved pro-regenerative role for the FGF signaling in the formation of the glial bridge and, hence, in axonal regeneration in the spinal cord.

2.4.2. The Brain

Aging, brain injury or neurodegenerative conditions such as Alzheimer's disease (AD) and Parkinson's disease cause a major loss of neural cells. After brain injury, glial cells present in the neurogenic niches have the potential to proliferate. However, a reactive gliosis also occurs, producing a glial scar that inhibits this proliferation and hampers neurogenesis. The zebrafish brain has an incredible capacity of regeneration that can be partially explained by its numerous neurogenic niches and by the capacity of radial cells in the parenchyma to form new neurons. Depending on the type of injury and its localization and severity, different mechanisms of regeneration can be activated. This topic has been recently reviewed [68,81,82]. In this section, we focus on two different models of zebrafish brain injury/neurodegeneration that lead to mechanistic translation in mammalian models. In the zebrafish stab lesion assay (Table 1), the parenchyma of the telencephalon is surgically injured but leaves the neurogenic niches intact, allowing radial cells to proliferate, migrate and generate new neurons [83]. Kizil et al. 2012b showed that the expression of the zinc finger transcription factor Gata3 is induced in radial cells in response to injury [43] where its activity is necessary to properly activate their proliferation, neurogenesis and to promote migration of the newborn neurons, specifically in an injury context [43]. Human/mouse astrocytes fail to induce *Gata3* in response to injury. To mimic injury conditions, scratches have been performed in 2D and 3D cultures of human astrocytes. However, though *Gata3* delivery increased the number of neuronal progenitors, they could not achieve neurogenesis [84]. These results show that *Gata3* enhances the neurogenic potential of human astrocytes but is not sufficient.

To study the mechanisms of brain plasticity in response to neurodegeneration, a zebrafish model of Alzheimer's-disease-like (AD) has been developed [44] (Table 1). A hallmark of AD is the accumulation of β-amyloid Ab42 aggregates in the brain. Injection of Ab42 peptides coupled with a cell peptide transporter (transportan) into the zebrafish brain lead to neurodegeneration [44]. In contrast to mammals, neurodegeneration triggers radial/astroglia cell proliferation and neurogenesis in zebrafish. Transcriptomic profiling of this zebrafish model showed that *gata3* does not seem to be involved but pinpointed immune signaling pathways upregulated in response to Ab42-mediated neurodegeneration. This uncovered the specific upregulation of the anti-inflammatory interleukin-4 (IL4)/STAT6 pathway and its beneficial action on glial cell proliferation in the AD-like model. In contrast, this pathway is not activated in mammals. Furthermore, IL4 overexpression in healthy zebrafish could increase brain progenitor proliferation and neurogenesis [44]. Papadimitriou et al. 2018 later developed a 3D-culture model of human astrocytes and neural stem cells and examined the effect of IL4 as these cells naturally express the IL4 receptor. Interestingly, the inhibitory effect of Ab42 peptide on proliferation capacities could be rescued by treatment with IL4 [85]. However, in an in vivo mouse model of AD, the expression of the IL4 receptor could not be detected in astrocytes [45] and its artificial delivery led to astrocyte death [45]. The authors hypothesized that the mammalian brain evolved to avoid hyper-proliferation by establishing a non-permissive environment for cells expressing the IL4 receptor.

To summarize, thanks to two different zebrafish models of brain regeneration, mediators of brain plasticity with favorable potential in mammalian models were identified though the complexity of the mammalian brain, which has evolved rigid barriers to repress regeneration in order to, presumably, avoid tumorigenesis.

2.4.3. The Retina

Photoreceptor death characterizes retinal degeneration and eye diseases like diabetic retinopathy, retinitis pigmentosa or glaucoma, leading to loss of vision and even to complete and untreatable blindness. A promising strategy to restore sight would be to activate endogenous regeneration of photoreceptors within the retina. Exploiting regenerative capacities of amphibians and fish, researchers revealed several cellular sources to regrow new photoreceptors. Among them, we can cite the retinal pigment epithelium (in amphibians but not in fish), the ciliary margin (the region which contains the retinal stem cells in fish and amphibians) and the Müller glia [86]. The Müller cells (MCs) constitute the major glial cells spread through the entire retina and are conserved from fish to mammals. Their function is to maintain retinal homeostasis and structure. During retinal development, the MCs are the latest cells to arise from retinal multipotent progenitors. MCs share molecular signatures with late retinal progenitor cells [87], leading to the hypothesis that MCs could be progenitors with a glial function. In response to retinal injury, MCs undergo reactive gliosis, i.e., change in morphology, dedifferentiation and proliferation [88,89]. However, this proliferation is rapidly inhibited in mammals, resulting in scar formation and preventing regeneration. On the other hand, zebrafish MCs can differentiate into new retinal neurons after replication [47] and restore vision. Assuming that this regenerative capacity is present in mammals but dormant, researchers focused on key factors specifically expressed or induced in zebrafish but not in mammals. The most tangible example is the case of achaete scute-like family bHLH transcription factor 1a (ASCL1a). In response to surgical injury, *ascl1a* expression is induced in the zebrafish retina and is necessary for MC proliferation and thus regeneration [90], while *Ascl1* is not expressed in the mammalian retina. In order to test if *Ascl1* expression can stimulate the neurogenic potential of mammalian MCs, *Ascl1* has been overexpressed in ex vivo explants of mice MCs, which enabled their dedifferentiation into retinal progenitors [91]. Furthermore, while *Ascl1* expression driven in vivo by transgenesis in mice retina did not affect the uninjured retina, it could activate regeneration after injury induced by N-methyl D-aspartate (NMDA) or excessive light [92] (Table 1). However, only juvenile mice were able to generate new retinal neurons, showing that *Ascl1* is important but not sufficient to induce retinal regeneration in adult mammals [92]. Epigenetic regulations were proposed to underlie the age-dependent regenerative capacities as the *Ascl1* target genes are accessible in juvenile MCs but less accessible in adult MCs [92]. Supporting this hypothesis, *Ascl1* overexpression in MCs combined with an eraser of epigenetic marks, the histone deacetylase inhibitor trichostatin-A, could stimulate photoreceptor regeneration after injury in adult mice [48]. Importantly, the regenerated cells responded to light [48], demonstrating functional recovery. Nevertheless, this mechanism of regeneration did not involve MC proliferation [48] and rather suggested direct transdifferentiation of MCs into retinal neurons, which could possibly lead to MC depletion. This could be overcome by the combined overexpression of *Ascl1* and *Lin28*. Lin28a is an RNA binding protein expressed in response to retinal injury in zebrafish [93] but not in mice [46]. *lin28a* expression is also necessary for retinal regeneration in zebrafish [93]. Combined *ascl1a* and *lin28a* overexpression mimics a regenerative response in the zebrafish retina without injury [46]. While *ascl1a* or *lin28a* expression alone does not impact the retinal phenotype, their combination induces MC proliferation and differentiation into several types of retinal neurons [46]. In the NMDA mice model of retinal injury, *Ascl1* and *Lin28* co-overexpression enhances MC proliferation in young mice [46] compared to *Ascl1* overexpression alone [92]. These studies taking advantage of the regenerative capacities of zebrafish revealed that Ascl1 and Lin28 are pieces to unlock the regeneration potential of mammalian MCs.

3. Conclusions

A question often asked to biomedical researchers using the zebrafish as a model organism is how a fish can help patients. Many studies point out that the zebrafish anatomy and physiology share many features with mammals and this is exemplified by the rapid expansion of zebrafish disease models. This review seeks to bring an answer to how zebrafish could benefit regenerative medicine by emphasizing the transposable potential of the zebrafish regenerative abilities. All the studies highlighted here share a common workflow

(Figure 1) such as drug and genetic screenings to enable the identification of regulators of regeneration first in zebrafish [28,31–33,43]. An important trait of these studies is the versatility of a few zebrafish injury models that allow us to tackle different regenerative processes. It is for example the case of the pancreas and the liver where the zebrafish NTR model is almost exclusively employed in contrast to the various mice models of injury that are used to cover regeneration from different cellular sources (Table 1) [31,33,67]. The NTR model is also exploited to study regeneration in the heart and the brain and is continuously improving [94–97]. Although this relatively simple model provides valuable clues about regeneration, zebrafish models recapitulating more closely the disease will determine how zebrafish regenerate in such settings, therefore further increasing our understanding of regeneration and the success of transposition to mammals. A critical step of the workflow is to choose the most relevant mammalian model of injury to further explore the zebrafish discoveries (Table 1). Another key aspect is to ensure that modulating the mechanisms identified in zebrafish can improve the function of regenerated cells in vivo in mammal models.

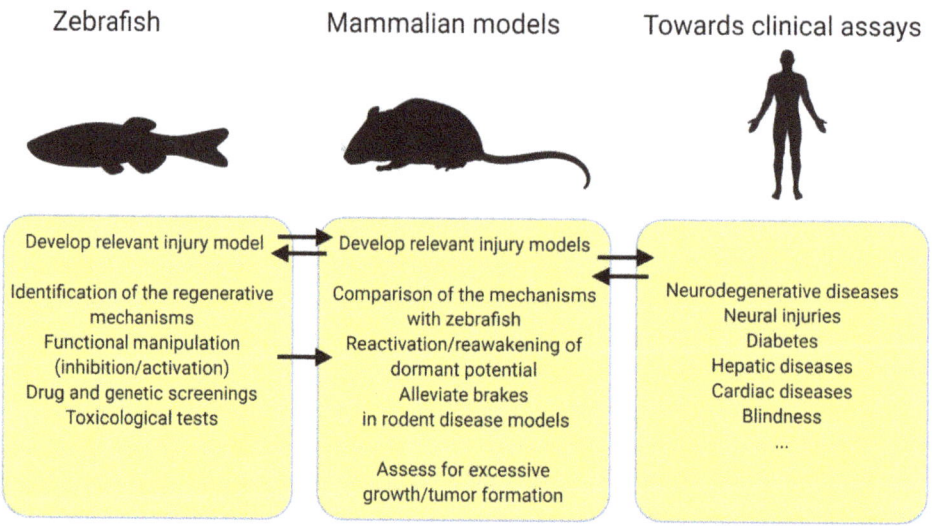

Figure 1. Workflow from zebrafish to mammals. Created with Biorender.com.

Altogether, these studies support the idea that regenerative mechanisms are relatively well conserved even in species with low regenerative capacities, but they are repressed. It can be assumed that mammals have evolved in a way to safeguard against hyper-proliferation to prevent tissue overgrowth and tumorigenesis while maintaining functionality. In this respect, polyploidization is a common feature of many mammalian tissues during aging, homeostasis and cancer. Polyploidy has also emerged to play a role in heart regeneration [18]. Similar to cardiomyocytes, many cell types in mammals such as hepatocytes also become polyploid after birth. Although the significance for liver regeneration is poorly understood, it is likely to play a role [98,99]. It would be interesting to assess the effect of polyploidy in hepatocyte regeneration in zebrafish.

Two other major types of obstacles involve the immune system/inflammation and epigenetic regulations (Figure 2). Repressing a prolonged inflammatory response improves regenerative responses in the mammalian brain or spinal cord. The immune system/inflammatory response differs between organisms able to regenerate and those which cannot [100]. In organisms unable to regenerate, the immune response is generally sustained. On the other hand, the zebrafish immune response is transient, as observed in the heart [101,102] and the spinal cord [74]. This environment favors a proper regenerative response without scarring. Another obstacle to regeneration is the epigenetic repression or the loss of enhancers of pro-regenerative genes [103] as it is the case in the heart, the liver and the retina (Figure 2).

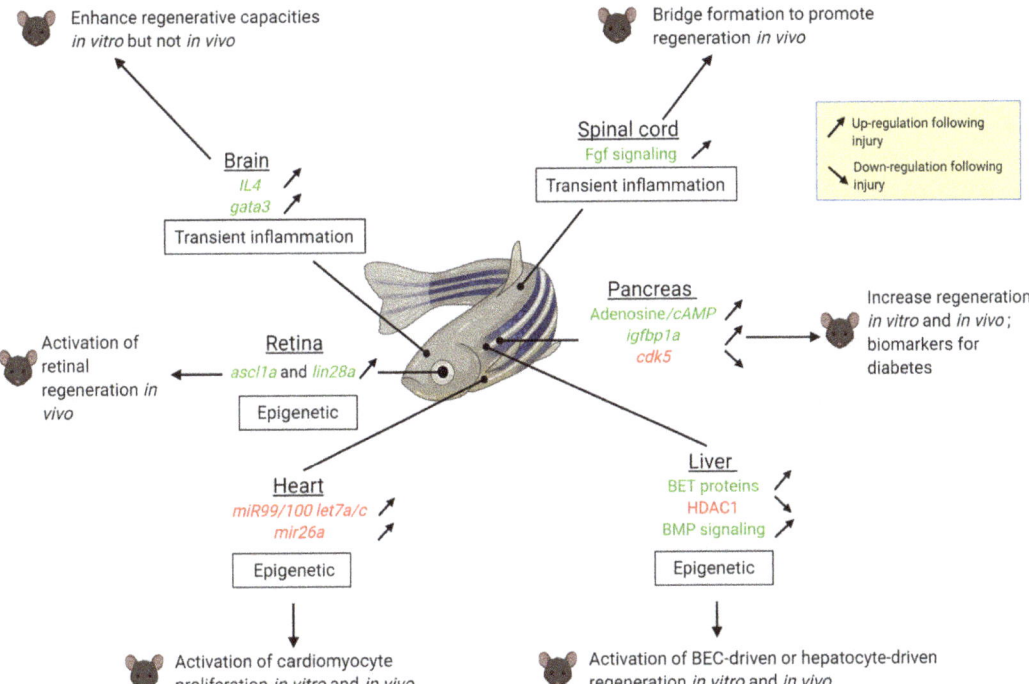

Figure 2. Summary of regenerative mechanisms identified in zebrafish which are able to awake the regenerative potential in mammals in the brain, the spine, the retina, the pancreas, the liver and the heart. The up-headed (vs. back-headed) arrows mean that the expression is upregulated (vs. downregulated) in zebrafish after injury. Factors highlighted in green exert positive effect in regeneration, those in red impair regeneration. Created with Biorender.com.

In addition to help decipher the mechanisms of regeneration, the studies performed in zebrafish also illustrate its great amenability to preclinical drug testing. To promote tissue repair, transplantation-free (or cell-free) therapies rely on administration of soluble factors, vesicles or microRNA that can be first tested in zebrafish for their efficiency and toxicity.

Even if the path is still long before we are able to overcome these obstacles and to offer beneficial treatments to patients, the zebrafish is a powerful model to help elucidate universal mechanisms of regeneration and to give clues about how and why more complex vertebrates erected barriers dampening this potential. The versatility of zebrafish enables the development of innovative models of regeneration and of novel technologies such as scRNAseq associated with CRISPR/Cas9 barcode editing for fine cell lineage tracing [104] and a growing number of genetic and metabolic reporter tools enabling non-toxic and non-invasive in vivo imaging to follow organ reconstruction and functional recovery. Associated with its regenerative capacity, all these assets confer the zebrafish with undeniable advantages over other preclinical models that will certainly accelerate research in regenerative medicine.

Funding: This work was supported by the National Belgian Funds for Scientific Research FNRS-FRS (I.M.), the FRIA PhD fellowship program (L.M.) and the Belgian FNRS under EOS Project No. 30826052 (M.A.D.).

Institutional Review Board Statement: Not applicable.

Informed Consent Statement: Not applicable.

Acknowledgments: We thank Bernard Peers, Marianne Voz and Jérémie Zappia for critically reading the manuscript.

Conflicts of Interest: The authors declare no conflict of interest.

Abbreviations

AD	Alzheimer's disease
APAP	N-acetyl-p-aminophenol
ASCL1	Achaete Scute-Like family bHLH transcription factor 1
BECs	Biliary Epithelial Cells
BET	Bromodomain and Extra-Terminal proteins
BMP	Bone Morphogenetic Protein
CDE	Choline-Deficient Ethionine-supplemented
CNS	Central Nervous System
DTA	Diphtheria Toxin Subunit A
DTR	Diphtheria Toxin Receptor
FGF	Fibroblast Growth Factor
HDAC1	Histone Deacetylase 1
Igf	insulin-like growth factor
igfbp1	Igf binding-protein 1
IL4	interleukin-4
LEN	lepb-linked enhancer
LPCs	Liver Progenitors Cells
MCs	Müller cells
miRNAs	micro RNAs
NECA	50-N-ethylcarboxamidoadenosine
NMDA	N-methyl D-Aspartate
NTR	Nitroreductase
PDL	Pancreatic Duct Ligation
PIAA	(E)-3-(3-phenylbenzo[c]isoxazol-5-yl) acrylic acid
STZ	StrepToZotocin
T1D	Type 1 Diabetes
T2D	Type 2 Diabetes

References

1. Elliott, S.A.; Sánchez Alvarado, A. Planarians and the History of Animal Regeneration: Paradigm Shifts and Key Concepts in Biology. In *Planarian Regeneration. Methods in Molecular Biology*; Humana Press: New York, NY, USA, 2018; Volume 1774, ISBN 9781493978021.
2. Maden, M. The evolution of regeneration—Where does that leave mammals? *Int. J. Dev. Biol.* **2018**, *62*, 369–372. [PubMed]
3. Gemberling, M.; Bailey, T.J.; Hyde, D.R.; Poss, K.D. The zebrafish as a model for complex tissue regeneration. *Trends Genet.* **2013**, *29*, 611–620. [CrossRef] [PubMed]
4. Kinth, P.; Mahesh, G.; Panwar, Y. Mapping of zebrafish research: A global outlook. *Zebrafish* **2013**, *10*, 510–517. [CrossRef] [PubMed]
5. Mehta, A.S.; Singh, A. Insights into regeneration tool box: An animal model approach. *Dev. Biol.* **2019**, *453*, 111–129. [CrossRef]
6. Marques, I.J.; Lupi, E.; Mercader, N. Model systems for regeneration: Zebrafish. *Development* **2019**, *146*, dev167692. [CrossRef]
7. Howe, K.; Clark, M.D.; Torroja, C.F.; Torrance, J.; Muffato, M.; Collins, J.E.; Humphray, S.; Mclaren, K.; Matthews, L.; Mclaren, S.; et al. The zebrafish reference genome sequence and its relationship to the human genome. *Nature* **2014**, *496*, 498–503. [CrossRef]
8. Roth, G.A.; Johnson, C.; Abajobir, A.; Abd-Allah, F.; Abera, S.F.; Abyu, G.; Ahmed, M.; Aksut, B.; Alam, T.; Alam, K.; et al. Global, Regional, and National Burden of Cardiovascular Diseases for 10 Causes, 1990 to 2015. *J. Am. Coll. Cardiol.* **2017**, *70*, 1–25. [CrossRef]

9. Bergmann, O.; Bhardwaj, R.D.; Bernard, S.; Zdunek, S.; Barnabé-Heider, F.; Walsh, S.; Zupicich, J.; Alkass, K.; Buchholz, B.A.; Druid, H.; et al. Evidence for cardiomyocyte renewal in humans. *Science* **2009**, *324*, 98–102. [CrossRef]
10. Hashimoto, H.; Olson, E.N.; Bassel-Duby, R. Therapeutic approaches for cardiac regeneration and repair. *Nat. Rev. Cardiol.* **2018**, *15*, 585–600. [CrossRef]
11. Poss, K.D.; Wilson, L.G.; Keating, M.T. Heart Regeneration in Zebrafish. *Science* **2002**, *298*, 2188–2190. [CrossRef]
12. Raya, A.; Koth, C.M.; Büscher, D.; Kawakami, Y.; Itoh, T.; Raya, R.M.; Sternik, G.; Tsai, H.-J.; Rodríguez-Esteban, C.; Izpisúa-Belmonte, J.C. Activation of Notch signaling pathway precedes heart regeneration in zebrafish. *Proc. Natl. Acad. Sci. USA* **2003**, *100* (Suppl. 1), 11889–11895. [CrossRef] [PubMed]
13. Chablais, F.; Veit, J.; Rainer, G.; Jaźwińska, A. The zebrafish heart regenerates after cryoinjury-induced myocardial infarction. *BMC Dev. Biol.* **2011**, *11*, 21. [CrossRef] [PubMed]
14. González-Rosa, J.M.; Martín, V.; Peralta, M.; Torres, M.; Mercader, N. Extensive scar formation and regression during heart regeneration after cryoinjury in zebrafish. *Development* **2011**, *138*, 1663–1674. [CrossRef] [PubMed]
15. Rubin, N.; Harrison, M.R.; Krainock, M.; Kim, R.; Lien, C.-L. Recent advancements in understanding endogenous heart regeneration-insights from adult zebrafish and neonatal mice. *Semin. Cell Dev. Biol.* **2016**, *58*, 34–40. [CrossRef]
16. Porrello, E.R.; Mahmoud, A.I.; Simpson, E.; Hill, J.A.; Richardson, J.A.; Olson, E.N.; Sadek, H.A. Transient regenerative potential of the neonatal mouse heart. *Science* **2011**, *331*, 1078–1080. [CrossRef]
17. Jopling, C.; Sleep, E.; Raya, M.; Martí, M.; Raya, A.; Izpisúa Belmonte, J.C. Zebrafish heart regeneration occurs by cardiomyocyte dedifferentiation and proliferation. *Nature* **2010**, *464*, 606–609. [CrossRef]
18. González-Rosa, J.M.; Sharpe, M.; Field, D.; Soonpaa, M.H.; Field, L.J.; Burns, C.E.; Burns, C.G. Myocardial Polyploidization Creates a Barrier to Heart Regeneration in Zebrafish. *Dev. Cell* **2018**, *44*, 433–446.e7. [CrossRef]
19. Li, F.; Wang, X.; Capasso, J.M.; Gerdes, A.M. Rapid Transition of Cardiac Myocytes from Hyperplasia to Hypertrophy During Postnatal Development. *J. Mol. Cell. Cardiol.* **1996**, *28*, 1737–1746. [CrossRef]
20. Soonpaa, M.H.; Kim, K.K.; Pajak, L.; Franklin, M.; Field, L.J. Cardiomyocyte DNA synthesis and binucleation during murine development. *Am. J. Physiol.* **1996**, *271*, H2183–H2189. [CrossRef]
21. Mollova, M.; Bersell, K.; Walsh, S.; Savla, J.; Das, L.T.; Park, S.-Y.; Silberstein, L.E.; Dos Remedios, C.G.; Graham, D.; Colan, S.; et al. Cardiomyocyte proliferation contributes to heart growth in young humans. *Proc. Natl. Acad. Sci. USA* **2013**, *110*, 1446–1451. [CrossRef]
22. Vivien, C.J.; Hudson, J.E.; Porrello, E.R. Evolution, comparative biology and ontogeny of vertebrate heart regeneration. *NPJ Regen. Med.* **2016**, *1*, 16012. [CrossRef]
23. Green, R.A.; Paluch, E.; Oegema, K. Cytokinesis in Animal Cells. *Annu. Rev. Cell Dev. Biol.* **2012**, *28*, 29–58. [CrossRef]
24. Porrello, E.R.; Mahmoud, A.I.; Simpson, E.; Johnson, B.A.; Grinsfelder, D.; Canseco, D.; Mammen, P.P.; Rothermel, B.A.; Olson, E.N.; Sadek, H.A. Regulation of neonatal and adult mammalian heart regeneration by the miR-15 family. *Proc. Natl. Acad. Sci. USA* **2013**, *110*, 187–192. [CrossRef]
25. Aguirre, A.; Montserrat, N.; Zacchigna, S.; Nivet, E.; Hishida, T.; Krause, M.N.; Kurian, L.; Ocampo, A.; Vazquez-Ferrer, E.; Rodriguez-Esteban, C.; et al. In vivo activation of a conserved microRNA program induces robust mammalian heart regeneration. *Cell Stem Cell* **2014**, *15*, 589–604. [CrossRef]
26. Russell, J.O.; Ko, S.; Saggi, H.S.; Singh, S.; Poddar, M.; Shin, D.; Monga, S.P. Bromodomain and Extraterminal (BET) Proteins Regulate Hepatocyte Proliferation in Hepatocyte-Driven Liver Regeneration. *Am. J. Pathol.* **2018**, *188*, 1389–1405. [CrossRef]
27. Choi, T.; Khaliq, M.; Tsurusaki, S.; Ninov, N.; Stainier, D.; Tanaka, M.; Shin, D. Bmp Signaling Governs Biliary-Driven Liver Regeneration in Zebrafish via Tbx2b and Id2a. *Hepatology* **2017**, *66*, 1616–1630. [CrossRef]
28. Ko, S.; Choi, T.; Russell, J.O.; So, J.; Shin, D. Bromodomain and extraterminal (BET) proteins regulate biliary-driven liver regeneration. *J. Hepatol.* **2016**, *64*, 316–325. [CrossRef]
29. Ko, S.O.; Russell, J.; Tian, J.; Gao, C.; Kobayashi, M.; Feng, R.; Yuan, X.; Shao, C.; Ding, H.; Poddar, M.; et al. Hdac1 Regulates Differentiation of Bipotent Liver Progenitor Cells During Regeneration via Sox9b and Cdk8. *Gastroenterology* **2019**, *156*, 187–202.e4. [CrossRef]
30. Lu, W.Y.; Bird, T.G.; Boulter, L.; Tsuchiya, A.; Cole, A.M.; Hay, T.; Guest, R.V.; Wojtacha, D.; Man, T.Y.; Mackinnon, A.; et al. Hepatic progenitor cells of biliary origin with liver repopulation capacity. *Nat. Cell Biol.* **2015**, *17*, 973–983. [CrossRef]
31. Andersson, O.; Adams, B.A.; Yoo, D.; Ellis, G.C.; Gut, P.; Anderson, R.M.; German, M.S.; Stainier, D.Y.R. Adenosine Signaling Promotes Regeneration of Pancreatic b Cells In Vivo. *Cell Metab.* **2012**, 885–894. [CrossRef]
32. Xu, J.; Jia, Y.F.; Tapadar, S.; Weaver, J.D.; Raji, I.O.; Pithadia, D.J.; Javeed, N.; García, A.J.; Choi, D.S.; Matveyenko, A.V.; et al. Inhibition of TBK1/IKKε Promotes Regeneration of Pancreatic β-cells. *Sci. Rep.* **2018**, *8*, 1–14. [CrossRef]
33. Lu, J.; Liu, K.; Schulz, N.; Karampelias, C.; Charbord, J.; Hilding, A.; Rautio, L.; Bertolino, P.; Östenson, C.; Brismar, K.; et al. IGFBP 1 increases β-cell regeneration by promoting α- to β-cell transdifferentiation. *EMBO J.* **2016**, *35*, 2026–2044. [CrossRef]
34. Ye, L.; Robertson, M.A.; Hesselson, D.; Stainier, D.Y.R.; Anderson, R.M. Glucagon is essential for alpha cell transdifferentiation and beta cell neogenesis. *Development* **2015**, *142*, 1407–1417. [CrossRef]
35. Kopp, J.L.; Dubois, C.L.; Schaffer, A.E.; Hao, E.; Shih, H.P.; Seymour, P.A.; Ma, J.; Sander, M. Sox9+ ductal cells are multipotent progenitors throughout development but do not produce new endocrine cells in the normal or injured adult pancreas. *Development* **2011**, *138*, 653–665. [CrossRef]

36. Solar, M.; Cardalda, C.; Houbracken, I.; Martín, M.; Maestro, M.A.; De Medts, N.; Xu, X.; Grau, V.; Heimberg, H.; Bouwens, L.; et al. Pancreatic Exocrine Duct Cells Give Rise to Insulin-Producing β Cells during Embryogenesis but Not after Birth. *Dev. Cell* **2009**, *17*, 849–860. [CrossRef]
37. Xu, X.; D'Hoker, J.; Stangé, G.; Bonné, S.; De Leu, N.; Xiao, X.; Van De Casteele, M.; Mellitzer, G.; Ling, Z.; Pipeleers, D.; et al. β Cells Can Be Generated from Endogenous Progenitors in Injured Adult Mouse Pancreas. *Cell* **2008**, *132*, 197–207. [CrossRef]
38. Al-Hasani, K.; Pfeifer, A.; Courtney, M.; Ben-Othman, N.; Gjernes, E.; Vieira, A.; Druelle, N.; Avolio, F.; Ravassard, P.; Leuckx, G.; et al. Adult duct-lining cells can reprogram into β-like cells able to counter repeated cycles of toxin-induced diabetes. *Dev. Cell* **2013**, *26*, 86–100. [CrossRef]
39. Chera, S. Diabetes Recovery By Age-Dependent Conversion of Pancreatic δ-Cells. *Nature* **2014**, *514*, 503–507. [CrossRef]
40. Thorel, F.; Nepote, V.; Avril, I.; Kohno, K.; Desgraz, R.; Chera, S.; Herrera, P.L.; Népote, V.; Kohno, K.; Desgraz, R. Conversion of Adult Pancreatic alpha-cells to Beta-cells after Extreme Beta Cell Loss. *Nature* **2010**, *464*, 1149–1154. [CrossRef]
41. Becker, T.; Wullimann, M.F.; Becker, C.G.; Bernhardt, R.R.; Schachner, M. Axonal regrowth after spinal cord transection in adult zebrafish. *J. Comp. Neurol.* **1997**, *377*, 577–595. [CrossRef]
42. Goldshmit, Y.; Frisca, F.; Pinto, A.R.; Pébay, A.; Tang, J.-K.K.Y.; Siegel, A.L.; Kaslin, J.; Currie, P.D. Fgf2 improves functional recovery-decreasing gliosis and increasing radial glia and neural progenitor cells after spinal cord injury. *Brain Behav.* **2014**, *4*, 187–200. [CrossRef] [PubMed]
43. Kizil, C.; Kyritsis, N.; Dudczig, S.; Kroehne, V.; Freudenreich, D.; Kaslin, J.; Brand, M. Regenerative Neurogenesis from Neural Progenitor Cells Requires Injury-Induced Expression of Gata3. *Dev. Cell* **2012**, *23*, 1230–1237. [CrossRef] [PubMed]
44. Bhattarai, P.; Thomas, A.K.; Cosacak, M.I.; Papadimitriou, C.; Mashkaryan, V.; Froc, C.; Reinhardt, S.; Kurth, T.; Dahl, A.; Zhang, Y.; et al. IL4/STAT6 Signaling Activates Neural Stem Cell Proliferation and Neurogenesis upon Amyloid-β42 Aggregation in Adult Zebrafish Brain. *Cell Rep.* **2016**, *17*, 941–948. [CrossRef] [PubMed]
45. Mashkaryan, V.; Siddiqui, T.; Popova, S.; Cosacak, M.I.; Bhattarai, P.; Brandt, K.; Govindarajan, N.; Petzold, A.; Reinhardt, S.; Dahl, A.; et al. Type 1 Interleukin-4 Signaling Obliterates Mouse Astroglia in vivo but Not in vitro. *Front. Cell Dev. Biol.* **2020**, *8*, 114. [CrossRef] [PubMed]
46. Elsaeidi, F.; Macpherson, P.; Mills, E.A.; Jui, J.; Flannery, J.G.; Goldman, D. Notch suppression collaborates with Ascl1 and Lin28 to unleash a regenerative response in fish retina, but not in mice. *J. Neurosci.* **2018**, *38*, 2246–2261. [CrossRef] [PubMed]
47. Fausett, B.V.; Goldman, D. A role for alpha1 tubulin-expressing Müller glia in regeneration of the injured zebrafish retina. *J. Neurosci.* **2006**, *26*, 6303–6313. [CrossRef]
48. Jorstad, N.L.; Wilken, M.S.; Grimes, W.N.; Wohl, S.G.; Vandenbosch, L.S.; Yoshimatsu, T.; Wong, R.O.; Rieke, F.; Reh, T.A. Stimulation of functional neuronal regeneration from Müller glia in adult mice. *Nature* **2017**, *548*, 103–107. [CrossRef]
49. Hodgkinson, C.P.; Dzau, V.J. Conserved MicroRNA Program as Key to Mammalian Cardiac Regeneration. *Circ. Res.* **2015**, *116*, 1109–1111. [CrossRef]
50. Crippa, S.; Nemir, M.; Ounzain, S.; Ibberson, M.; Berthonneche, C.; Sarre, A.; Boisset, G.; Maison, D.; Harshman, K.; Xenarios, I.; et al. Comparative transcriptome profiling of the injured zebrafish and mouse hearts identifies miRNA-dependent repair pathways. *Cardiovasc. Res.* **2016**, *110*, 73–84. [CrossRef]
51. Kang, J.; Hu, J.; Karra, R.; Dickson, A.L.; Tornini, V.A.; Nachtrab, G.; Gemberling, M.; Goldman, J.A.; Black, B.L.; Poss, K.D. Modulation of tissue repair by regeneration enhancer elements. *Nature* **2016**, *532*, 201–206. [CrossRef]
52. Bersell, K.; Arab, S.; Haring, B.; Kühn, B. Neuregulin1/ErbB4 signaling induces cardiomyocyte proliferation and repair of heart injury. *Cell* **2009**, *138*, 257–270. [CrossRef] [PubMed]
53. Begeman, I.J.; Kang, J. Transcriptional Programs and Regeneration Enhancers Underlying Heart Regeneration. *J. Cardiovasc. Dev. Dis.* **2018**, *6*, 2. [CrossRef] [PubMed]
54. Xiao, J.C.; Ruck, P.; Adam, A.; Wang, T.X.; Kaiserling, E. Small epithelial cells in human liver cirrhosis exhibit features of hepatic stem-like cells: Immunohistochemical, electron microscopic and immunoelectron microscopic findings. *Histopathology* **2003**, *42*, 141–149. [CrossRef] [PubMed]
55. So, J.; Kim, A.; Lee, S.H.; Shin, D. Liver progenitor cell-driven liver regeneration. *Exp. Mol. Med.* **2020**, *52*, 1230–1238. [CrossRef]
56. Ko, S.; Russell, J.O.; Molina, L.M.; Monga, S.P. Liver Progenitors and Adult Cell Plasticity in Hepatic Injury and Repair: Knowns and Unknowns. *Annu. Rev. Pathol. Mech. Dis.* **2020**, *15*, 23–50. [CrossRef]
57. Xia, J.; Zhou, Y.; Ji, H.; Wang, Y.; Wu, Q.; Bao, J.; Ye, F.; Shi, Y.; Bu, H. Loss of histone deacetylases 1 and 2 in hepatocytes impairs murine liver regeneration through Ki67 depletion. *Hepatology* **2013**, *58*, 2089–2098. [CrossRef]
58. Dor, Y.; Brown, J.; Martinez, O.I.; Melton, D.A. Adult pancreatic beta-cells are formed by self-duplication rather than stem-cell differentiation. *Nature* **2004**, *429*, 41–46. [CrossRef]
59. Pan, F.C.; Bankaitis, E.D.; Boyer, D.; Xu, X.; Van de Casteele, M.; Magnuson, M.A.; Heimberg, H.; Wright, C.V.E. Spatiotemporal patterns of multipotentiality in Ptf1aexpressing cells during pancreas organogenesis and injuryinduced facultative restoration. *Development* **2013**, *140*, 751–764. [CrossRef]
60. Tsuji, N.; Ninov, N.; Delawary, M.; Osman, S.; Roh, A.S.; Gut, P.; Stainier, D.Y.R. Whole organism high content screening identifies stimulators of pancreatic beta-cell proliferation. *PLoS ONE* **2014**, *9*, e104112. [CrossRef]
61. Basile, G.; Kulkarni, R.N.; Morgan, N.G. How, When, and Where Do Human β-Cells Regenerate? *Curr. Diabetes Rep.* **2019**, *19*, 48. [CrossRef]

62. Sharma, A.; Purohit, S.; Sharma, S.; Bai, S.; Zhi, W.; Ponny, S.R.; Hopkins, D.; Steed, L.; Bode, B.; Anderson, S.W.; et al. IGF-binding proteins in type-1 diabetes are more severely altered in the presence of complications. *Front. Endocrinol. (Lausanne)* **2016**, *7*, 2. [CrossRef] [PubMed]
63. Inada, A.; Nienaber, C.; Katsuta, H.; Fujitani, Y.; Levine, J.; Morita, R.; Sharma, A.; Bonner-Weir, S. Carbonic anhydrase II-positive pancreatic cells are progenitors for both endocrine and exocrine pancreas after birth. *Proc. Natl. Acad. Sci. USA* **2008**, *105*, 19915–19919. [CrossRef] [PubMed]
64. Ninov, N.; Hesselson, D.; Gut, P.; Zhou, A.; Fidelin, K.; Stainier, D.Y.R. Metabolic regulation of cellular plasticity in the pancreas. *Curr. Biol.* **2013**, *23*, 1242–1250. [CrossRef] [PubMed]
65. Ghaye, A.P.; Bergemann, D.; Tarifeño-Saldivia, E.; Flasse, L.C.; Von Berg, V.; Peers, B.; Voz, M.L.; Manfroid, I. Progenitor potential of nkx6.1-expressing cells throughout zebrafish life and during beta cell regeneration. *BMC Biol.* **2015**, *13*, 70. [CrossRef]
66. Delaspre, F.; Beer, R.L.; Rovira, M.; Huang, W.; Wang, G.; Gee, S.; Del Carmen Vitery, M.; Wheelan, S.J.; Parsons, M.J. Centroacinar cells are progenitors that contribute to endocrine pancreas regeneration. *Diabetes* **2015**, *64*, 3499–3509. [CrossRef]
67. Liu, K.C.; Leuckx, G.; Sakano, D.; Seymour, P.A.; Mattsson, C.L.; Rautio, L.; Staels, W.; Verdonck, Y.; Serup, P.; Kume, S.; et al. Inhibition of Cdk5 promotes β-cell differentiation from ductal progenitors. *Diabetes* **2018**, *67*, 58–70. [CrossRef]
68. Jurisch-Yaksi, N.; Yaksi, E.; Kizil, C. Radial glia in the zebrafish brain: Functional, structural, and physiological comparison with the mammalian glia. *Glia* **2020**, *68*, 2451–2470. [CrossRef]
69. Asher, R.A.; Morgenstern, D.A.; Fidler, P.S.; Adcock, K.H.; Oohira, A.; Braistead, J.E.; Levine, J.M.; Margolis, R.U.; Rogers, J.H.; Fawcett, J.W. Neurocan is upregulated in injured brain and in cytokine-treated astrocytes. *J. Neurosci.* **2000**, *20*, 2427–2438. [CrossRef]
70. Stichel, C.C.; Hermanns, S.; Luhmann, H.J.; Lausberg, F.; Niermann, H.; D'Urso, D.; Servos, G.; Hartwig, H.G.; Müller, H.W. Inhibition of collagen IV deposition promotes regeneration of injured CNS axons. *Eur. J. Neurosci.* **1999**, *11*, 632–646. [CrossRef]
71. McKeon, R.J.; Schreiber, R.C.; Rudge, J.S.; Silver, J. Reduction of neurite outgrowth in a model of glial scarring following CNS injury is correlated with the expression of inhibitory molecules on reactive astrocytes. *J. Neurosci.* **1991**, *11*, 3398–3411. [CrossRef]
72. Goldshmit, Y.; Sztal, T.E.; Jusuf, P.R.; Hall, T.E.; Nguyen-Chi, M.; Currie, P.D. Fgf-dependent glial cell bridges facilitate spinal cord regeneration in zebrafish. *J. Neurosci.* **2012**, *32*, 7477–7492. [CrossRef] [PubMed]
73. Cigliola, V.; Becker, C.J.; Poss, K.D. Building bridges, not walls: Spinal cord regeneration in zebrafish. *Dis. Models Mech.* **2020**, *13*, 5. [CrossRef] [PubMed]
74. Ghosh, S.; Hui, S.P. Axonal regeneration in zebrafish spinal cord. *Regeneration* **2018**, *5*, 43–60. [CrossRef] [PubMed]
75. Reimer, M.M.; Kuscha, V.; Wyatt, C.; Sörensen, I.; Frank, R.E.; Knüwer, M.; Becker, T.; Becker, C.G. Sonic hedgehog is a polarized signal for motor neuron regeneration in adult zebrafish. *J. Neurosci.* **2009**, *29*, 15073–15082. [CrossRef]
76. Goldshmit, Y.; Frisca, F.; Kaslin, J.; Pinto, A.R.; Tang, J.-K.K.Y.; Pébay, A.; Pinkas-Kramarski, R.; Currie, P.D. Decreased anti-regenerative effects after spinal cord injury in spry4-/- mice. *Neuroscience* **2015**, *287*, 104–112. [CrossRef]
77. Tsai, M.-C.; Shen, L.-F.; Kuo, H.-S.; Cheng, H.; Chak, K.-F. Involvement of acidic fibroblast growth factor in spinal cord injury repair processes revealed by a proteomics approach. *Mol. Cell. Proteom.* **2008**, *7*, 1668–1687. [CrossRef]
78. Kasai, M.; Jikoh, T.; Fukumitsu, H.; Furukawa, S. FGF-2-responsive and spinal cord-resident cells improve locomotor function after spinal cord injury. *J. Neurotrauma* **2014**, *31*, 1584–1598. [CrossRef]
79. Sakai, K.; Yamamoto, A.; Matsubara, K.; Nakamura, S.; Naruse, M.; Yamagata, M.; Sakamoto, K.; Tauchi, R.; Wakao, N.; Imagama, S.; et al. Human dental pulp-derived stem cells promote locomotor recovery after complete transection of the rat spinal cord by multiple neuro-regenerative mechanisms. *J. Clin. Investig.* **2012**, *122*, 80–90. [CrossRef]
80. Nagashima, K.; Miwa, T.; Soumiya, H.; Ushiro, D.; Takeda-Kawaguchi, T.; Tamaoki, N.; Ishiguro, S.; Sato, Y.; Miyamoto, K.; Ohno, T.; et al. Priming with FGF2 stimulates human dental pulp cells to promote axonal regeneration and locomotor function recovery after spinal cord injury. *Sci. Rep.* **2017**, *7*, 13500. [CrossRef]
81. Zambusi, A.; Ninkovic, J. Regeneration of the central nervous system-principles from brain regeneration in adult zebrafish. *World J. Stem Cells* **2020**, *12*, 8–24. [CrossRef]
82. Lange, C.; Brand, M. Vertebrate brain regeneration—A community effort of fate-restricted precursor cell types. *Curr. Opin. Genet. Dev.* **2020**, *64*, 101–108. [CrossRef] [PubMed]
83. Kroehne, V.; Freudenreich, D.; Hans, S.; Kaslin, J.; Brand, M. Regeneration of the adult zebrafish brain from neurogenic radial glia-type progenitors. *Development* **2011**, *138*, 4831–4841. [CrossRef] [PubMed]
84. Celikkaya, H.; Cosacak, M.I.; Papadimitriou, C.; Popova, S.; Bhattarai, P.; Biswas, S.N.; Siddiqui, T.; Wistorf, S.; Nevado-Alcalde, I.; Naumann, L.; et al. GATA3 promotes the neural progenitor state but not neurogenesis in 3D traumatic injury model of primary human cortical astrocytes. *Front. Cell. Neurosci.* **2019**, *13*, 23. [CrossRef] [PubMed]
85. Papadimitriou, C.; Celikkaya, H.; Cosacak, M.I.; Mashkaryan, V.; Bray, L.; Bhattarai, P.; Brandt, K.; Hollak, H.; Chen, X.; He, S.; et al. 3D Culture Method for Alzheimer's Disease Modeling Reveals Interleukin-4 Rescues Aβ42-Induced Loss of Human Neural Stem Cell Plasticity. *Dev. Cell* **2018**, *46*, 85–101.e8. [CrossRef] [PubMed]
86. Langhe, R.; Pearson, R.A. Rebuilding the Retina: Prospects for Müller Glial-mediated Self-repair. *Curr. Eye Res.* **2020**, *45*, 349–360. [CrossRef] [PubMed]
87. Roesch, K.; Jadhav, A.P.; Trimarchi, J.M.; Stadler, M.B.; Roska, B.; Sun, B.B.; Cepko, C.L. The transcriptome of retinal Müller glial cells. *J. Comp. Neurol.* **2008**, *509*, 225–238. [CrossRef]

88. Cepko, C.; Dyer, M.A. Control of Müller glial cell proliferation and activation following retinal injury. *Nat. Neurosci.* **2000**, *3*, 873–880.
89. Hamon, A.; Roger, J.E.; Yang, X.J.; Perron, M. Müller glial cell-dependent regeneration of the neural retina: An overview across vertebrate model systems. *Dev. Dyn.* **2016**, *245*, 727–738. [CrossRef]
90. Fausett, B.V.; Gumerson, J.D.; Goldman, D. The proneural basic helix-loop-helix gene Ascl1a is required for retina regeneration. *J. Neurosci.* **2008**, *28*, 1109–1117. [CrossRef]
91. Pollak, J.; Wilken, M.S.; Ueki, Y.; Cox, K.E.; Sullivan, J.M.; Taylor, R.J.; Levine, E.M.; Reh, T.A. ASCL1 reprograms mouse Müller glia into neurogenic retinal progenitors. *Development* **2013**, *140*, 2619–2631. [CrossRef]
92. Ueki, Y.; Wilken, M.S.; Cox, K.E.; Chipman, L.; Jorstad, N.; Sternhagen, K.; Simic, M.; Ullom, K.; Nakafuku, M.; Reh, T.A. Transgenic expression of the proneural transcription factor Ascl1 in Müller glia stimulates retinal regeneration in young mice. *Proc. Natl. Acad. Sci. USA* **2015**, *112*, 13717–13722. [CrossRef] [PubMed]
93. Ramachandran, R.; Fausett, B.V.; Goldman, D. Ascl1A regulates Muller glia dedifferentiation and retina regeneration via a Lin-28 dependent, let7 miRNA signaling pathway. *Nat. Cell Biol.* **2010**, *7*, 1959–1967.
94. Pisharath, H.; Rhee, J.M.; Swanson, M.A.; Leach, S.D.; Parsons, M.J. Targeted ablation of beta cells in the embryonic zebrafish pancreas using E.coli nitroreductase. *Mech. Dev.* **2007**, *124*, 218–229. [CrossRef] [PubMed]
95. Curado, S.; Anderson, R.M.; Jungblut, B.; Mumm, J.; Schroeter, E.; Stainier, D.Y.R. Conditional targeted cell ablation in zebrafish: A new tool for regeneration studies. *Dev. Dyn.* **2007**, *236*, 1025–1035. [CrossRef] [PubMed]
96. Bergemann, D.; Massoz, L.; Bourdouxhe, J.; Carril Pardo, C.A.; Voz, M.L.; Peers, B.; Manfroid, I. Nifurpirinol: A more potent and reliable substrate compared to metronidazole for nitroreductase-mediated cell ablations. *Wound Repair Regen.* **2018**, *26*, 238–244. [CrossRef] [PubMed]
97. Sharrock, A.; Mulligan, T.; Hall, K.; Williams, E.; White, D.; Zhang, L.; Matthews, F.; Nimmagadda, S.; Washington, S.; Le, K.; et al. NTR 2.0: A rationally-engineered prodrug converting enzyme with substantially enhanced efficacy for targeted cell ablation. *bioRxiv* **2020**, 1–26. [CrossRef]
98. Wilkinson, P.D.; Alencastro, F.; Delgado, E.R.; Leek, M.P.; Weirich, M.P.; Otero, P.A.; Roy, N.; Brown, W.K.; Oertel, M.; Duncan, A.W. Polyploid Hepatocytes Facilitate Adaptation and Regeneration to Chronic Liver Injury. *Am. J. Pathol.* **2019**, *189*, 1241–1255. [CrossRef]
99. Donne, R.; Saroul-Aïnama, M.; Cordier, P.; Celton-Morizur, S.; Desdouets, C. Polyploidy in liver development, homeostasis and disease. *Nat. Rev. Gastroenterol. Hepatol.* **2020**, *17*, 391–405. [CrossRef]
100. Julier, Z.; Park, A.J.; Briquez, P.S.; Martino, M.M. Promoting tissue regeneration by modulating the immune system. *Acta Biomater.* **2017**, *53*, 13–28. [CrossRef]
101. Lai, S.L.; Marín-Juez, R.; Moura, P.L.; Kuenne, C.; Lai, J.K.H.; Tsedeke, A.T.; Guenther, S.; Looso, M.; Stainier, D.Y.R. Reciprocal analyses in zebrafish and medaka reveal that harnessing the immune response promotes cardiac regeneration. *Elife* **2017**, *6*, 1–20. [CrossRef]
102. Ryan, R.; Moyse, B.R.; Richardson, R.J. Zebrafish cardiac regeneration-looking beyond cardiomyocytes to a complex microenvironment. *Histochem. Cell Biol.* **2020**, *154*, 533–548. [CrossRef] [PubMed]
103. Suzuki, N.; Ochi, H. Regeneration enhancers: A clue to reactivation of developmental genes. *Dev. Growth Regen.* **2020**, 1–12. [CrossRef] [PubMed]
104. Zafar, H.; Lin, C.; Bar-Joseph, Z. Single-cell lineage tracing by integrating CRISPR-Cas9 mutations with transcriptomic data. *Nat. Commun.* **2020**, *11*, 305. [CrossRef] [PubMed]

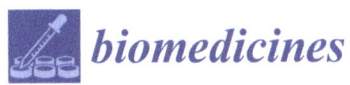

Article

Functional Role of the RNA-Binding Protein Rbm24a and Its Target *sox2* in Microphthalmia

Lindy K. Brastrom [1], C. Anthony Scott [2], Kai Wang [3] and Diane C. Slusarski [1,*]

[1] Department of Biology, University of Iowa, Iowa City, IA 52245, USA; melinda-brastrom@uiowa.edu
[2] Mercury Data Science, Houston, TX 77098, USA; anthony@mercuryds.com
[3] Department of Biostatistics, University of Iowa, Iowa City, IA 52245, USA; kai-wang@uiowa.edu
* Correspondence: diane-slusarski@uiowa.edu

Abstract: Congenital eye defects represent a large class of disorders affecting roughly 21 million children worldwide. Microphthalmia and anophthalmia are relatively common congenital defects, with approximately 20% of human cases caused by mutations in *SOX2*. Recently, we identified the RNA-binding motif protein 24a (Rbm24a) which binds to and regulates *sox2* in zebrafish and mice. Here we show that morpholino knockdown of *rbm24a* leads to microphthalmia and visual impairment. By utilizing sequential injections, we demonstrate that addition of exogenous *sox2* RNA to *rbm24a*-deplete embryos is sufficient to suppress morphological and visual defects. This research demonstrates a critical role for understanding the post-transcriptional regulation of genes needed for development.

Keywords: *rbm24a*; *sox2*; post-transcriptional regulation; vision; visual assay; microphthalmia; RNA binding protein; zebrafish

1. Introduction

Congenital eye defects represent a large class of disorders affecting roughly 21 million children worldwide [1]. Defects can affect every part of the eye from the retina to the lens, but can also include the eye as a whole. Microphthalmia, a smaller than normal eye(s), and anophthalmia, a lack of an eye(s), are both relatively common congenital defects affecting between 1 in 7000 and 1 in 30,000 live births, respectively [2–5].

Mutations in SRY (sex determining region Y)-box2 *(SOX2)* account for approximately 20% of human anophthalmia cases [6]. As a transcription factor, SOX2, often in cooperation with a partner transcription factor, is responsible for the regulation of many genes and is one of the Yamanaka reprogramming factors that regulates pluripotency [7–9]. Thus, understanding the regulation of *SOX2* is crucial. While the transcriptional regulation of *SOX2* has been explored, only recently has the post-transcriptional aspect of its regulation been appreciated [10].

Previously, we identified the RNA-binding protein, RBM24, as a post-transcriptional regulator of *Sox2* [11,12]. Consistent with *SOX2*'s known role in microphthalmia and anophthalmia in human patients, knockdown and knockout *Rbm24*-deficient mice and zebrafish often displayed eye defects including microphthalmia and/or anophthalmia [12,13]. In addition to its role in eye development, *rbm24a* knockdown, mutation, and overexpression are also associated with cardiac defects. Previous inquiries found *Rbm24* mutant mice to be embryonic lethal, dying between E7.5 and E14.5. The embryonic lethality observed is thought to be cardiomyopathy due to numerous cardiovascular malformations, which included ventricular septum defects, reduced trabeculation and compaction, dilated atria and ventricle chambers, thinner atrioventricular endocardial cushions, sarcomere disarray, and fibrosis [12,14–16]. Most previous research focused on the cardiac phenotypes associated with *rbm24a* depletion.

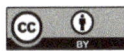

It is challenging to study global factors such as Rbm24a due to their wide-ranging impacts on a multitude of target RNAs. We chose to focus on a single proposed RNA target, *sox2*, to perform more in-depth analyses as to the relationship between Rbm24a and *sox2*. To do so, we analyzed the expression pattern of *rbm24a* and found, consistent with previous studies in zebrafish, *Xenopus*, mice, and chick, its expression in the somites, heart, and lens in a spatiotemporal manner [11,14,17–23]. To study the role of *rbm24a* in zebrafish development, we performed morpholino knockdown and CRISPR mutagenesis which phenocopied previously reported morphants and mutants [19,20,23]. We next performed sequential injection of *rbm24a* morpholino and exogenous *sox2* RNA to determine the extent to which *sox2* can suppress the *rbm24a*-depleted microphthalmia. We found phenotypic suppression of the *rbm24a*-induced microphthalmia. We also performed a visual assay which tests for light/dark detection on these embryos and found partial visually functional rescue by *sox2* RNA. This work highlights the study of post-transcriptional modification and their target RNAs during eye development.

2. Experimental Section

2.1. Animal Care

Zebrafish are maintained in standard conditions under the approval of the University of Iowa Institutional Animal Care and Use Committee (#8071513, 13 August 2018). Embryos are collected from natural spawning and raised between 28 and 30 °C. No more than 50 embryos are kept per 100 mm plate. Embryo plates are cleaned of dead daily and water changes are made as needed.

2.2. Microinjection

Embryos at the 1–2 cell stage were injected with either a translation-blocking *rbm24a* morpholino (0.6–1.2, 1–1.3, or 1.7–2 ng), splice-blocking *rbm24a* morpholino, or AltR CRISPR construct (3 nL). The morpholinos were ordered from Gene Tools. *rbm24a* AUG MO sequence: 5′-GCATCCTCACGAAACGCTCAAGTGC-3′. *rbm24a* SB MO sequence: 5′-TTGATATAATCCTCACCTGGCTGCA-3′. The AltR crRNA was ordered from IDT [24]. *rbm24a* AltR crRNA sequence: 5′-GGACUUUCCAGUCUGUCUGUGUUUUAGAGCUAUGCU-3′. RNA for *rbm24a* (100–400 pg), *sox2* (200–300 pg), and EGFP (200–300 pg) was generated from cDNA that was cloned into the pCR8/GW/TOPO vector (*rbm24a*, *sox2*; Invitrogen, Carlsbad, CA, USA) or pCS2 + (EGFP, RZPD) before linearized templates were transcribed using the SP6 Ambion mMessage mMachine kit (Invitrogen, Carlsbad, CA, USA). *rbm24a* and *sox2* RNAs have N-terminal Myc tags. *sox2* RNA lacks a 3′ UTR. Microinjection needles were measured via a capillary tube to ensure dosages fell in the aforementioned ranges. Sequential injections were performed utilizing the same needle between morpholino-injected embryos (morpholino-only and morpholino with RNA) and RNA-injected embryos (RNA-only and morpholino with RNA) to ensure consistent dosage between experimental groups. An app was used to calculate the amount of construct injected (https://play.google.com/store/apps/details?id=com.canthonyscott.microinjectioncalc&hl=en_US). When noted, sequential injections were performed on a single day per set and involved the usage of the same clutch of eggs, needle, and dosage for all embryos injected.

2.3. Mutagenesis Detection

Uninjected and injected embryos underwent gDNA extraction at 2–4 dpf. Briefly, 20 µL of 50 mM NaOH per embryo was added before embryos were heated at 95 °C for 15 min. Samples were cooled and neutralized with 1 µL of 1 M Tris pH 8.0 per 10 µL of NaOH. The resulting gDNA underwent PCR amplification before being sequenced and insertion/deletion (indels) detection was performed utilizing Synthego ICE [25]. *rbm24a*-Forward-5′-ATGCATACCACGCAAAAGGAC-3′, *rbm24a*-Reverse-5′-CAGTCTGTCTGTCGGTAATCA-3′.

2.4. Automated Startle Response

The automated vision startle response, VIZN, was performed on 5 or 6 days post-fertilization (dpf) larvae as previously described [26]. Phenotypically normal larvae were first tested for the ability to swim by being prodded to ensure touch responsiveness and swimming ability, before being sorted and placed in 48-well plates.

2.5. Statistical Analysis

Data in tables were analyzed statistically with Fisher's exact test implement in R [27]. VIZN assays were statistically analyzed by Mann–Whitney.

3. Results

3.1. Mutation of rbm24a Leads to Microphthalmia and Cardiomyopathy

Zebrafish *rbm24a* is expressed in the developing heart, somites, and lens [19,20,22]. Translation and splice-blocking morpholino knockdown leads to dose-dependent defects, with lower doses exhibiting microphthalmia, while higher doses display microphthalmia and cardiac defects leading to edema (Supplemental Figure S1). We previously analyzed the microphthalmia phenotype both morphologically and histologically [13]. To validate the usage of the morpholino, we aimed to generate an *rbm24a* mutant. Similar to other organisms, including mice and humans, the zebrafish Rbm24a contains two domains: the RNA recognition motif (RRM) and an Alanine-rich region. The RRM domain spans exons 1 and 2 and is the domain responsible for binding to target RNAs. This domain is highly conserved, with 96.2% identity shared between zebrafish and humans. The Alanine-rich region is in exon 4 and has an unknown function in Rbm24a (Figure 1). Due to the key role of the RRM domain, we designed a CRISPR site in exon 1 which was a predicted null mutation (Figure 1). We performed CRISPR knockout and found phenotypes similar to those of morpholino knockdown. Most CRISPR-injected F0 embryos displayed microphthalmia (small eye(s)) and cardiac edema (fluid around the heart) which is consistent with the expression pattern of *rbm24a*, previously reported morphant phenotypes, and previously reported mutant phenotypes (Figure 1B–E) [19,20,23]. We extracted genomic DNA (gDNA) from both uninjected and CRISPR-injected F0, amplified the region flanking the target cut site, and sequenced the products. We next used Synthego ICE to determine the nature and frequency of indels [25]. Analysis of the CRISPR-injected F0 mutants showed an indel frequency between 20% and 24% when compared to the uninjected control embryos (Figure 1F). There is a statistically significant difference between the phenotypes of uninjected control and CRISPR-injected F0 embryos ($p < 1 \times 10^{-16}$) (Table 1).

3.2. rbm24a RNA Suppression of rbm24a Morpholino Knockdown

Due to the high number of CRISPR injected F0 embryos exhibiting both microphthalmia and cardiac edema, we chose to utilize a low dose of translation-blocking morpholino in order to generate microphthalmia-only *rbm24a* knockdown phenotypes. When compared to uninjected embryos, morphant embryos injected with a low dose (1–1.3 ng) displayed only microphthalmia, while embryos injected at a higher dose (1.7–2 ng) phenocopied the CRISPR-injected F0 embryos with both microphthalmia and cardiac edema (Figure 2A–C').

Table 1. Number of phenotypes associated with uninjected control and CRISPR-injected F0 embryos.

	Uninjected	*rbm24a* CRISPR F0
Normal	83	4
Microphthalmia		0
Microphthalmia and CVD [1]		28
CVD		1
Other [2]	1	1
Total	84	34

[1] CVD stands for cardiovascular defect. [2] Other is a category reserved for phenotypes that do not fall under the above categories. They are frequently trunk defects.

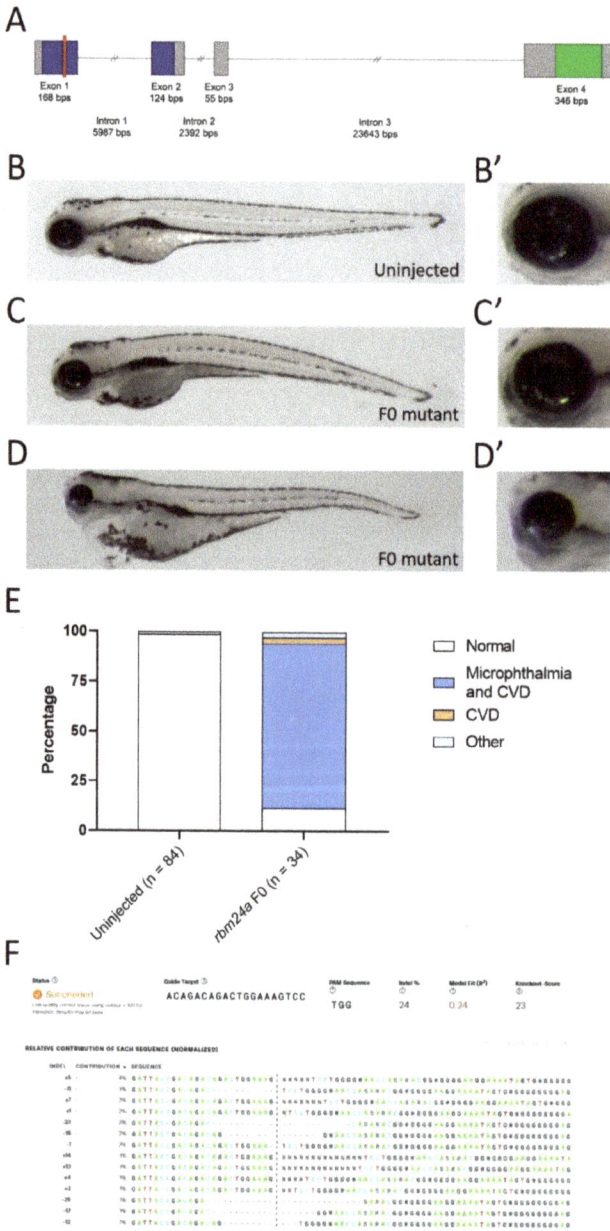

Figure 1. Mutation of rbm24a phenocopies morpholino knockdown. (**A**) Schematic for genetic structure of Rbm24a, with the RNA recognition motif (RRM) in blue and the Ala-rich region in green. The red line indicates the site of the Alt-R CRISPR/Cas0 mutation. (**B**) Uninjected control 4 dpf embryo with wild type morphology. (**B′**) Detail of eye shown in B. (**C**) and (**D**) are Alt-R CRISPR/Cas9-injected embryos showing the variation of the phenotypes. (**C′**) and (**D′**) are detail of eyes found in C and D, respectively. (**E**) Graph of uninjected and CRISPR-injected F0 embryos. (**F**) Synthego ICE analysis of mutations found in F0 mutants. Indels are listed. Images taken at 33×.

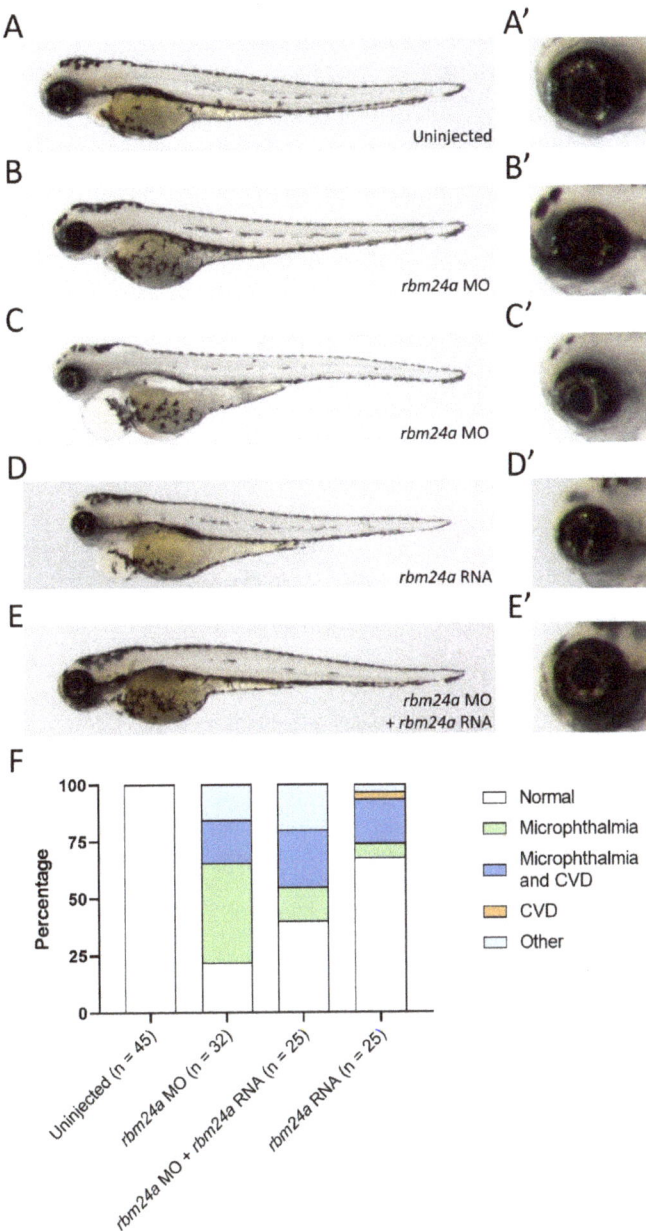

Figure 2. Suppression of *rbm24a* morpholino knockdown with *rbm24a* RNA. (**A**) Uninjected 4 dpf embryo with wild type morphology, (**A'**) detail of eye in A. (**B**) Knockdown of *rbm24a* at low doses leads to microphthalmia, (**B'**) detail of eye in B, while (**C**) is a higher dose showing microphthalmia with cardiac edema, (**C'**) detail of eye in C. (**D**) Injection of *rbm24a* RNA yields phenotypes similar to higher dose knockdown, (**D'**) detail of eye in D. (**E**) Sequential injection of *rbm24a* morpholino and *rbm24a* RNA suppresses the phenotypes, (**E'**) detail of eye in E. (**F**) Graph of phenotypes. Images taken at 33×.

As an additional confirmation of the *rbm24a* knockdown phenotype, we next determined the extent to which exogenous *rbm24a* RNA can suppress the knockdown defects. We modified the *rbm24a* RNA construct so the morpholino could not bind to this exogenous *rbm24a* RNA. When injected alone, *rbm24a* RNA led to an overexpression phenotype very similar to the *rbm24a* knockdown phenotype (100–400 pg; Figure 2D–D'). The similarity of the *rbm24a* knockdown and overexpression phenotypes poses a challenge for phenotypic suppression studies, yet when we performed sequential injections of *rbm24a* morpholino and *rbm24a* RNA, we demonstrated phenotypic suppression (Figure 2E–E'). In morpholino knockdown alone, approximately 20% of the embryos were phenotypically normal, while the remaining 80% of embryos displayed defects. When embryos were sequentially injected with *rbm24a* morpholino and *rbm24a* RNA, the number with normal morphology doubled to nearly 40%, resulting in partial suppression of the knockdown microphthalmia defect ($p = 0.0745$) (Figure 2F, Table 2). The overlapping phenotypes generated by two different morpholinos, the suppression of the knockdown phenotype by exogenous *rbm24a* RNA, and the phenotypic similarity between the CRISPR-injected and morphant embryos indicate that the phenotypes observed are specific to *rbm24a*.

Table 2. Number of phenotypes associated with uninjected, *rbm24a* knockdown, *rbm24a* knockdown with *rbm24a* RNA, and *rbm24a* RNA alone.

	Uninjected	*rbm24a* MO	*rbm24a* MO + *rbm24a* RNA	*rbm24a* RNA
Normal	45	7	10	21
Microphthalmia		14	4	2
Microphthalmia and CVD		6	6	6
CVD				1
Other		5	5	1
Total	45	32	25	31

3.3. EGFP RNA Does Not Suppress rbm24a Morpholino Knockdown Phenotypes

Rbm24a is an RNA-binding protein. Therefore, we sought to determine if any exogenous RNA was sufficient to suppress the *rbm24a* knockdown phenotype. We utilized EGFP RNA as a control for RNA injection. EGFP is not naturally found in zebrafish and should have no function. Additionally, we can check for successful injection by screening embryos for EGFP fluorescence (Figure 3A). When compared to uninjected control embryos, both embryos injected with *rbm24a* morpholino (1.7–2 ng) and embryos injected with both *rbm24a* morpholino and EGFP RNA (200–300 pg) showed similar phenotypes, including many with microphthalmia and microphthalmia with cardiac edema (Figure 3B–D'). Injection of EGFP RNA alone yielded a phenotype similar to the uninjected control group (Figure 3E–E'). The number of normal embryos in both the uninjected group and EGFP RNA group is almost identical ($p = 0.1050$), while the number and nature of the affected embryos in both the *rbm24a* knockdown and *rbm24a* knockdown with EGFP RNA are also very similar ($p = 0.5884$) (Figure 3F, Table 3). Taken together, these data suggest that *rbm24a* knockdown defects cannot be suppressed by sequential injection of an unrelated exogenous RNA.

Table 3. Number of phenotypes associated with uninjected, *rbm24a* knockdown, *rbm24a* knockdown with EGFP RNA, and EGFP RNA alone.

	Uninjected	*rbm24a* MO	*rbm24a* MO + EGFP RNA	EGFP RNA
Normal	63	2	1	28
Microphthalmia	2	6	10	2
Microphthalmia and CVD		13	6	
CVD				
Other		4	9	
Total	63	25	26	30

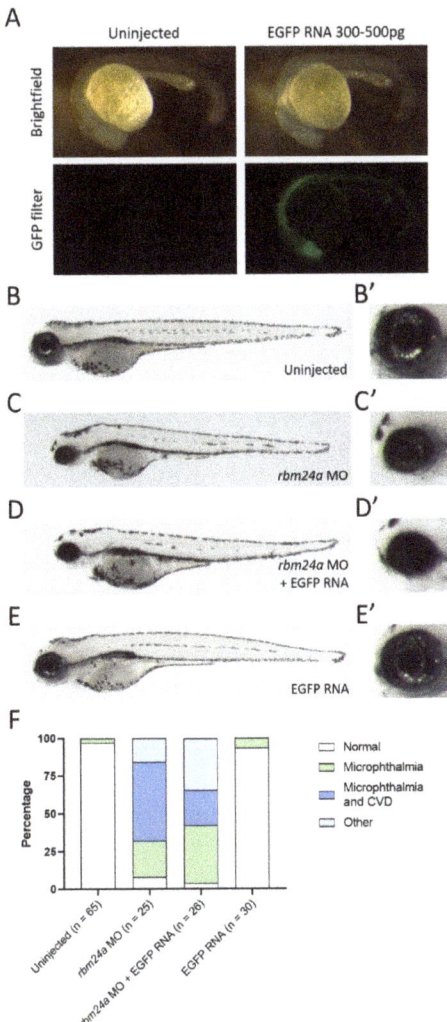

Figure 3. EGFP RNA does not suppress *rbm24a* knockdown. (**A**) Uninjected and EGFP RNA-injected 1 dpf embryos are shown in both brightfield (top) and with a GFP filter (bottom). (**B**) Uninjected 4 dpf embryo with wild type morphology, (**B′**) detail of eye in B. (**C**) *rbm24a* knockdown embryos display microphthalmia with cardiac edema, (**C′**) detail of eye in C. (**D**) Sequential injection of *rbm24a* morpholino and EGFP RNA yields phenotypes similar to knockdown alone, (**D′**) detail of eye in D. (**E**) EGFP RNA-injected embryos are morphologically wild type, (**E′**) detail of eye in E. (**F**) Graph of phenotypes. Image A taken at 62×. Images B-E′ taken at 33×.

3.4. sox2 RNA Phenotypically Suppresses rbm24a Morpholino-Induced Microphthalmia

We previously identified *sox2* as a target of Rbm24a in both zebrafish and mouse models [12]. In that study, we demonstrated that loss of *rbm24a* led to decreased levels of *sox2*. We hypothesize that supplying exogenous *sox2* RNA would supplement the reduced endogenous *sox2* RNA levels. We previously identified the binding site in the 3′ UTR of *Sox2* for RBM24 via mouse cell culture studies [12]. Thus, we generated a zebrafish *sox2* RNA construct which lacked the 3′ UTR to prevent Rbm24a binding (referred to as *sox2*

RNA). To test the functional role of *sox2* as a target of Rbm24a, we performed sequential injection of *rbm24a* morpholino followed by *sox2* RNA. Knockdown of *rbm24a* (1.7–2 ng) generated embryos with microphthalmia or microphthalmia with cardiac edema when compared against the uninjected control (Figure 4A–B').

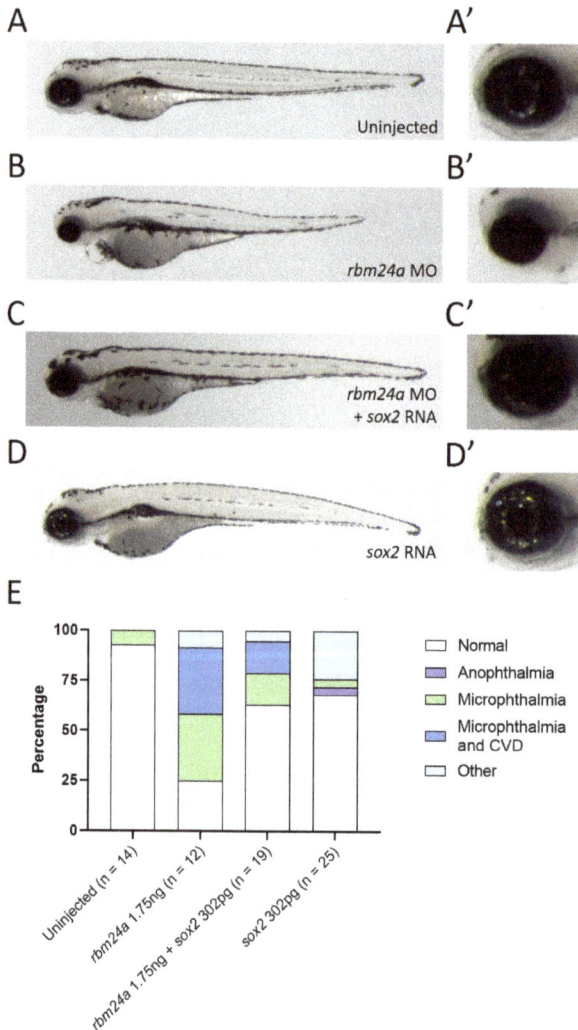

Figure 4. Exogenous *sox2* can suppress *rbm24a*-associated microphthalmia. (**A**) Uninjected 4 dpf embryo with wild type morphology, (**A'**) detail of eye in A. (**B**) Knockdown of *rbm24a* at low doses leads to microphthalmia, (**B'**) detail of eye in B. (**C**) Sequential injection of *rbm24a* morpholino and *sox2* RNA results in a phenotype more similar to wild type than *rbm24a* morphant, (**C'**) detail of eye in C. (**D**) Injection of sox2 RNA alone results in wild type morphology, (**D'**) detail of eye in D. (**E**) Graph of phenotypes. Images taken at 33×.

In contrast, embryos sequentially injected with both *rbm24a* morpholino and *sox2* RNA (200–300 pg) were often normal in morphology (Figure 4C–C'). Injection of *sox2* RNA alone also generated mostly phenotypically normal embryos (Figure 4D–D'). A majority of uninjected, *rbm24a* morpholino and *sox2* RNA-injected, and *sox2* RNA-injected embryos were morphologically normal with some exceptions in both injection groups. The *rbm24a* knockdown embryos displayed more embryos with microphthalmia or microphthalmia with cardiac edema when compared to the *rbm24a* knockdown with *sox2* RNA, indicating that injection of exogenous *sox2* RNA can partially suppress the *rbm24a* knockdown phenotype (Figure 4E, Table 4).

Table 4. Number of phenotypes associated with uninjected, *rbm24a* knockdown, *rbm24a* knockdown with *sox2* RNA, and *sox2* RNA alone.

	Uninjected	*rbm24a* MO	*rbm24a* MO + *sox2* RNA	*sox2* RNA
Normal	13	3	12	17
Microphthalmia				2
Microphthalmia and CVD		4	3	
CVD				
Other	1	5	4	6
Total	14	12	17	25

3.5. EGFP RNA Does Not Functionally Suppress rbm24a-Induced Visual Defects

We next wanted to determine the functional role of *rbm24a* in vision. Previously, we demonstrated that morpholino knockdown of *rbm24a* impacts the startle response in a dose-dependent manner [13]. When 5 to 6 days post-fertilization zebrafish larvae are exposed to an interruption of a constant light source, they perform a characteristic escape response which can be tracked with motion detection cameras and software. We utilized the automated startle response assay (VIZN) which generates five interruptions in light and records the zebrafish movement in response to the interruption in light [26]. Uninjected control larvae responded roughly four out of five times, indicating that they are visually responsive to the stark change in light in the startle response assay. Our previous studies indicated that low-dose knockdown of *rbm24a* maintained light detection [13]. For this study, we utilized a mid-range dose of *rbm24a* morpholino to better evaluate the effectiveness of RNA suppression. For all of our vision assays, we only utilized larvae that were touch responsive with a characteristic swimming response and had no cardiac edema. These *rbm24a* morphant larvae responded to the automated startle response assay (VIZN) significantly fewer times (approximately two out of five times) than the uninjected control (Figure 5). When sequentially injected with both *rbm24a* morpholino and EGFP RNA, larvae had a similar response to the *rbm24a* morpholino-alone larvae and responded about two out of five times. The difference between the *rbm24a* morpholino-only and *rbm24a* morpholino with EGFP RNA was not significantly different. The larvae injected with only EGFP RNA responded roughly four out of five times. There was no significant difference between the uninjected control and EGFP RNA-alone groups (Figure 5).

3.6. sox2 RNA Partially Functionally Suppresses rbm24a-Induced Visual Defects

We next investigated the extent to which *sox2* RNA can restore visual functionality to *rbm24a* knockdown larvae. We performed VIZN on the uninjected control and *rbm24a* knockdown larvae. Uninjected control larvae responded approximately four out of five times, indicating that they are visually responsive to the startle response assay (Figure 6). As stated previously, we purposely utilized a dose of *rbm24a* morpholino which resulted in larvae responding statistically significantly fewer times (roughly two out of five) than the uninjected control. Sequential injection of *rbm24a* morpholino and *sox2* RNA larvae responded significantly more times (about three out of five) than *rbm24a* morpholino-injected larvae. However, the *rbm24a* morpholino and *sox2* RNA larvae were also statistically significantly different from the uninjected control larvae. Larvae injected with only *sox2* RNA responded similarly (about four out of five times) to the uninjected control (Figure 6). Taken together, these data indicate *sox2* partially restores visual function in *rbm24a* morpholino knockdown larvae.

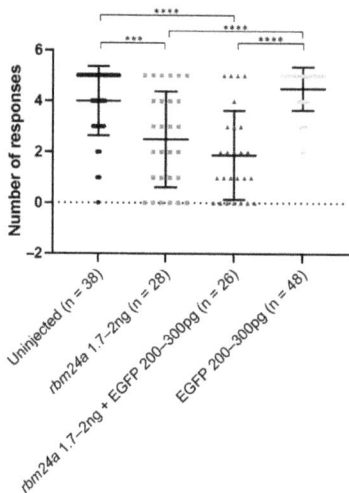

Figure 5. EGFP RNA does not improve visual function of *rbm24a* knockdown embryos. Automated startle response assay (VIZN) was performed on uninjected, *rbm24a* knockdown, *rbm24a* knockdown with EGFP RNA, and EGFP RNA larvae. Knockdown of *rbm24a* inhibits visual function, which was statistically significant compared to uninjected. Addition of EGFP RNA to *rbm24a* knockdown does not statistically significantly increase visual function when compared to *rbm24a* knockdown alone. Injection of EGFP RNA alone does not statistically significantly alter visual function from uninjected. Mann–Whitney *** $p < 0.001$, **** $p < 0.0001$. Nonsignificant interactions not shown.

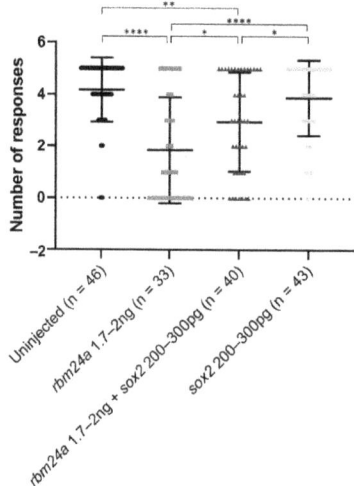

Figure 6. Injection of *sox2* RNA can partially restore visual function by VIZN to *rbm24a* knockdown embryos. VIZN was performed on uninjected, *rbm24a* knockdown, *rbm24a* knockdown with *sox2* RNA, and *sox2* RNA larvae. Knockdown of *rbm24a* statistically significantly inhibits visual function when compared to uninjected. Addition of *sox2* RNA to *rbm24a* knockdown statistically significantly improves visual function when compared to *rbm24a* knockdown, but not to the same level as uninjected. Injection of *sox2* RNA alone does not statistically significantly alter visual function from uninjected. Mann–Whitney * $p < 0.05$, ** $p < 0.01$, **** $p < 0.0001$. Nonsignificant interactions not shown.

4. Discussion

Our previous research indicated *sox2* as a target for Rbm24a and suggests that Rbm24a binds to and stabilizes the *sox2* mRNA transcript [12]. Localization data indicate that *rbm24a* is expressed exclusively in the lens. This suggests that Rbm24a binds to and regulates lens-expressed *sox2* in the lens [17–21,28]. When knocked down via morpholino or mutated via CRISPR, the levels of Rbm24a are depleted which leads to a decrease in the stability and amount of *sox2* mRNA. One possibility is that the reduced levels of *sox2*, a proliferative factor, lead to decreased lens vesicle size. Due to coordinated development between the lens vesicle and optic cup via reciprocal induction, the optic cup develops in tandem with the lens vesicle and results in microphthalmia (Figure 7).

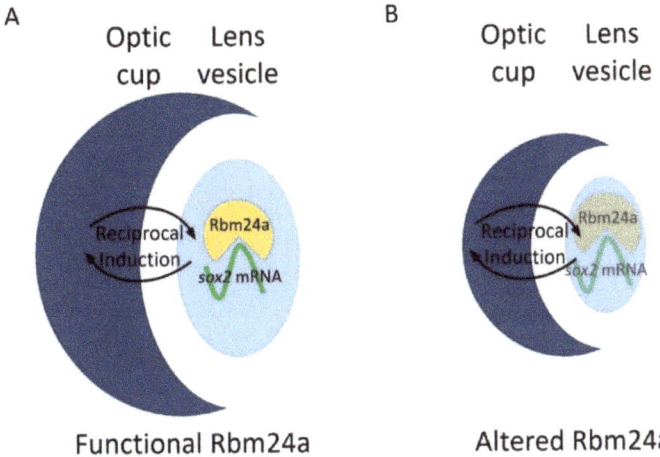

Figure 7. Model for Rbm24a in zebrafish eye development. (**A**) Functional Rbm24a is found in the developing lens of zebrafish. There, the protein acts to bind to and stabilize *sox2* mRNA. This interaction leads to the development of a normal sized lens and, with reciprocal induction signaling between the lens and retina, the retina also develops normally to size-match the lens. (**B**) With either knockdown or mutation of *rbm24a*, there is lessened Rbm24a protein in the lens which in turn cannot stabilize as many *sox2* mRNA molecules (represented as transparent shapes). The lack of the correct amount of *sox2*, a proliferative factor, causes the lens to develop smaller than normal. However, reciprocal induction has not been affected, which leads to the lens and retina developing small in tandem.

Recently, a zebrafish TALEN mutant for *rbm24a* has been published which phenocopies both our morpholino knockdown and CRISPR-injected F0 defects [23]. In the Shao et al. 2020 study, the authors suggest that microphthalmia is the result of a cardiac morphological defect leading to poor blood flow to the eye. We hypothesized that the microphthalmia was due to target RNA disruption by decreased *rbm24a* expression. In our previously published studies, we identified that RBM24 binds to *Sox2* in mouse cell cultures [12]. From this, we hypothesized that knockdown of *rbm24a* with the addition of exogenous *sox2* would suppress the microphthalmia phenotype. We found that sequential knockdown of *rbm24a* and the addition of exogenous *sox2* RNA generated a phenotype more similar to that of uninjected control embryos than *rbm24a* knockdown (Figure 4A–C'). Our data indicate *sox2* is a main contributor to the *rbm24a*-induced microphthalmia. In terms of the previous study by Shao et al., it is possible that the TALEN mutant was not a null mutation which could have allowed for some function in the lens. Additionally, the utilization of heterotypic parabiosis allows for the potential transfer of more than just blood (including hormones, signaling molecules, etc.) between embryos. It is possible that the transfer of these biomolecules could have played a role in suppressing the microphthalmia phenotype [23]. Follow-up studies utilizing an organ-specific driver would resolve this contrast.

We occasionally observed cardiovascular defects in the *sox2* overexpression embryos, perhaps stemming from the ubiquitous overexpression of *sox2*. Ubiquitously expressed exogenous *sox2* may be able to substitute for cardiac members of the SOX family including *Sox6* which has been shown to be a cardiomyocyte regulator in murine cells, *Sox9* which is involved in heart valve development in mice, and *Sox17* which has been shown to be essential for specification of cardiac mesoderm in mouse cell cultures [29–31]. In the future, an eye-specific promoter could be utilized to allow for the study of *rbm24a*/*sox2* interactions with specificity to the eye.

In this study, we demonstrated that knockdown and mutation of the RNA-binding motif protein 24a gene, *rbm24a*, leads to microphthalmia at low-dose knockdown and microphthalmia with cardiac edema at increased knockdown doses. Additionally, we demonstrated that the microphthalmia induced by *rbm24a* functionally impacted the visual capabilities of the larvae, as knockdown fish performed worse in a visual behavior study. Previously, we identified *sox2* as a target of Rbm24a [12]. When sequentially injected, exogenous *sox2* RNA is able to phenotypically and partially functionally suppress the *rbm24a* knockdown larvae. This shows functional validation of a suspected target RNA by an RNA-binding protein. This work broadly demonstrates the key role RNA-binding proteins and post-transcriptional modification plays during development. It also highlights that genes not associated with disease, such as *rbm24a*, can impact a well-studied disease-associated gene (*sox2*), making it critical to better understand post-transcriptional regulation and the potential impacts of RNA-binding proteins and their associated target RNAs.

Supplementary Materials: The following are available online at https://www.mdpi.com/2227-9059/9/2/100/s1, Figure S1: Knockdown of *rbm24a* yields dose-dependent phenotypes at 4 days post-fertilization.

Author Contributions: Conceptualization, L.K.B. and D.C.S.; methodology, L.K.B.; investigation, L.K.B.; resources, C.A.S.; statistical analysis, L.K.B. and K.W.; writing—original draft preparation, L.K.B. and D.C.S.; writing—review and editing, L.K.B., C.A.S., and D.C.S.; project administration, D.C.S.; funding acquisition, D.C.S. All authors have read and agreed to the published version of the manuscript.

Funding: This research was funded by the American Heart Association, grant number 17GRNT33670684.

Institutional Review Board Statement: Zebrafish are maintained in standard conditions under the approval of the University of Iowa Institutional Animal Care and Use Committee (#8071513, 13 August 2018).

Informed Consent Statement: Not applicable.

Data Availability Statement: Data sharing not applicable.

Acknowledgments: The authors would like to thank Douglas Houston, Sheila Baker, Michael Dailey, and Bryan Phillips for their suggestions and expertise.

Conflicts of Interest: The authors declare no conflict of interest.

References

1. Johnson, G.J.; Minassian, D.C.; Weale, R.A.; West, S.K. *The Epidemiology of Eye Disease*; Arnold: London, UK, 2003.
2. Graw, J. The genetic and molecular basis of congenital eye defects. *Nat. Rev. Genet.* **2003**, *4*, 876–888. [CrossRef] [PubMed]
3. Shah, S.P.; Taylor, A.E.; Sowden, J.C.; Ragge, N.K.; Russell-Eggitt, I.; Rahi, J.S.; Gilbert, C.E. Anophthalmos, microphthalmos, and typical coloboma in the United Kingdom: A prospective study of incidence and risk. *Investig. Ophthalmol. Vis. Sci.* **2011**, *52*, 558–564. [CrossRef] [PubMed]
4. Kong, L.; Fry, M.; Al-Samarraie, M.; Gilbert, C.; Steinkuller, P.G. An update on progress and the changing epidemiology of causes of childhood blindness worldwide. *J. Am. Assoc. Pediatric Ophthalmol. Strabismus* **2012**, *16*, 501–507. [CrossRef] [PubMed]
5. Reis, L.M.; Semina, E.V. Conserved genetic pathways associated with microphthalmia, anophthalmia, and coloboma. *Birth Defects Res. Part C Embryo Today Rev.* **2015**, *105*, 96–113. [CrossRef]

6. Fantes, J.; Ragge, N.K.; Lynch, S.-A.; McGill, N.I.; Collin, J.R.O.; Howard-Peebles, P.N.; Hayward, C.; Vivian, A.J.; Williamson, K.; van Heyningen, V. Mutations in SOX2 cause anophthalmia. *Nat. Genet.* **2003**, *33*, 462–463. [CrossRef]
7. Takahashi, K.; Yamanaka, S. Induction of pluripotent stem cells from mouse embryonic and adult fibroblast cultures by defined factors. *Cell* **2006**, *126*, 663–676. [CrossRef]
8. Zhou, Q.; Chipperfield, H.; Melton, D.A.; Wong, W.H. A gene regulatory network in mouse embryonic stem cells. *Proc. Natl. Acad. Sci. USA* **2007**, *104*, 16438–16443. [CrossRef]
9. Kondoh, H.; Lovell-Badge, R. *Sox2: Biology and Role in Development and Disease*; Academic Press: London, UK, 2015.
10. Wu, J.; Belmonte, J.C.I. The molecular harbingers of early mammalian embryo patterning. *Cell* **2016**, *165*, 13–15. [CrossRef]
11. Lachke, S.A.; Ho, J.W.; Kryukov, G.V.; O'Connell, D.J.; Aboukhalil, A.; Bulyk, M.L.; Park, P.J.; Maas, R.L. iSyTE: Integrated Systems Tool for Eye gene discovery. *Investig. Ophthalmol. Vis. Sci.* **2012**, *53*, 1617–1627. [CrossRef]
12. Dash, S.; Brastrom, L.K.; Patel, S.D.; Scott, C.A.; Slusarski, D.C.; Lachke, S.A. The master transcription factor SOX2, mutated in anophthalmia/microphthalmia, is post-transcriptionally regulated by the conserved RNA-binding protein RBM24 in vertebrate eye development. *Hum. Mol. Genet.* **2020**, *29*, 591–604. [CrossRef]
13. Brastrom, L.K.; Scott, C.A.; Dawson, D.V.; Slusarski, D.C. A high-throughput assay for congenital and age-related eye diseases in zebrafish. *Biomedicines* **2019**, *7*, 28. [CrossRef] [PubMed]
14. Yang, J.; Hung, L.-H.; Licht, T.; Kostin, S.; Looso, M.; Khrameeva, E.; Bindereif, A.; Schneider, A.; Braun, T. RBM24 is a major regulator of muscle-specific alternative splicing. *Dev. Cell* **2014**, *31*, 87–99. [CrossRef] [PubMed]
15. Zhang, M.; Zhang, Y.; Xu, E.; Mohibi, S.; de Anda, D.M.; Jiang, Y.; Zhang, J.; Chen, X. Rbm24, a target of p53, is necessary for proper expression of p53 and heart development. *Cell Death Differ.* **2018**, *25*, 1118–1130. [CrossRef] [PubMed]
16. Liu, J.; Kong, X.; Zhang, M.; Yang, X.; Xu, X. RNA binding protein 24 deletion disrupts global alternative splicing and causes dilated cardiomyopathy. *Protein Cell* **2019**, *10*, 405–416. [CrossRef] [PubMed]
17. Fetka, I.; Radeghieri, A.; Bouwmeester, T. Expression of the RNA recognition motif-containing protein SEB-4 during Xenopus embryonic development. *Mech. Dev.* **2000**, *94*, 283–286. [CrossRef]
18. Oberleitner, S. Seb4—An RNA-Binding Protein as a Novel Regulator of Myogenesis during Early Development in Xenopus laevis. Ph.D. Dissertation, Ludwig Maximilian University of Munich, Munich, Germany, 2008.
19. Maragh, S.; Miller, R.A.; Bessling, S.L.; McGaughey, D.M.; Wessels, M.W.; De Graaf, B.; Stone, E.A.; Bertoli-Avella, A.M.; Gearhart, J.D.; Fisher, S. Identification of RNA binding motif proteins essential for cardiovascular development. *BMC Dev. Biol.* **2011**, *11*, 1–13. [CrossRef]
20. Maragh, S.; Miller, R.A.; Bessling, S.L.; Wang, G.; Hook, P.W.; McCallion, A.S. Rbm24a and Rbm24b are required for normal somitogenesis. *PLoS ONE* **2014**, *9*, e105460. [CrossRef]
21. Grifone, R.; Saquet, A.; Xu, Z.; Shi, D.L. Expression patterns of Rbm24 in lens, nasal epithelium, and inner ear during mouse embryonic development. *Dev. Dyn.* **2018**, *247*, 1160–1169. [CrossRef]
22. Wagner, D.E.; Weinreb, C.; Collins, Z.M.; Briggs, J.A.; Megason, S.G.; Klein, A.M. Single-cell mapping of gene expression landscapes and lineage in the zebrafish embryo. *Science* **2018**, *360*, 981–987. [CrossRef]
23. Shao, M.; Lu, T.; Zhang, C.; Zhang, Y.-Z.; Kong, S.-H.; Shi, D.-L. Rbm24 controls poly (A) tail length and translation efficiency of crystallin mRNAs in the lens via cytoplasmic polyadenylation. *Proc. Natl. Acad. Sci. USA* **2020**, *117*, 7245–7254. [CrossRef]
24. Vakulskas, C.A.; Dever, D.P.; Rettig, G.R.; Turk, R.; Jacobi, A.M.; Collingwood, M.A.; Bode, N.M.; McNeill, M.S.; Yan, S.; Camarena, J. A high-fidelity Cas9 mutant delivered as a ribonucleoprotein complex enables efficient gene editing in human hematopoietic stem and progenitor cells. *Nat. Med.* **2018**, *24*, 1216. [CrossRef] [PubMed]
25. Roginsky, J. Analyzing CRISPR Editing Results: Synthego Developed a Tool Called ICE to Be More Efficient Than Other Methods. *Genet. Eng. Biotechnol. News* **2018**, *38*, S24–S26. [CrossRef]
26. Scott, C.A.; Marsden, A.N.; Slusarski, D.C. Automated, high-throughput, in vivo analysis of visual function using the zebrafish. *Dev. Dyn.* **2016**, *245*, 605–613. [CrossRef]
27. Team, R.C. *R: A Language and Environment for Statistical Computing*; The R Foundation: Vienna, Austria, 2017.
28. Poon, K.L.; Tan, K.T.; Wei, Y.Y.; Ng, C.P.; Colman, A.; Korzh, V.; Xu, X.Q. RNA-binding protein RBM24 is required for sarcomere assembly and heart contractility. *Cardiovasc. Res.* **2012**, *94*, 418–427. [CrossRef] [PubMed]
29. Cohen-Barak, O.; Yi, Z.; Hagiwara, N.; Monzen, K.; Komuro, I.; Brilliant, M.H. Sox6 regulation of cardiac myocyte development. *Nucleic Acids Res.* **2003**, *31*, 5941–5948. [CrossRef] [PubMed]
30. Garside, V.C.; Cullum, R.; Alder, O.; Lu, D.Y.; Vander Werff, R.; Bilenky, M.; Zhao, Y.; Jones, S.J.; Marra, M.A.; Underhill, T.M. SOX9 modulates the expression of key transcription factors required for heart valve development. *Development* **2015**, *142*, 4340–4350. [CrossRef] [PubMed]
31. Liu, Y.; Asakura, M.; Inoue, H.; Nakamura, T.; Sano, M.; Niu, Z.; Chen, M.; Schwartz, R.J.; Schneider, M.D. Sox17 is essential for the specification of cardiac mesoderm in embryonic stem cells. *Proc. Natl. Acad. Sci. USA* **2007**, *104*, 3859–3864. [CrossRef]